Histamine and H_2 Antagonists in Inflammation and Immunodeficiency

ALLERGIC DISEASE AND THERAPY

Series Editor

David G. Tinkelman

Atlanta Allergy Clinic

Atlanta, Georgia

Volume 1 Histamine and H_2 Antagonists in Inflammation and Immunodeficiency, *edited by Ross E. Rocklin*

Additional Volumes in Preparation

Childhood Allergic Rhinitis and Sinusitus, *edited by David G. Tinkelman and Charles K. Naspitz*

Histamine and H_2 Antagonists in Inflammation and Immunodeficiency

edited by

Ross E. Rocklin
Boehringer Ingelheim Pharmaceuticals, Inc.
Ridgefield, Connecticut
and
New England Medical Center Hospital
Boston, Massachusetts

MARCEL DEKKER, INC. New York and Basel

Library of Congress Cataloging-in-Publication

Histamine and H_2 antagonists in inflammation and immunodeficiency /
edited by Ross E. Rocklin.
p. cm. -- (Allergic disease and therapy)
ISBN 0-8247-8280-1
1. Immunodeficiency. 2. Inflammation. 3. Histamine--Immunology.
4. Histamine--Receptors. 5. Histamine--Antagonists. I. Rocklin,
Ross E. (Ross Elliot), II. Series.
[DNLM: 1. Histamine--immunology. 2. Histamine H_2 Receptor
Blockaders--immunology. 3. Immunologic Diseases--physiopathology.
4. Inflammation--physiopathology. QV 157 H6732]
QR188.35.H57 1990
616'.0473--dc20
DNLM/DLC
for Library of Congress 89-23765
CIP

This book is printed on acid-free paper.

MARCEL DEKKER, INC.
270 Madison Avenue, New York, New York 10016

Current printing (last digit):
10 9 8 7 6 5 4 3 2 1

PRINTED IN THE UNITED STATES OF AMERICA

Dedicated with affection to my wife Suzanne,
my children Jeremy and Alexander, and,
last but not least, my parents

Series Introduction

Allergic disease and its therapy has long been a topic of discussion. The development of theories on the cause of allergic symptoms has consumed volumes of medical literature dealing with virtually all organ systems. From these postulations have come practical approaches to the diagnosis and management of allergic disorders. Despite the continuum of medical "breakthroughs," the answers to many of the questions relating to allergy remain unknown.

In this series, Allergic Disease and Therapy, the authors will attempt to concisely put forth reviews of past approaches as well as the most up-to-date information relating to a variety of different allergic states. Basic scientists, clinical researchers, and experts will combine their efforts to establish rational approaches to the diagnosis and management of the complex allergic problems of today. This will be a multidisciplinary approach by individuals spanning the globe in an effort to cover these topics from many different perspectives. From the genetics laboratories where complex questions concerning the role of certain gene pools in the development of immunologic competence are being studied to the research facilities of pharmaceutical companies where new products are being tested, this series will address many unanswered questions in the rapidly growing field of allergy and immunology. The goal of the series is to provide the practitioner with the background knowledge and tools with which to approach the allergic problems that are so common in today's society.

David G. Tinkelman, M.D.

Foreword

This book renders up-to-date several exciting lines of investigation concerning the capacity of histamine to modulate, and of histamine type II antagonists to augment, inflammatory and immune responses. In this foreword I will attempt to place these lines of investigation into perspective.

In order for histamine to modulate immune and inflammatory reactions in vivo, it must be available at inflammatory sites. In man, the only cells that contain stored histamine are also the only cells that bear high affinity IgE receptors, or FceRI. These cells are tissue mast cells and circulating basophils, the principal effector cells of immediate hypersensitivity reactions. In addition to these stores of histamine, relatively large quantities of the molecule can be synthesized rapidly, presumably by mast cell precursors in the hematopoietic tissue of mice and other species. Both GM-CSF and IL-3 induce this rapid synthesis and release of histamine. The relative importance of newly synthesized histamine is unknown, but histamine secreted from mature basophils and mast cells is likely to represent the major source of the molecule.

Allergic reactions require an induction stage in which antigen stimulates the production of specific IgE antibody. These antibody molecules will bind to the surface IgE receptors on mast cells and basophils. Subsequently, antigen, by crosslinking the IgE molecules, crosslinks the IgE receptors, leading to secretion of the stored histamine. Other stimuli, ranging from complement-derived anaphylatoxins to cytokines, can also induce histamine secretion. The secreted histamine has a variety of biological effects, all mediated by binding to specific histamine receptors. The classical effects of histamine, which result in pathophysiologic changes similar to those occurring during allergic reactions, are via histamine type I receptors, and include the induction of both smooth muscle contraction and edema. (Edema is produced by contraction of the endothelial cells of postcapillary venules.)

Several important developments from the 1970s to the present have led to a reconsideration of the role of histamine in inflammation and immunity. First, several autacoids, including catecholamines, prostaglandins, adenosine, and histamine have been shown to modulate the activities of several immune and inflammatory effector cells, such as human basophils and rodent cytotoxic T lymphocytes. Second, histamine was shown to act on distinct types of receptors, as a team headed by Nobel laureate Sir James Black defined histamine-type II receptors on the basis of new, specific antagonists. (Now, a third histamine receptor has been defined, that mediates inhibition of histamine production and release from the central nervous system and peripheral sites. The role of histamine type III receptors in inflammation and immunity is as yet undefined.) Histamine acting on histamine type II receptors has been shown to activate adenylate cyclase and to have actions similar to other autacoids that activate adenylate cyclase. These actions include the inhibition of inflammatory and immune cell effector functions. Third, histamine, as distinct from other autacoids, has functional effects on distinct cell subsets. As examples, histamine inhibits the activity of mouse spleen but not mouse peritoneal cytoxic T lymphocytes; and histamine increases cAMP levels in human suppressor T lymphocytes more than in other lymphocyte subsets. Fourth, the functional activity of histamine is unique in certain diseases states. For example, histamine fails to activate suppressor T cells of atopic individuals, while it does activate suppressor cells of normals. The observations that histamine has distinct actions on different cell subsets and in cells from patients with certain diseases argue that histamine may have a specialized role, and that histamine antagonists may be therapeutically useful for blocking the unique effects of histamine. A fifth line of investigation is based on the observation that histamine type II antagonists are immunostimulatory. For example, the excess suppressor cell activity in patients with common variable hypogammaglobulinemia is reversed by the histamine type II antagonist, cimetidine. A reasonable interpretation of these data is that the histamine type II antagonists are immunostimulatory because they block the effects of endogenous histamine. Thus, histamine may be an important endogenous immunosuppressive agent, and in specific disease states its immunosuppressive activity may be excessive. Therefore, the histamine type II antagonists may have significant therapeutic benefit, particularly since they are relatively safe agents.

There remains a number of unresolved issues concerning the role of histamine in inflammation and immunity. The immunomodulatory effects of histamine in most systems are quite modest. The therapeutic utility of histamine type II antagonists remains generally unproven. The mechanism of some of the described effects of histamine are unknown, because many in vitro systems yield opposing effects, and because some reagents that would be most useful for defining these effects, such as monoclonal antibodies to histamine receptors, are not available. Surprisingly, immunostimulatory effects of histamine type II antagonists have been easier to demonstrate in vivo than in vitro. It is possible that the antagonists do not act in vivo by blocking the effects of endogenous histamine, but act independently of histamine.

This book presents a well-chosen selection of investigators who have been studying histamine, inflammation, and immunity. It accurately describes the present understanding of the field, and it provides convincing evidence that histamine-mediated immunomodulation is important in certain in vitro and in vivo situations, and even in some clinical settings. The future of these investigations may lie in the development of newer antagonists that have even more specific effects on unique cell subsets. Such agents, if they are relatively safe and significantly immunostimulatory, will be useful therapeutic options.

Lawrence M. Lichtenstein, M.D.
The Johns Hopkins University
School of Medicine
Baltimore, Maryland

Preface

Traditionally, histamine has been considered a mediator whose release in certain tissues results in either the production of the symptoms of allergic disease, gastric acid, or neurotransmission. It has only been in the past 15 years that the role of histamine as a modulator of the immune response has been appreciated. The latter has come about primarily through the observation that receptors for histamine are also present on immunocompetent lymphoid cells (T and B lymphocytes) and leukocytes (neutrophils, eosinophils, basophils, and monocytes/macrophages). Thus, the release of histamine within the local milieu of an emerging immune/inflammatory response may potentially modify, in either a positive or a negative way, the development of that reaction. The outcome of such reactions is determined to some extent by the type of histamine receptors present on the tissues or cells involved. In general, stimulation of histamine type I (H_1) receptors leads to enhanced pro-inflammatory events, while stimulation of histamine type II (H_2) receptors is associated with down-regulation of immune/inflammatory responses.

The purpose of this book is twofold: to review the experimental evidence that documents the ability of histamine to influence a panoply of T and B lymphoid cell functions in vitro and in vivo in both animal models and in humans, and to present preliminary studies describing the ability of H_2 antagonists to augment immune responses in immunocompromised patients. The book is organized into four parts. The authors in Part I present data from in vivo and in vitro animal (mouse and guinea pig) and human studies that describe the ability of histamine to regulate T lymphocyte proliferative, lymphokine producing, and cytotoxic responses as well as granulocyte function. Potential mechanisms by which histamine achieves these regulatory effects are also addressed in terms of stimulation of suppressor T cells, signal transduction, and the generation of second messengers. That abnormalities in histamine-receptor bearing suppressor T lymphocyte function may be present in patients with diseases whose pathogenesis is characterized by immune dysregulation is proposed by authors in Part II.

The clinical extension of Parts I and II—the potential use of H_2 antagonists to augment immune responses—is presented in Part III. Here a wide array of clinical entities is described in which the immune response may be compromised, and in which the in vivo administration of an H_2 antagonist has lead to the restoration of that response. This has included primary and acquired immunodeficiency states, postsurgical effects, burn shock, transplantation, and malignancy. While these results are very exciting and may ultimately lead to potential new therapeutic indications for H_2 antagonists, it should be emphasized that these are preliminary, uncontrolled studies and require controlled clinical trials to properly document these observations. Finally, in Part IV, Dr. Melmon provides some insight into what the future may yield in terms of potential new drugs with selective actions on the immune system.

The authors who have provided chapters in this book have been active investigators in this field and have made significant contributions to its progress through the years. Their fine efforts have resulted in an up-to-date overview of this field and its potential clinical implications. I thank them for their participation in this endeavor and in particular, I am grateful to Dr. Dennis J. Beer, who also helped me with the organization of the book.

Ross E. Rocklin, M.D.

Contents

Contributors

Francesca T. Aweeka, Pharm. D. University of California, San Francisco, California

Alison M. Badger, Ph.D. Smith Kline & French Laboratories, King of Prussia, Pennsylvania

Mark Ballow, M.D.* University of Connecticut Health Center, School of Medicine, Farmington, Connecticut

Dennis J. Beer, M.D. Boston University School of Medicine, Boston, Massachusetts

Jeffrey S. Berman, M.D. Boston University School of Medicine, Boston, Massachusetts

John Bernardo, M.D. Boston University School of Medicine, Boston, Massachusetts

---

**Present affiliation*: The Children's Hospital of Buffalo, and State University of New York at Buffalo, Buffalo, New York

Joseph V. Boykin, Jr., M.D. Medical College of Virginia, Richmond, Virginia

Norbert H. Brockmeyer, M.D. University Clinic, Essen, Federal Republic of Germany

William W. Busse, M.D. University of Wisconsin Medical School, Madison, Wisconsin

David M. Center, M.D. Boston University School of Medicine, Boston, Massachusetts

William W. Cruikshank, M.D. Boston University School of Medicine, Boston, Massachusetts

William B. Ershler, M.D. University of Wisconsin, Madison, Wisconsin

Michele A. Gadd, M.D. University of California, San Diego Medical Center, San Diego, California

John G. Gambertoglio, Pharm.D. University of California, San Francisco, California

Marvin R. Garovoy, M.D. University of California, San Francisco, California

Don E. Griswold, Ph.D. Smith Kline & French Laboratories, King of Prussia, Pennsylvania

Nabil Hanna, Ph.D. Smith Kline & French Laboratories, King of Prussia, Pennsylvania

John F. Hansbrough, M.D., F.A.C.S. University of California, San Diego Medical Center, San Diego, California

Joseph L. Jorizzo, M.D. Bowman Gray School of Medicine of Wake Forest University, Winston-Salem, North Carolina

Manzoor M. Khan, M.S. Ph.D. Stanford University School of Medicine, Palo Alto, California

Nancy H. Manson, Ph.D. University of Virginia, Charlottesville, Virginia

Kenneth L. Melmon, M.D. Stanford University School of Medicine, Stanford, California

Madhavan P. N. Nair, Ph.D. University of Michigan, Ann Arbor, Michigan

George Poste, M.D. Smith Kline & French Laboratories, King of Prussia, Pennsylvania

Ross E. Rocklin, M.D. Boehringer Ingelheim Pharmaceuticals, Inc., Ridgefield, Connecticut, and New England Medical Center Hospital, Boston, Massachusetts

Stanley A. Schwartz, M.D., Ph.D. University of Michigan, Ann Arbor, Michigan

Julie B. Sedgwick, Ph.D. University of Wisconsin Medical School, Madison, Wisconsin

Tina B. Smith, M.D. Bowman Gray School of Medicine of Wake Forest University, Winston-Salem, North Carolina

Arthur C. Theodore, M.D. Boston University School of Medicine, Boston, Massachusetts

Robert Volpé, M.D., F.R.C.P. (C), F.A.C.P. University of Toronto and The Wellesley Hospital, Toronto, Ontario, Canada

William B. White, M.D. University of Connecticut Health Center, School of Medicine, Farmington, Connecticut

Histamine and H_2 Antagonists in Inflammation and Immunodeficiency

Part I
Influence of Histamine on Immunologic and Inflammatory Responses

1

Histamine Modulation of Murine Suppressor Cell Function

ALISON M. BADGER, DON E. GRISWOLD, GEORGE POSTE, and NABIL HANNA *Smith Kline & French Laboratories, King of Prussia, Pennsylvania*

I. INTRODUCTION

The immune system is controlled by a complicated system of positive and negative regulatory control networks involving a variety of cell types and soluble factors. Suppressor cells, in particular suppressor T cells (T_S), are responsible for much of the negative regulation of immune responsiveness. Suppressor-cell function was first described in a murine system by Gershon and Kondo in 1970 (1). They demonstrated that adoptive transfer of spleen cells from mice made tolerant to sheep red blood cells (SRBCs) caused specific unresponsiveness in naive recipients. Although the predominating suppressor cell in immune regulation is classically a T cell, other cell types, including B cells (2) and macrophages (3) can have suppressor cell functions. In addition, a population of null cells, or "natural" suppressor cells, has been described which have a controlling influence on antigen responsiveness, and may be implicated in the induction of tolerance (4).

Suppressor cells can be modulated in vitro by diverse stimuli, including antigen, mitogen, and antigen-antibody complexes and, as described in this chapter, by histamine. Histamine modulation of immunocompetent cells occurs via interaction with specific receptors on the cell surface (5,6), and it has been reported that functional histamine receptors are distributed nonrandomly on certain murine lymphocyte subpopulations (7-9). The evaluation of the effects of autacoids such as histamine, and its agonists/antagonists, on suppressor-cell function and activation is complicated, however, by significant variation depending on the precise in vitro and in vivo systems employed to evaluate such activity. Histamine has been shown to activate and to inhibit the generation of suppressor cells, and the role of histamine type I (H_1), histamine type II (H_2), or an unclassified category of histamine-binding receptors in mediating these effects is unclear.

Histamine, in keeping with the concept that agents that increase cyclic adenosine monophosphate (cAMP) levels in lymphocytes have a negative modulatory effect, blocks induction of antigen-induced suppressor cells for antibody formation, and this effect is abrogated by the histamine type I antagonist diphenhydramine (10). In contrast, several investigators have reported that activation of suppressor cells by histamine is mediated via histamine type II receptors in both human and murine systems, and this interaction appears to be dissociated from an elevation of cAMP (see reviews in Refs. 6 and 11).

These observations illustrate the complexity of analyzing the effects of histamine on immune regulation. It is important to note that much of the evidence implicating a histamine type II receptor interaction in suppressor cell modulation is circumstantial and stems from observations showing that histamine type II receptor antagonists can abrogate the activity of these cells.

This chapter reviews studies on the modulation of murine suppressor cell function by histamine in vitro and in vivo and discusses the putative receptor interactions involved.

II. MODULATION OF SUPPRESSOR CELLS REGULATING HUMORAL IMMUNITY

Interest in the role of histamine and histamine receptor-bearing lymphocytes in the regulation of humoral and cell-mediated immunity stems from the original observations of Melmon et al. (12-14). They showed that histamine and other vasoactive amines inhibited antibody synthesis to sheep red blood cells (SRBCs), and inhibition was correlated with increases in intracellular cyclic AMP levels. These investigators also demonstrated that a subpopulation of spleen cells adhered to histamine, coupled via rabbit serum albumin to sepharose beads (H-RSA-S) (15). Subsequent studies revealed that passage of spleen cells over these histamine affinity columns resulted in the depletion of a population(s) of cells that regulated antibody production to SRBCs (16). Adoptive transfer of the histamine nonadherent cell population into irradiated syngeneic mice showed that the recipient animals had a significantly greater response to antigen than animals receiving the unfractionated cells, indicating that a suppressor-cell population(s) had been removed. A similar result was obtained when histamine column-fractionated thymocytes were injected together with unfractionated bone marrow cells. In contrast, no enhancing effect was observed when fractionated marrow cells were mixed with unseparated thymocytes (16). The binding of cells to H-RSA-S columns was not due simply to the charge of the beads, since the immunoregulatory suppressor-cell subset did not bind to poly-L-lysine-RSA-S columns.

Similar studies were performed with spleen cells from animals that had been tolerized with high doses of soluble components derived from a hypotonic lysis of SRBCs (17). In these experiments, antigen-specific suppression of both the T cell-independent immunoglobulin M (IgM) and the T cell–dependent IgG response was obtained. However, only IgG unresponsiveness could be adoptively transferred, and passage of spleen cells from unresponsive mice over H-RSA-S columns abrogated the adoptive transfer of IgG unresponsiveness. Identification of the suppressor cells as T cells was confirmed by showing that anti-Thy 1.2 antibody and complement abrogated the effect. The suppressive effect was antigen specific and did not affect responsiveness to horse or chicken red blood cells (17).

Suppressor T cells that inhibit in vitro plaque-forming responses against SRBCs are also induced by incubation with the mitogen concanavalin A (Con A). The Con A-activated suppressor cells have been characterized as Thy 1.2^+, Ly 2.3^+ and to be histamine receptor positive (18). The expression of histamine receptors was deduced from the finding that suppressor T cells activated by Con A were significantly depleted by fractionation on H-RSA-S columns, whereas fractionation of normal cells followed by exposure to Con A had no effect on subsequent suppressor T-cell induction. Direct addition of histamine (5×10^{-4}-5×10^{-8} M) to Con A precultures had no effect on suppressor T-cell generation. This suggested that the immunomodulatory activity of histamine was expressed at the effector stage rather than the induction of suppressor T-cell activation by Con A. These results contrast with those of Schwartz et al. (19), in which the generation of T cells by Con A that suppressed cytotoxic T lymphocyte (CTL) responses were inhibited by a high concentration (10^{-3} M) of histamine (see below). These results suggest a differential sensitivity within suppressor T-cell subpopulations to signals mediated by histamine, allowing a cytotoxic suppressor cell to be inhibited, whereas a suppressor cell of antibody responsiveness is unaffected.

The use of immobilized histamine affinity H-RSA-S columns for selective depletion of regulatory subsets of lymphocytes warrants comment. Although the evidence that suppressor cells bind to these columns is convincing, there is some doubt as to the exact role of histamine receptors in binding to these conjugates. This concern applies particularly to those studies in which discordant influences of histamine columns on cell-mediated cytotoxicity and humoral antibody production are observed (reviewed in Refs. 6, 11, and 20).

The studies reviewed so far describe histamine-mediated modulation of suppressor cells in vitro. A similar regulatory role for histaminergic regulation of suppressor cells in vivo has yet to be demonstrated. Szewczuk et al. evaluated the inhibitory effect of histamine on immune reactivity of LAF_1 mice to trinitrophenylated bovine-γ-globulin (TNP-BGG), but failed to detect suppressor cell activity in spleen cell populations (21). The results suggested that histamine in combination with antigen induced the formation of auto-anti-idiotypic antibodies which were involved in the normal regulation of the immune response to TNP-BGG. Studies in our laboratory also provide evidence that histamine can have an inhibitory effect on antibody synthesis by a mechanism(s) other than induction of suppressor cells. We have demonstrated that histamine injected into BALB/c mice 24 hr after sensitization with Con A results in marked suppression of antibody to SRBCs injected 2 hr later (22). This effect was strain, but not major histocompatibility complex (MHC) specific, and did not occur with the T-independent antigen polyvinylpyrolidone (PVP). This would suggest a direct effect of histamine on B cells rather than T-suppressor cells. In addition, no evidence of induction of suppressor cells was detected when the spleen cells were explanted and cultured in vitro in coculture assays. We hypothesized that this suppression was due to histamine type I-mediated release of adrenocorticotrophic hormone (ACTH) with the subsequent action of corticosterone on B cells (22). Evidence to support this interpretation was provided by the demonstration that ACTH and corticosterone could mimic the effects of histamine, and that drugs that ablate adrenocortical cell function abrogated the effects of histamine (22).

III. MODULATION OF SUPPRESSOR CELLS REGULATING CELL-MEDIATED IMMUNITY

A variety of cell types are involved in the manifestation of delayed-type hypersensitivity (DTH) responses, including mast cells and basophils. These cells contain significant quantities of histamine and are known to degranulate at local sites of DTH (23). It is estimated that local histamine concentrations as high as 10^{-3} M may occur, and that this local release of transiently high levels of histamine, while having no significant vasoactive effects in the mouse, may have considerable immunomodulatory effects (24).

In vivo studies have provided circumstantial evidence to support an immunoregulatory role for histamine in DTH responses (25,26). The responses are complex in that hyporesponsive DTH reactions are augmented and normal DTH responses are inhibited. This bidirectional effect suggests an action of histamine on regulatory cells such as modulation of suppressor-cell activity. This regulatory effect was demonstrated in an in vitro system in which histamine (10^{-3} M) was shown to inhibit the activation of suppressor cells by Con A. The population of cells activated by Con A and inhibited by histamine was Thy 1.2^+ and Ly 2.3^+ (19). In a different experimental system, histamine treatment of spleen cells from animals tolerized to trinitrobenzene sulfonic acid (TNBS) resulted in the genesis of cells that inhibited the production of TNP-altered self-specific CTL (27). These latter findings may be more relevant to the in vivo situation in that the cells were incubated with concentrations of histamine that might be expected to exist in vivo (10^{-4}-10^{-5} M) and the cells were washed free of histamine prior to their addition to the culture system.

In contrast to the observations on the effects of histamine-reactive suppressor cells on antibody production, passage of spleen cells over H-RSA-S columns prior to their sensitization for T cell–mediated cytotoxic activity did not enhance responsiveness. When spleen cells from normal BALB/c mice were passed over these columns prior to sensitization with irradiated C57/BL6 stimulator cells, the cytotoxic potential of the unretained cells against EL-4 cells was depleted or significantly reduced (20). Thus, cells that are adherent to histamine columns may have regulatory influences on the generation of antibody responses, but not on the generation of cytotoxic reactions. However, it is difficult to compare the effects of histamine columns on cell-mediated versus humoral immunity unless a common antigen is utilized and a common in vitro or in vivo model is adopted for generating the response.

Histamine has also been shown to inhibit the generation of secondary cytotoxic T-lymphocyte responses in vitro toward allogeneic P815 mastocytoma cells (28). This activity appeared to be mediated via histamine type II receptors, since the effect could be mimicked by the histamine type II agonist, dimaprit, and reversed by the histamine type II antagonist, cimetidine. Although the authors attribute the activity to histamine effects on suppressor cells, data on isolated suppressor cell populations were not presented.

Additional studies describing the effects of histamine on the activation of suppressor cells in vitro indicated that these cells inhibit the response of murine spleen cells to PHA but not LPS (29). The cells activated by histamine are removed on H-RSA-S columns and are Ly 2 positive. In this system, it appears that the suppressive activity is mediated by a soluble factor elaborated by histamine-activated cells (30). This suppressor factor has an approximate molecular weight of 45,000–68,000 daltons, it adheres to H-RSA-S columns, and its production is inhibited by histamine type II receptor, but not by histamine type I receptor antagonists. In studies to evaluate the mechanism of action of suppression, it was shown that histamine-induced inhibition of the lymphocyte responses to PHA as well as the activity of the histamine-induced suppressor factor were both blocked by the prostaglandin synthesis inhibitors indomethacin and Ro 205720

(30). These findings illustrate yet another facet of the role of vasoactive amines in the regulation of murine suppressor cells via an interaction between histamine and prostaglandins.

The suppressor cells identified in these experiments exert a negative regulatory effect, and their removal often results in marked augmentation of immune responses (31). Another class of suppressor cells has been described which exert a positive effect on immune responsiveness, and thus "oppose" suppressor cell activity. They have been named contrasuppressor cells and their activity referred to as contrasuppression (32,33). Experiments have been described which indicate that both interferon (34) and histamine (27) can activate both suppressor and contrasuppressor cell populations. Studies with histamine were carried out with spleen cells tolerized with TNBS. The functional activity of these cells was measured by their ability to regulate normal cell-mediated lympholysis (CML) to TNP-modified self (27). When such cells were incubated with histamine, suppressor cells became evident in the cultures, but their appearance was often variable and the cells gave unusual dose-response curves. Further investigation of the effects of histamine revealed that the histamine type II agonist dimaprit was a more efficient inducer of suppressor cells than histamine, whereas the histamine type I agonist [2-(2-pyridyl)-ethylamine dihydrochloride] (PEA) had a greater effect on contrasuppressor cells. Regulatory cells preincubated with PEA blocked the suppressive effect of regulatory cells preincubated with dimaprit (Fig. 1). The activity of these PEA-activated contrasuppressor cells could be abrogated by treatment with anti–I-J antibody and complement, thereby resembling the contrasuppressor cell populations described in other experimental systems (27).

Although histamine enhances suppressor-cell function in vitro, and this suppression can be abrogated either totally or partially with specific histamine type II receptor antagonists, more convincing evidence of the role of histamine in immunomodulation comes from in vivo studies. In many models the effect of histamine type II antagonists has been inferred but not proven, and the results are often conflicting. We have demonstrated an immunodulatory effect of histamine on suppressor-cell function in vivo by evaluating the effect of histamine type II antagonists on the induction and expression of hapten-specific suppressor T cells (35). These studies were carried out using an adoptive transfer model where the role of antigen-specific suppressor cells has been well defined. The intravenous injection of dinitrobenzene sulfonic acid ($DNBSO_3$) results in an antigen-specific tolerance mediated by multiple mechanisms that include T_S and clonal deletion. The adoptive transfer of splenic suppressor cells from these tolerized animals results in the inability of the recipient mice to respond to a sensitizing dose of dinitrofluorobenzene (DNFB). These T_S cells act during the afferent phase of the immune response in that they suppress sensitization but have no effect on the elicitation of DTH in previously sensitized mice (36, 37). Treatment of the tolerized donor mice with the H_2 antagonists cimetidine and ranitidine produces moderate but significant inhibition of T_S cell induction,

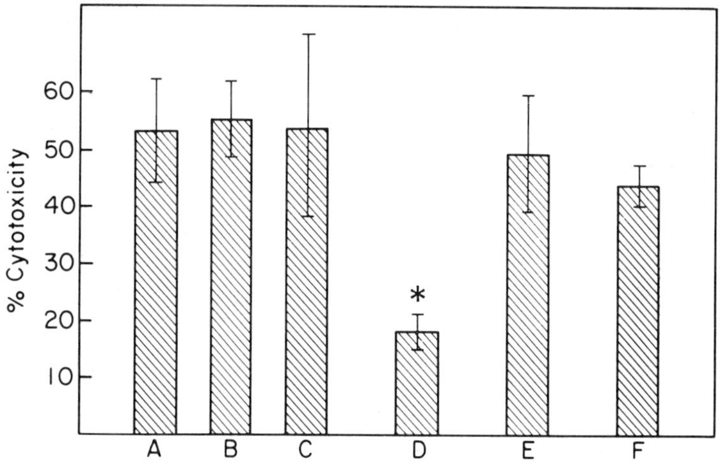

Figure 1 Synthetic histamine agonists induce opposing regulatory activities in different aliquots of cells from mice made tolerant with TNBS. Regulatory cells were divided into 2 aliquots. Prior to being combined and then added or added alone to 5-day CML cultures of normal B6AF, responder cells and TNP-labeled stimulator cells, the aliquots were preincubated for 60 min at 37°C as follows: bar A, no regulatory cells added (control); bar B, aliquot 1 preincubated in medium; bar C, aliquot 2 preincubated with 0.1 mM PEA; bar D, aliquot 1 preincubated with 1 mM dimaprit; bar E, aliquot 1 preincubated with 0.1 mM PEA; bar F, aliquot 1 preincubated with 1 mM dimaprit and then combined with aliquot 2 that was preincubated with 0.1 mM PEA. After 5 days, the cells were harvested and incubated with [^{51}Cr]-labeled TNP target cells for 4 hr, and then percentage toxicity was determined. Results are shown as mean ± SD, % cytotoxicity is shown in parenthesis. *Significantly different ($p < 0.01$) from controls. (From Ref. 27, used with permission.)

as shown by the enhanced response to DNFB in spleen cell recipients (35). However, definitive dose-response relationships are not observed (Table 1). A more impressive abrogation of suppressor cells is seen when histamine type II antagonists are assayed for their effects on the expression of adoptively transferred spleen cells. A dose-related inhibition of suppression is observed with both cimetidine and ranitidine. At doses of 10-25 mg/kg both compounds completely abrogate the expression of the transferred T_S cells (Fig. 2). Neither antagonist has any effect on the optimal response to DNFB in normal animals sensitized and challenged with DNFB, and they also fail to affect the response to DNFB in tolerized mice (35). Similar studies by Sahasrabudhe (38) have confirmed our findings with cimetidine in this model demonstrating inhibition of the expression as opposed to the induction of T_S cells, and he also demonstrated the antigenic specificity of the phenomenon.

Table 1 Effect of H_2 Antagonists and an Inactive Structurally Related Cimetidine Congener on $DNBSO_3$ T_S Induction

Treatment of donor[a] (mg/kg)	Response of recipient to DNFB[b]	Percent suppression
None (normal cell control)	65.3 ± 3.4	–
$DNBSO_3$ i.v.	14.0 ± 2.2	78.5
$DNBSO_3$ + cimetidine		
25	32.8 ± 5.2[c]	49.7
12.5	39.1 ± 5.2[c]	40.0
6.25	20.5 ± 3.3	68.6
$DNBSO_3$ + ranitidine		
25	23.8 ± 6.7	63.5
12.5	29.0 ± 4.7[d]	55.6
6.25	20.0 ± 2.4	69.3
$DNBSO_3$ + norburimamide		
25	9.1 ± 1.9	86.1

[a]BALB/c mice were treated with the compounds indicated (orally, twice daily) from 1 day before tolerization to 7 days after. Spleen cells (80–100 × 10^6/recipient) were transferred into naive recipients (seven mice/group). They were immediately sensitized and 5 days later were challenged with DNFB.
[b]Data expressed in microliters of edema (mean t ± SEM).
[c]Significantly different from tolerant control ($p < 0.001$).
[d]Significantly different from tolerant control ($p < 0.05$).
Source: Modified from Ref. 35, used with permission.

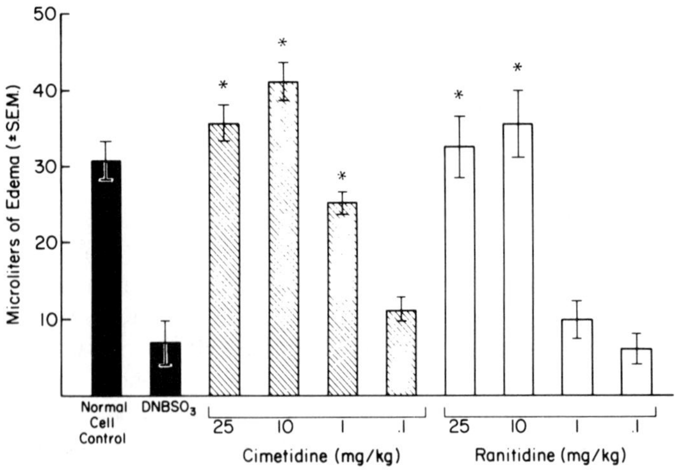

Figure 2 BALB/c mice were treated with indicated drugs from 1 day before adoptive transfer of tolerized spleen cells (80–100 × 10^6/mouse) to day +5. Recipients were immediately sensitized and 5 days later were challenged with DNFB. Edema was read plethysmographically 24 hr after challenge. *Significantly different from tolerant control ($p < 0.001$).

We have also examined the ability of histamine type II antagonists to inhibit the immune suppression mediated by different types of murine T_S cells. The suppressor cells induced by intravenous injection of $DNBSO_3$ are Lyt 2^+ T cells (35). A population of T_S is also induced by ultraviolet (UV) irradiation, and these cells exhibit the Lyt 1^+ phenotype (39,40). We have demonstrated that the histamine type II antagonists cimetidine and oxmetidine are able to inhibit the expression of both T_S populations (41). Much higher doses of cimetidine than oxmetidine were required to produce similar restoration of the response to DNFB (Table 2). In these studies, evidence that the modulating effects were specific for histamine type II receptor antagonists was provided by the fact that the histamine type I antagonist diphenhydramine was ineffective in both the $DNBSO_3$ and the UV-induced suppressor cell models. In contrast to the results with $DNBSO_3$ and UV-induced suppressor cells, we were unable to modulate the activity of suppressor cells induced by high-dose SRBC with these histamine type II antagonists (41).

Evidence for a role for histamine in modulating suppressor cells in vivo is also provided by studies using a system in which suppressor cells are induced by the intravenous inoculation of BALB/c mice with DNP-coupled syngeneic spleen cells. The adoptive transfer of spleen or lymph node cells from these animals results in a reduction in ear swelling after contact sensitization with DNFB in syngeneic recipients. Cimetidine treatment of the donor animals with 50 mg/kg intraperitoneally 2 days before, or on the day of suppressor cell induction, resulted in a diminished capacity to transfer functional suppressor-cell activity (42). These studies, like our own (35), demonstrate the ability of treatment with cimetidine to inhibit suppressor cells in vivo. However, in this study the effect of cimetidine in the recipients of adoptively transferred spleen cells was not evaluated.

In contrast, Mekori et al. (43) were unable to demonstrate an immunomodulatory action of cimetidine and ranitidine on antigen-specific suppressor T cell–mediated tolerance to DNFB in BALB/c mice when they were administered during the induction or the effector stage. The lack of effect of cimetidine in this model of antigen-specific tolerance is difficult to explain. However, there are several differences in the model systems used, including the use of female as opposed to male mice, intraperitoneal versus oral dosing and different dosing schedules, and the use of x-irradiated recipients (43). This ineffectiveness of histamine type II antagonists was in contrast to these compounds' ability to counteract the nonspecific immunosuppression of contact sensitivity induced by burns. In this model, therapy with cimetidine or ranitidine was also shown to be effective in preserving normal helper/inducer and suppressor/cytotoxic lymphocyte populations. Evaluation of the frequencies of splenic helper (Ly 1^+)- and suppressor (Ly 2^+)-positive cells following cimetidine therapy normalized the helper:suppressor T-cell ratios, whereas treatment of unburned animals had no effect (44).

Table 2. The Effects of High Doses of Oxmetidine, Cimetidine, and Diphenhydramine on UV-induced Suppressor Cells

Experiment	Treatment[a] (mg/kg)	DNFB response µl Paw Edema ± SEM	Percent restoration	p Value
1	DNFB control	97.6 ± 2.9		
	UV control	55.8 ± 6.3		
	Oxmetidine			
	50	91.8 ± 2.2	86.1	<0.001
	25	86.5 ± 5.5	73.4	<0.01
	12.5	73.7 ± 9.3	42.8	NS
	Diphenhydramine			
	40	61.7 ± 7.6	14.1	NS[b]
	20	67.4 ± 7.6	27.7	NS
	10	50.2 ± 8.9	0.0	NS
2	DNFB control	64.8 ± 9.1		
	UV control	28.0 ± 2.0		
	Cimetidine			
	400	51.2 ± 7.7	63.0	<0.001
	200	57.7 ± 7.5	80.7	<0.001
	100	30.2 ± 3.0	6.0	NS

[a]BALB/c mice were treated with the indicated drugs beginning 1 day before the adoptive transfer of UV-tolerized spleen cells (80–100 × 10^6/mouse). Recipients were immediately sensitized and were challenged with DNFB 5 days later. Edema was measured plethysmographically 24 hr after challenge.

[b]Not statistically significant.

Source: Modified from Ref. 41, used with permission.

IV. HISTAMINE REGULATION OF NATURAL SUPPRESSOR CELLS

A population of suppressor cells known as natural suppressor (NS) cells are also known to be modulated by histamine. These cells suppress the in vitro mixed leukocyte culture reaction and graft-vs.-host disease. They have been identified in the spleens of neonatal mice (45), and of adult mice recovering from total lymphoid irradiation (46), whole-body irradiation (47), syngeneic marrow transplantation (48), and cyclophosphamide therapy (49). Natural suppressor cells may have a key role in the induction of immune tolerance. They can inhibit the antigen-specific cytolytic arm of alloreactive immune responses without affecting the antigen-specific suppressor-cell arm (4). These cells are viewed as being related to natural killer cells in that they are found in the "null" cell population, they lack antigen specificity, and carry out their effector function without antigenic stimulation. However, they appear to differ with regard to function (for review see Ref. 4). Recent evidence with cloned NS cells indicates that these cells may be members of the T-cell lineage that express the α, β, and γ genes of the T-cell antigen receptor (50).

Naturally occurring suppressor cells as well as long-term cultures of these cells inhibit mixed lymphocyte reactions in vitro (4,46). The suppressor fucntion of NS cells is enhanced by preincubation with histamine (10^{-4} M) for 4 hr before the washed NS cells are added to responder and stimulator cells in mixed lymphocyte cultures (MLRs). The histamine-induced effects occur in the absence of proliferation as the NS cells are irradiated prior to culture. The action of histamine on these NS cells is a histamine type I receptor-mediated event, and is inhibited by the histamine type I receptor antagonists mepyramine (10^{-6} M) and pyrobutamine (10^{-7} M), but cimetidine (10^{-5} M) does not alter the suppressor-enhancing action of histamine. No effect is seen on suppression if histamine is incorporated into the MLR coculture assay (8). These results are interesting in light of the fact that in the murine T-suppressor cell system histamine activates contrasuppressor cells via a histamine type I-mediated effect (27). Using the radioligand histamine type I antagonist, [^{3}H]pyrilamine, a single, specific binding site for [^{3}H]pyrilamine has been shown to exist on NS cells (51).

Mast cells represent a major storage site for histamine, and large numbers of mast cells have been found in the vicinity of NS cells in neonatal mouse spleens (52). The influence of mast cells on NS cell function has been evaluated by examining the effect of mast cells and mast cell supernatants on NS activity. Incubation of a clone of NS cells with a mast cell supernatant for 4 hr before they are added to an MLR results in enhanced suppression of the MLR. Enhanced suppression is also observed when the mast cells themselves are added to the MLR. Enhanced suppressor-cell activity was histamine type I receptor mediated, and indicates that mast cells may be major modulators of NS cell function (52). These authors have also investigated the modulatory effects of a number of congener derivatives and conjugates of histamine on NS activity. Some compounds showed selective effects on natural suppressor cells in that they were inactive on myocardial tissue, whereas other compounds were selectively active on the myocardium (53).

Enhancement of the suppressive effects of NS cells by histamine is independent of changes in intracellular cAMP concentrations. Stimulation of histamine type II receptors by histamine results in accumulation of cAMP that is blocked by cimetidine (10^{-5} M), but this accumulation does not result in an enhancement of suppressor-cell function. In addition, treatment of these cells with two cAMP-elevating agents, isoproterenol and forskolin, does not result in augmentation of their suppressor activity (8). On the other hand, stimulation of histamine type I receptors enhances the suppressor potential of NS cells in the absence of an accumulation of cAMP. Two histamine type I receptor antagonists, mepyramine (10^{-6} M) and pyrobutamine (10^{-7} M), each competitively block histamine activation of the NS cells (8).

V. SUPPRESSOR CELLS IN TUMOR IMMUNITY

There are several studies indicating that suppressor cells may play a role in the immunosuppression observed during tumor growth (reviewed in Ref. 54). This suppression may involve the suppression of specific antitumor immunity or general nonspecific suppression of immunologic competence or both. There is also evidence from murine tumor models that the suppressor cell subsets bear histamine receptors, and that histamine agonists/antagonists modulate tumor immunity. In one study, spleen cells from C57BL/6 mice bearing metastatic Lewis lung carcinoma (3LL) were shown to contain a population of cells that adhered to H-RSA-S columns. These cells enhanced tumor growth when mixed with tumor cells and inoculated into syngeneic mice. The cells that failed to adhere to the H-RSA-S columns had no effect on tumor growth (55,56).

If histamine receptor–bearing suppressor cells play a role in tumor progression, it is not unreasonable to believe that selective inactivation of these cells could be of therapeutic benefit. This hypothesis has been tested by investigating the effects of the histamine type II antagonist cimetidine in C57BL/6 mice bearing the Lewis lung carcinoma (57). Flow cytometric analysis showed that the number of histamine type II receptor–bearing cells in the spleens of tumor-bearing animals increases steadily after tumor inoculation. This increase is associated with an increase in histamine-activated suppression in vitro. Animals treated with cimetidine have less histamine-activated suppressor-cell function and decreased in vivo metastatic spread of tumor as well as prolonged survival compared to controls (57).

Using a Cloudman melanoma tumor model, Nordlund et al. (58) have demonstrated that tumor cells can activate either helper/inducer or T_S cells, and the rate of growth of the tumor is a reflection of this complex interplay. Which of these cell populations predominates depends on the dose of melanoma tumor antigen associated with the original tumor inoculum. Induction of suppressor cells enhances tumor growth, and this effect can be adoptively transferred with splenocytes (58,59). Immunosuppression (thymectomy and treatment with antilymphocyte serum) of these animals also results in marked acceleration of tumor growth. Histamine treatment accelerates tumor growth, but only in normal animals, and has little effect on tumor growth in immunocompromised hosts. Cimetidine treatment tends to increase tumor growth in normal hosts, but significant suppression of tumor growth occurs in immunosuppressed animals (60). As these animals are known to have augmented suppressor-cell activation these data are consistent with a modulation of histamine-dependent suppressor cells.

In an additional model, described by Babayan et al. (61), ingestion of N-(4-(5-nitro-2-furyl)-2-thiazoyl)formamide (FANFT) causes the development of transitional cell carcinoma of the bladder in C3H/HeJ mice. The primary growth of this tumor when implanted in the footpad and its subsequent metastasis to the lung correlates with the development of increased numbers of suppressor cells as characterized by the expression of surface histamine type II receptors. The appearance of these suppressor cells in the spleen is maximal 4 weeks following tumor implantation. These cells then migrate from the spleen to the peripheral blood, and this event parallels the growth and metastasis of this tumor.

VI. CONCLUSIONS

The studies reviewed in this chapter demonstrate the complexity of the pharmacologic effects of histamine, an endogenous physiologic modulator, on immune suppressor cell function in vitro and in vivo. Although the evidence for a role of histamine in the activation of suppressor cells cannot be disputed, a variety of mechanisms could explain the immunoregulatory role of this autacoid. One of the reasons for the conflicting opinions on the role of histamine on murine suppressor-cell populations may be the result of working with heterogeneous target cell populations. The pharmacologic effects of autacoids such as histamine on unseparated cell populations in vitro are difficult to interpret, especially when cells other than T cells bear histamine receptors and will certainly respond to the presence of the autacoid. In addition, the potential for both an immunosuppressive and an immunostimulatory role for histamine must be emphasized. This depends heavily upon the model being used, the interacting cell types, and the surface histamine receptors involved, all of which result in a complex process of immunoregulation.

Considerable emphasis has been placed on the hypothesis that suppressor T cells bear histamine type II receptors, and that pharmacologic manipulation of these receptors will result in either positive or negative regulatory effects on the immune system. Although a considerable volume of proof exists that supports this concept, it is possible that simple blockade of histamine type II receptors may not be responsible for the loss of T-suppressor cell effector function in vivo. A study by Descotes et al. suggests, in fact, that the immunologic effects of cimetidine may be mediated through the imidazole moiety and is not solely a function of histamine type II receptor blockade (62).

Much of the controversy surrounding the concept of histamine type II receptor-mediated immunoregulation would be resolved if histamine receptors could be well defined on lymphocyte subpopulations. However, direct identification and subtyping of histamine receptors on specific subsets of immune cells has proved difficult. Traditional radioligand-binding assays have met with limited success for several reasons (6). Whole-cell assays are problematic owing to internalization of ligand and high levels of nonspecific binding. Membrane-binding assays require purification of significant quantities of lymphocyte subpopulations to provide interpretable results. While high affinity [^{3}H]pyrilamine binding to lymphocytes has been described, similar high-affinity histamine type II selective ligands have not yet been identified. Protein conjugates of histamine (6) or related ligands (63,64) potentially offer multivalent high-affinity reagents compatible with flow cytometric identification of subpopulation-specific binding. However, the current consensus in both murine and human systems is that such reagents do not exhibit sufficient binding selectivity. The need for selective and specific binding assays remains crucial to further progress in defining the cell types and histamine receptor subtypes which mediate the immunologic effects of this autacoid.

It is clear that additional studies are required to better define the mechanism(s) by which histamine exerts its modulatory effects on suppressor cells and the receptor interactions involved. With this knowledge it might then be possible to pharmacologically manipulate this population of cells and to modify immune responses for experimental and therapeutic benefit.

REFERENCES

1. Gershon, R. K., and K. Kondo, Cell interactions in the induction of tolerance: The role of thymic lymphocytes. Immunology 21:903–914 (1970).
2. Gilbert, K. M., and M. K. Hoffman, Suppressor B lymphocytes. Immunol. Today 4:253–255 (1983).
3. Allison, A. C., Mechanisms by which activated macrophages inhibit lymphocyte responses. Immunol. Rev. 40:3–27 (1978).

4. Strober, S., Natural suppressor cells, neonatal tolerance and total lymphoid irradiation. Exploring obscure relationships, Annu. Rev. Immunol. 2:219–237 (1984).
5. Plaut, M., and W. Roszkowski, Lymphocyte subpopulations bearing histamine receptors. In Histamine Receptors, (Yellin, T. O., Ed.), Spectrum, Holliswood, New York (1979), pp. 361–376.
6. Beer, D. J., and R. E. Rocklin, Histamine modulation of lymphocyte biology: Membrane receptors, signal transduction, and functions, Crit. Rev. Immunol. 7 (1):55–91 (1987).
7. Melmon, K. L., R. E. Rocklin, and R. P. Rosenkranz, Autacoids as modulators of the inflammatory and immune response, Am. J. Med. 71:100–106 (1981).
8. Khan, M. M., K. L. Melmon, C. G. Fathman, B. Hertel-Wulff, and S. Strober, The effects of autacoids on cloned murine lymphoid cells: Modulation of IL-2 secretion and the activity of natural suppressor cells. J. Immunol. 134: 4100–4106 (1985).
9. Kahn, M. M., P. Sansoni, E. G. Engleman, and K. L. Melmon, Pharmacologic effects of autacoids on subsets of T cells. Regulation of expression/function of histamine 2 receptors by a subset of suppressor cells, J. Clin. Invest. 75: 1578–1583 (1985).
10. Mozes, E., Y. Weinstein, H. R. Bourne, K. L. Melmon, and G. M. Shearer, *In vitro* correction of antigen-induced immune suppression: Effects of histamine, dibutyryl cyclic AMP and cholera toxin, Cell. Immunol. 11:57–63 (1974).
11. Plaut, M., Histamine and immune responses. In Pharmacology of Histamine Receptors (Ganellin, C. R., and Parsons, M. E., Eds.), Wright, PSG, Littleton, Massachusetts (1982), pp. 392–435.
12. Melmon, K. L., H. R. Bourne, and Y. Weinstein, Receptors for histamine can be detected on the surface of selected leukocytes, Science 177:707–709 (1972).
13. Melmon, K. L., H. R. Bourne, Y. Weinstein, G. M. Shearer, J. Kram, and S. Bauminger, Hemolytic plaque formation by leukocytes *in vitro*, control by vasoactive hormones, J. Clin. Invest. 53:13–21 (1974).
14. Melmon, K. L., Y. Weinstein, G. M. Shearer, H. R. Bourne, and S. Bauminger, Separation of specific antibody-forming mouse cells by their adherence to insolubilized endogenous hormones, J. Clin. Invest. 53:22–30 (1974).
15. Shearer, G. M., K. L. Melmon, Y. Weinstein, and M. Sela, Regulation of antibody response by cells expressing histamine receptors, J. Exp. Med. 136:1302–1307 (1972).
16. Shearer, G. M., Y. Weinstein, and K. L. Melmon, Enhancement of immune response potential of mouse lymphoid cells fractionated over insolubilized conjugated histamine columns, J. Immunol. 113:597–607 (1974).
17. Segal, S., K. L. Melmon, and Y. Weinstein, Isolation of suppressor T-lymphocytes adherent to histamine-conjugated albumin and their role in suppression of IgG responses to SRBC, Cell. Immunol. 59:171–180 (1981).

18. Orme, I., and F. L. Shand, Concanavalin A-induced alteration of surface marker expression on murine T cells, Int. J. Immunopharmacol. 4:137–142 (1982).
19. Schwartz, A., S. Sutton, P. W. Askenase, and R. K. Gershon, Histamine inhibition and concanavalin-A induced suppressor T-cell activation, Cell. Immunol. 60:426–439 (1981).
20. Shearer, G. M., E. Simpson, Y. Weinstein, and K. L. Melmon, Fractionation of lymphocytes involved in the generation of cell-mediated cytotoxicity over insolubilized conjugated histamine columns, J. Immunol. 118:756–761 (1977).
21. Szewczuk, M. R., R. J. Campbell, and J. W. Smith, Evidence for histamine-induced auto-anti-idiotypic antibody immunoregulation *in vivo*, Cell. Immunol. 65:152–165 (1981).
22. Badger, A. M., D. E. Griswold, M. J. DiMartino, and G. Poste, Inhibition of antibody synthesis by histamine in concanavalin A-treated mice: The possible role of glucocorticosteroids, J. Immunol. 129:1017–1022 (1982).
23. Askenase, P. W., S. Bursztajn, M. D. Gershon, and R. K. Gershon, T cell dependent mast cell degranulation and release of serotonin in murine delayed-type hypersensitivity, J. Exp. Med. 152:1358–1374 (1980).
24. Schwartz, A., P. W. Askenase, and R. K. Gershon, The effects of locally injected vasoactive amines on the elicitation of delayed-type hypersensitivity, J. Immunol. 118:159–165 (1977).
25. Askenase, P. W., A. Schwartz, J. N. Siegel, and R. D. Gershon, Role of histamine in the regulation of cell-mediated immunity, Int. Arch. Allergy Appl. Immunol. 66 (Suppl. 1):225–233 (1981).
26. Griswold, D. E., S. Alessi, and D. T. Walz, Stimulation of contact sensitivity to oxazolone by disodium cromoglycate, Int. Arch. Allergy Appl. Immunol. 69:93–97 (1982).
27. Siegel, J. N., A. Schwartz, P. W. Askenase, R. K. Gershon, T cell suppression and contrasuppression induced by histamine H_2 and H_1 receptor agonists respectively, Proc. Natl. Acad. Sci. U.S.A. 79:5052–5056 (1982).
28. French, S., Walker, M., Susskind, B., and R. Faanes, Modulation of *in vitro* cellular immune responses by histamine agonists or antagonists in murine species, Arzneimmitelforsch./Drug Res. 35:390–394 (1985).
29. Suzuki, S., and R. Huchet, Mechanism of histamine-induced inhibition of lymphocyte response to mitogens in mice, Cell. Immunol. 62:396–405 (1981).
30. Suzuki, S., and R. Huchet, Properties of histamine-induced suppressor factor in the regulation of lymphocyte response to PHA in mice, Cell. Immunol. 68:349–358 (1982).
31. Cantor, H., and R. K. Gershon, Immunological circuits: Cellular composition, Fed. Proc. Am. Soc. Exp. Biol. 38:2058–2064 (1979).
32. Gershon, R. K., D. D. Eardley, S. Durum, D. R. Green, F. W. Shen, K. Yamauchi, H. Cantor, and D. B. Murphy, Contrasuppression: A novel immunoregulatory activity, J. Exp. Med. 153:1533–1546 (1981).

33. Yamauchi, K., D. R. Green, D. D. Eardley, D. B. Murphy, and R. K. Gershon, Immunoregulatory circuits that modulate responsiveness to suppressor cell signals: Failure of B10 mice to respond to suppressor factors can be overcome by quenching the contrasuppressor cell circuit, J. Exp. Med. 153: 1547–1561 (1981).
34. Knop, J., R. Stremmer, C. Neuman, E. DeMaeyer, and E. Macher, Interferon inhibits the suppressor T cell response of delayed-type hypersensitivity, Nature 296:757–759 (1982).
35. Griswold, D. E., S. Alessi, A. M. Badger, G. Poste, and N. Hanna, Inhibition of T suppressor cell expression by histamine type 2 (H_2) receptor antagonist, J. Immunol. 132:3054–3057 (1984).
36. Claman, H. N., S. D. Miller, M. Sy, and J. W. Moorhead, Suppressive mechanisms involving sensitization and tolerance in contact allergy, Immunol. Rev. 40:105–132 (1980).
37. Phanaphak, P., J. W. Moorhead, and H. N. Claman, Tolerance and contact sensitivity to DNFB in mice. III Transfer of tolerance with "suppressor T cells," J. Immunol. 113:1230–1236 (1974).
38. Sahasrabudhe, D. M., C. S. McCune, R. W. O'Donnell, and E. C. Henshaw, Inhibition of suppressor T lymphocytes (T_S) by cimetidine, J. Immunol. 138:2760–2763 (1987).
39. Ullrich, S. E., and M. L. Kripke, Mechanisms in the suppression of tumor rejection produced in mice by repeated UV irradiation, J. Immunol. 133: 2786–2790 (1984).
40. Granstein, R. D., J. A. Parrish, and D. J. McAuliffe, C. Waltenbaugh, and M. I. Greene, Immunologic inhibition of ultraviolet radiation-induced tumor suppressor cell activity, Science 224:615–617 (1984).
41. Griswold, D. E., S. Alessi, A. M. Badger, G. Poste, and N. Hanna, Differential sensitivity of T suppressor cell expression to inhibition by histamine type 2 receptor antagonists, J. Immunol. 137:1811–1815 (1986).
42. Jin, Z., A. Kumar, R. P. Cleveland, D. L. Murphy, and D. B. Kaufman, Inhibition of suppressor cell function by cimetidine in a murine model, Clin. Immunol. Immunopathol. 38:350–356 (1986).
43. Mekori, Y. A., E. M. Bender, R. Zapata-Sirvent, J. F. Hansbrough, and H. N. Claman, The effect of histamine receptor antagonists on specific and nonspecific suppression of experimental contact sensitivity, J. Allergy Clin. Immunol. 76:90–96 (1985).
44. Zapata-Sirvent, R. L., and J. F. Hansbrough, Postburn immunosuppression in an animal model. III. Maintenance of normal splenic helper and suppressor lymphocyte subpopulations by immunomodulating drugs, Surgery 97:721–727 (1985).
45. Oseroff, A., S. Okada, and S. Strober, Natural suppressor (NS) cells found in the spleen of neonatal mice and adult mice given total lymphoid irradiation (TLI) express the null surface phenotype, J. Immunol. 132:101–110 (1984).
46. Hertel-Wulff, B., S. Okada, A. Oseroff, and S. Strober, *In vitro* propagation and cloning of murine natural suppressor (NS) cells, J. Immunol. 133:2791–2796 (1984).

47. Waer, M., K. K. Ang, E. van der Schueren, and M. Vandeputte, Allogeneic bone marrow transplantation in mice under total lymphoid irradiation: Influences of breeding conditions and strain of recipient mice, J. Immunol. 132:991-996 (1984).
48. Waer, M., K. K. Ang, E. van der Schueren, and M. Vandeputte, Increased incidence of murine graft versus host disease after allogeneic bone marrow transplantation by previous infusion of syngeneic bone marrow cells, Transplantation, 38:496-400 (1984).
49. Segre, M., E. Tomei, and D. Segre, Cyclophosphamide-induced suppressor cells in mice: Suppression of the antibody responses *in vitro* and characterization of the effector cells, Cell. Immunol. 91:443-454 (1985).
50. Hertel-Wulff, B., T. Lindstein, and R. Strober, Rearrangement and expression of T cell receptor genes in cloned murine natural suppressor cell lines, J. Exp. Med. 166:1168-1173 (1987).
51. Khan, M.M., A. L. Wilson, and K. L. Melmon, Characterization of histamine type 1 receptors on natural suppressor lymphoid cells, Biochem. Pharmacol. 36:3867-3871 (1987).
52. Khan, M. M., S. Strober, and K. L. Melmon, Regulatory effects of mast cells on lymphoid cells. The role of histamine type 1 receptors in the interaction between mast cells, helper T cells and natural suppressor cells, Cell. Immunol. 103:41-53 (1986).
53. Khan, M. M., D. Marr-Leisy, M. S. Verlander, M. R. Bristow, S. Strober, M. Goodman, and K. L. Melmon, The effects of derivatives of histamine on natural suppressor cells, J. Immunol. 137:308-314 (1986).
54. Schatten, S., R. D. Granstein, J. A. Drebin, and M. I. Greene, Suppressor T cells and the immune response to tumors, C.R.C. Crit. Rev. Immunol. 4:335-379 (1984).
55. Schechter, B., S. Segal, and M. Feldman, Generation of suppressor lymphocytes during sensitization in culture against a syngeneic tumor: Affinity chromatography on insolubilized histamine, J. Immunol. 120:1268-1273 (1978).
56. Schechter, B., S. Segal, and M. Feldman, Enhancing lymphocytes in spleens of tumor-bearing mice: Affinity chromatography on insolubilized histamine, Int. J. Cancer 20:239-246 (1977).
57. Osband, M. E., Y. J. Shen, M. Shlesinger, A. Brown, D. Hamilton, E. Cohen, P. Lavin, and R. McCaffery, Successful tumor immunotherapy with cimetidine in mice, Lancet 1:636-638 (1981).
58. Norlund, J. J., A. E. Ackles, and R. K. Gershon, Quantitative factors which determine the effect of the immune response on growth rate of Cloudman melanoma in DBA/2 mice, Cell Immunol. 56:258-272 (1980).
59. Norland, J. J., and R. K. Gershon, Splenic regulation of the clinical appearance of small tumors, J. Immunol. 114:1486-1490 (1975).
60. Norland, J. J., and P. W. Askenase, The effect of histamine, antihistamines and a mast cell stabilizer on the growth of Cloudman Melanoma cells in DBA/2 mice, J. Invest. Dermatol. 81:28-31 (1983).

61. Babayan, R. K., M. E. Osband, G. A. Caprinito, Z. S. Ho, E. B. Cohen, and R. J. Krane, The relationship of histamine H_2 receptor-bearing suppressor cells with the growth and metastasis of FANFT-induced bladder cancer, J. Surg. Oncol. 24:53–58 (1983).
62. Descotes, J., R. Tedone, and J. C. Evreux, Effects of cimetidine and ranitidine on delayed-type hypersensitivity, Immunopharmacology 6:31–35 (1983).
63. Muirhead, K., P. Bender, N. Hanna, and G. Poste, Binding of histamine and histamine analogs to lymphocyte subsets analyzed by flow cytometry, J. Immunol. 135:4120–4128 (1985).
64. Cohen, M. G., A. J. Munro, B. N. Dracott, R. I. Ife, and M. R. Vickers, Histamine receptors on leukocytes: The binding of histamine serum albumin conjugates is non-specific, Int. Arch. Allergy Appl. Immunol. 76:9–15 (1985).

2

Human Lymphocyte Responses

MANZOOR M. KHAN AND KENNETH L. MELMON *Stanford University School of Medicine, Stanford, California*

I. INTRODUCTION

Our knowledge of the function of histamine as an immunoregulatory autacoid is rapidly expanding (1-7). The presence of histamine in many tissues in which the immune response takes place (8-9) and its release during immune response lend credibility to the notion that histamine's role in the immune response could be an important one. Pepys (10) made the first report of an effect of histamine on the immune response in 1955. He found that injection of histamine into the site of a tuberculin skin test reduced the subsequent expression of the delayed hypersensitivity reaction. However, these observations that should have focused some attention on a possible immune modulatory role of histamine were not appreciated until 2 decades later. During the past 15 years, it has become apparent that in addition to histamine's role as a neurotransmitter, a mediator of inflammation, and a regulator of cardiovascular function it also is an immune modulator.

The work of Bourne et al. (11,12) and Plaut et al. (13) gave the initial indications that histamine exerted its immunoregulatory effects by causing accumulation of intracellular cyclic adenosine monophosphate (cAMP). These authors reported that certain autacoids, including histamine, suppressed T lymphocyte-mediated cytolysis and inhibited histamine release from basophils. The effects were correlated with the extent of the increase in cAMP content of lymphoid cells. Bourne et al. (14) proposed that certain hormones and mediators of inflammation act in vivo to regulate the character of inflammatory and immune responses. This cAMP-regulated effect is generally inhibitory (14).

Since these preliminary reports, investigators have characterized histamine receptors on immunocompetent cells, and have studied the role of histamine as a regulator of both humoral and cellular immune response (15-21). Histamine has been shown to suppress T-cell proliferation (22), to inhibit antibody production (23) and the cytolytic activity of natural killer and T cells (24,25), and to inhibit the secretion of lymphokines (26,27). Other immunoregulatory effects of histamine include suppression of complement production by monocytes (28,29), of lysosomal enzyme release by neutrophils (30), and of neutrophil chemotaxis (31). Histamine stimulates thymocyte maturation (32), eosinophil chemotaxis, and the expression of eosinophil complement receptors (33,34).

The mechanisms by which histamine exerts these effects on immune response have not been clearly established. In this chapter, we discuss the distribution of histamine receptors on lymphocyte subsets, the regulation of lymphokine production by histamine, and the effects of histamine on lymphokine secretion by immunocompetent cells.

II. CELL SURFACE RECEPTORS

Many bioregulators, including neurotransmitters, hormones, and growth factors, do not penetrate the plasma membrane of cells. Instead, like histamine, they interact with receptors at the cell surface, which in turn transduce the signals via a second messenger. In a wide variety of tissues, including smooth muscles, neurons, endocrine and exocrine glands, and lymphoid cells, histamine increases intracellular levels of transducers generated either by the phosphatidyl inositol or adenylate cyclase pathway. These two intracellular messengers are influenced by pharmacologically distinct histamine receptor subclasses, type I (H_1) and type II (H_2), respectively. Recently, a third class of histamine receptor (type III, H_3) has been reported on nerve endings (35,36). Whether H_3 receptors are present on lymphocytes remains to be seen.

So far, we know that histamine affects lymphocyte functions via type 1 and type 2 receptors. Stimulation of lymphocyte histamine type II receptors generates cAMP, which is responsible for a number of intracellular functions. Some histamine type II receptor-mediated effects on the immune system have been established. However, we know less about the function of lymphocytic histamine type I receptors.

Histamine receptors are not randomly expressed. Instead they are found on specific subsets of lymphocytes. If the receptors were equally distributed on all lymphocyte subsets, histamine would be unlikely to play an important role in modulating the immune response. The evidence for the presence of histamine receptors on lymphocytes has come from four types of experiments: (a) histamine protein conjugate-affinity columns, (b) measurement of intracellular cAMP by radioimmunoassay, (c) radioligand binding, and (d) flow cytometric analysis. Each technique has advantages and drawbacks. But, to date histamine type II receptors have not been satisfactorily demonstrated on lymphocytes or any other tissue by classic radioligand-binding techniques. Neither has the second messenger(s) for histamine type I receptors been clearly identified in lymphocytes. Finally, neither histamine type I nor type II receptors have been isolated for physiologic, biochemical, or pharmacologic characterization. In this section, we describe the known features of histamine types I and II receptors on human lymphocytes.

A. Histamine Type I Receptors on T-cell Subsets

[^{3}H]Pyrilamine (a histamine type I receptor antagonist) has been used to characterize histamine type I receptors on human lymphocytes. Before [^{3}H]pyrilamine was available, investigators attempted to define histamine receptors on lymphocytes by a number of techniques, including chemically coupling histamine to carrier proteins. The resultant conjugate was subsequently attached to sepharose beads and the beads were used as affinity attractants for cells with histamine receptors (37-39). While the results using the insolubilized conjugates as affinity attractants were of value, Cohen et al. (40) questioned the reliability of the approach in some settings. The result of the attraction was not easily reversible with histamine type II antagonists, and the adherent cells were not easily retrieved for subsequent experiments. The data suggested that not all binding was by receptor specificity. Ultimately, Casale et al. (41) used [^{3}H]pyrilamine to demonstrate the presence of histamine type I receptors on lymphocytes. Cameron et al. (42) reported a single specific binding site for [^{3}H]pyrilamine on human CD4 and CD8 subsets. The dissociation constants for [^{3}H]pyrilamine were 5 ± 6.6 nM for the helper T-cell (CD4) subset and 44.6 ± 49.4 nM for the suppressor-cell (CD8) subset. The suppressor T cells expressed higher numbers of histamine type I receptors (35,697 ± 15,468) than the helper T cells (6,838 ± 8,167). T cells incubated with mitogen for 48 hr had a higher affinity for [^{3}H]-pyrilamine, whereas the number of receptors per T cell was unchanged. In contrast, T cells stimulated for 48 hr with concanavalin A (Con A) or phythohemagglutinin (PHA) showed a greater than fourfold increase in the number of histamine type I receptors per cell, and a lower binding affinity for [^{3}H]pyrilamine.

Since histamine levels in plasma can be in the 100-300 pg/ml range (43) and reach 10–40 ng/ml after acute antigenic challenges (44), it appears that lymphocytes are exposed to 1-3 ng histamine. This amount, given the histamine type I-binding affinity, is enough to stimulate their type I receptors. However, the consequences of in vivo histamine type I receptor stimulation of lymphocytes have not been characterized.

B. Histamine Type II Receptors on T-cell Subsets

To date, histamine type II receptors have not been definitively demonstrated on human lymphocytes by specific and direct radioligand binding. Khan et al. (45) used cAMP radioimmunoassays to show that histamine type II receptor-mediated responses could be seen in CD4; CD8,9.3$^+$; and CD8,9.3$^-$ subsets of lymphocytes. These responses were characteristic for each cell type. The CD8,9.3$^-$ (suppressor) T cells produced more cAMP in response to histamine than did CD4 (helper) T cells. The CD8,9.3$^+$ (cytolytic T cells) produced even less. Khan et al. also analyzed the effects of mitogen stimulation of the T-lymphocyte subsets on the expression of histamine type II receptors. They reported that although basal cAMP levels remained unchanged after mitogen stimulation, the human CD4 subset exhibited a sevenfold increase in cAMP response to histamine. The response in the mixture of T cells, in the CD8$^+$ subset, and in the CD8,9.3$^-$ cells was enhanced twofold, twofold, and one and one-half-fold, respectively after mitogen stimulation. However, when suppressor T cells (CD8,9.3$^-$) were separated from cytolytic T cells (CD8,9.3$^+$), the CD8,9.3$^+$ cells showed a more than ninefold increase in cAMP response over their original nonmitogen-stimulated response level. These effects were blocked by histamine type II antagonists and not by type I antagonists. In the same experiments, neither histamine type I or type II antagonists blocked forskolin-induced cAMP accumulation. The degree of histamine-induced augmentation of cAMP response in mitogen-treated subsets was time dependent, and reached a plateau after 72 hr. The data suggest that the presence of human suppressor cells affected the response of mitogen-treated cytolytic and helper T-cell subsets. Thus, it appears that cell-cell interactions may be able to control receptor expression and/or function.

Several investigators have reported that the expression and function of histamine receptors on lymphocytes also are modulated by cells' commitment to a physiologic function or by exposure to antigen and/or drugs. For example, Lichtenstein (46) has suggested that effector T cells exposed to allogeneic target cells became more responsive to histamine as a function of time of exposure to the targets. Rozkowski et al. (19) showed that thymocytes are unresponsive to histamine. However, once exposed to corticosteroids in vivo, those cells resistant to the killing effects of steroid became responsive to histamine (i.e., accumulated cAMP upon stimulation with histamine). Melmon et al. (38) and Shearer et al. (47) have reported that precursor B cells are not likely to have histamine receptors, where as those committed to antibody production became responsive to histamine. Thus, the expression of both histamine types I and II receptors appears to be modulated by the cellular makeup of a particular immune response, the stage of the response, and the type (humoral or cell mediated) of response that is developing or is developed.

III. HISTAMINE-INDUCED LYMPHOKINES

Many investigators have focused on the pharmacologic effects of histamine on the immune function of suppressor lymphocytes. Histamine activates the precursors of suppressor T cells (CD8,9.3$^-$ subset) separated from fresh peripheral blood. This stimulation is blockable in a competitive manner by histamine type II antagonists, but not by type I antagonists (48). Incubation of the precursors of suppressor T cells with histamine for 30 sec was sufficient to initiate the activation of suppression, which maximized days later. Histamine-treated suppressor T cells inhibited both PHA-induced T-cell proliferation and pokeweed mitogen-induced B-cell proliferation. One possible mechanism of this histamine-mediated suppression of the immune response is via release of soluble factor(s) (lymphokines) by suppressor T cells.

A. Soluble Immune-Response Suppressor

Soluble immune response suppressor (SIRS) is an immunosuppressive protein produced by human and murine suppressor cells in response to treatment with a number of agonists. These agents include interferon, Con A, and histamine. This protein suppresses delayed hypersensitivity and plaque-forming cell (PFC) responses in vivo and PFC responses and tumor cell division in vitro (49-52). This lymphokine also is secreted in vitro by unstimulated lymphocytes from patients with steroid-responsive nephrotic syndrome (53), and is found in the serum from nephrotic patients (54). Murine SIRS has been purified to homogeneity. Experiments with human SIRS have determined that its antigenic, functional, and physical properties are similar to those of its murine analog (50-51).

Schnaper et al. (55) have reported that histamine-treated suppressor cells produced SIRS. In these experiments, a soluble product of lymphocytes treated with histamine (10^{-4} M) suppressed polyclonal immunglobulin (IgM) PFC responses of human splenocytes; this substance was antigenically, physically, and functionally similar to SIRS. The SIRS molecular weight in PBS is 110,000-160,000. Fractionation of the same supernatant in pyridine-acetic acid yielded suppressive activity in the 10,000-15,000-dalton range portions. Release of SIRS by histamine and by some unrelated agents was inhibited by the histamine type II antagonists cimetidine and ranitidine. This finding suggests that histamine has a role in SIRS production even when histamine itself was not used as the primary agonist. However, the precise role of histamine type II receptors in

SIRS synthesis and release and the relationship of other histamine-induced suppressor factor(s) to the SIRS pathway have not been established.

B. Histamine-induced Suppressor Factor

Histamine-induced suppressor factor (HSF) is secreted by T lymphocytes in response to graded doses of histamine (10^{-4}-10^{-9} M). T lymphocytes that secrete HSF belong to the CD8 subset and bear Fc receptors for IgG (T_T) (56-58). These T lymphocytes possess both histamine types I and II receptors, but the release of HSF is mediated by type II receptors alone.

Histamine-induced suppressor factor has been biochemically characterized. It consists of two species of acidic glycoproteins with molecular weights between 25,000 and 40,000. It is stable over a wide pH range (pH 3-10), and is sensitive to temperatures greater than 80°C. Expression of HSF requires cell-cell interactions between lymphocytes, monocytes, and their lymphokines (59-62). The release of HSF by T cells appears to be a unique effect of histamine and is not induced by other cAMP-elevating agents, including isoproterenol, prostaglandin E_1, and cholera toxin. The second messenger involved in transducing the signal for release of HSF has not been characterized. The second messenger in this system may be a specific histamine type II receptor-linked cAMP component (i.e., a cAMP component not linked to β-adrenergic or prostaglandin E receptors). Alternatively, the elevated cAMP in response to histamine may not be the actual stimulus to the synthesis and secretion of HSF.

C. Histamine-induced Soluble Suppressor Factor (HISSF)

Nair et al. (25,63) have reported that supernatants from cultures of peripheral blood lymphocytes (PBLs) that are stimulated with histamine (10^{-3}-10^{-8} M) for 24 hr contained HISSF. The soluble factor suppressed the natural killer activity of allogeneic PBLs. This HISSF-induced suppression was completely blocked by interferon or interleukin-2. Histamine type II receptor antagonists blocked the histamine-mediated secretion of HISSF. The natural killer-specific HISSF was produced by peripheral blood mononuclear cells, lymphocyte-depleted mononuclear cells, and T lymphocytes. It was not secreted by natural killer-enriched, Percoll-separated lymphocyte subpopulations, namely, large granular lymphocytes (LGLs). Furthermore, HISSF produced by peripheral blood lymphocytes suppressed the natural killer activity of large granular lymphocytes. The result indicates that LGLs are affected by nonspecific stimuli such as HISSF even though LGLs do not themselves produce HISSF.

Preliminary characterization of HISSF suggests that it has a molecular weight greater than 20,000. However, it is unclear whether HISSF is similar or identical to HSF or SIRS, or instead is a structurally, functionally, and antigenically distinct lymphokine (63).

D. Lymphocyte Migration Inhibitory Factors (LMIFs)

Histamine (10^{-4}-10^{-7} M) induces the secretion of two lymphocyte migration inhibitory factors (LMIFs). Both LMIFs are cationic proteins, but their molecular weights are different—one being 70,000-80,000 and the other 30,000-40,000. The high molecular weight LMIF is a glycoprotein with an isolelectric point of 8.5. Its biological activity is sensitive to heat and neuraminidase, but it is insensitive to trypsin digestion. The low molecular weight LMIF has an isoelectric point of 7.5, and its biological activity is destroyed by trypsin, but is unchanged by neuraminidase and heat treatment (64).

The release of LMIFs has been attributed to stimulation of histamine type I receptors. T lymphocytes that secrete LMIFs appear to belong to the CD4 subset, which includes helper and inducer T cells. These lymphokines are noncytotoxic inhibitors of T-lymphocyte migration (65). The second messenger linked to histamine type I receptors that stimulates the synthesis and release of LMIFs has not been identified.

E. Lymphocyte Chemoattractant Factor (LCF)

Chemoattractant lymphokines play a part in the generation of mononuclear cell infiltrates. Center et al. (66,67) have reported chemoattractant activity in supernatants from human lymphocytes stimulated by histamine. Human peripheral blood lymphocytes treated with histamine (10^{-4}-10^{-7} M) secreted LCF within 4 hr. The lymphokine did not have chemoattractant activity for neutrophils or monocytes. It is a cationic molecule with a molecular weight of 56,000 whose activity is abolished by neuraminidase and trypsin, but not after treatment with heat. The CD8 lymphocytes appear to secrete the lymphokine when their histamine type II receptors are stimulated (68).

IV. EFFECTS OF HISTAMINE ON LYMPHOKINE SECRETION

The mechanisms by which histamine inhibits the immune response have not been fully elucidated. The lymphokines that are secreted in response to histamine and that suppress the immune response in vitro models are described above. One of the inhibitory lymphokines, HSF, may initiate the release of prostaglandins (mainly PGE_2) from monocytes. These prostaglandins in turn may inhibit helper T-cell activity (61). Histamine may affect the immune response through suppressor T cells alone and/or by directly affecting other T-cell subsets. The latter possibility is supported by evidence that human helper and cytolytic T cells possess histamine receptors. In one murine model, it was found that histamine affected helper T-cell function in the absence of suppressor T cells (69).

In this section, we describe the direct inhibitory effects of histamine on production of interleukin-2 and interferon-γ by human helper T cells.

A. Interleukin-2

Interleukin-2 (IL-2, or T-cell growth factor) is a lymphokine that is synthesized and secreted by some T cells following their activation with antigen or mitogen. In order to produce IL-2, the secreting cells must be accompanied by monocyte-derived interleukin-1. Interleukin-2 permits long-term in vitro growth of helper and cytotoxic T cells. It also augments natural killer cell activity.

Histamine at 10^{-5} M inhibits the production of IL-2 by human T lymphocytes stimulated with staphylococcal enterotoxin A (SEA) in the presence of monocytes (26,27). Highly purified T cells stimulated with SEA in the absence of monocytes do not produce detectable levels of IL-2. The effects of histamine on IL-2 production are variable. The same investigators studied the effects of histamine on T cells (absent accessory cells), but using purified T cells that had been activated by Phorbol ester or phytohemagglutinin plus calcium ionophore A23187. Phorbol ester in combination with either PHA or A23187 stimulated production of IL-2. Histamine suppressed this production of IL-2 by about 50%. However, addition of exogenous IL-2 abolished the histamine-mediated effect. The substitution of monocytes with a B-cell lymphoma line produced similar results (26,27).

Dohlsten et al. also assessed whether CD8 cells participate in histamine's effects on CD4 cells. They reported that histamine substantially suppressed SEA-induced IL-2 secretion from CD4 cells even in the absence of CD8 cells. Reconstitution of the mixture of CD4 cells by adding the CD8 lymphocyte subset did not result in any change in histamine-induced suppression of IL-2 synthesis. The inhibitory effects of histamine on IL-2 synthesis by CD4 cells is mediated by histamine type II receptors.

B. Interferon-γ

Interferon is an antiviral agent with immunoregulatory effects that are in part produced by inhibition of cell growth. It has antitumor effects in certain leukemias, juvenile laryngeal papilloma, and intraepithelial neoplasia of the uterine cervix. Clinically, it is a prophylactic agent against the common cold, and may be used to ameliorate other viral diseases of man, such as hepatitis B and reactivated herpes simplex. The physiologic role of interferon-γ is under active study in several laboratories. Histamine suppresses the production of interferon-γ from human peripheral blood lymphocytes that are exposed to SEA. The inhibition is via histamine type II receptors. The effect of histamine on interferon-γ secretion was completely reversed by the addition of exogenous interleukin-2. These data suggest that histamine acts primarily at the level of interleukin-2 synthesis (26,27).

Dohlsten et al. (26,27) reported that a combination of histamine and the anti-Tac monoclonal antibody had an additive suppressive effect on production of interferon-γ. The synthesis of interferon-γ might be inhibited by interleukin-2 via its interaction with its low-affinity receptor. The production of interferon-γ by CD8 lymphocytes was not influenced by histamine in the presence of low levels of exogenously added IL-2. But the suppressive effect of histamine on interferon-γ production by CD4 lymphocytes and unseparated peripheral blood lymphocytes was completely abolished by high concentrations of interleukin-2. As was mentioned earlier, histamine induced very large increases in cAMP levels in mitogen-stimulated CD4 cells, but not in CD8 cells (43). According to Dohlsten et al. (26,27) this result may also explain why CD4 lymphocytes require more exogenous interleukin-2 to overcome the inhibitory effects of histamine on interferon-γ production than do CD8 lymphocytes.

The molecular mechanisms of histamine's effects on lymphokine secretion have not been determined. However, agents that elevate cAMP antagonize the increase in cytoplasmic calcium in mitogen-stimulated lymphocytes (70). This result suggests a possible molecular mechanism by which histamine suppresses IL-2 and interferon-γ production.

V. MODULATION OF HUMAN LYMPHOCYTE CELL SURFACE ANTIGENS

T cells regulate the immune response through "helper" and "suppressor" signals, and cytotoxic T cells that serve as the effector arm of cellular immunity. The presence of CD2 receptors on the cell surface distinguishes T lymphocytes from other lymphoid cells. T cells form rosettes with sheep red blood cells (SRBCs) because the CD2 receptors bind to certain monosaccharides present on the SRBC membrane. Human T cells can be divided into two subsets: the so-called suppressor/cytotoxic subsets (CD8) that includes both suppressor and cytotoxic T cells, and the CD4 subset that constitutes approximately 80% of T cells in the peripheral blood of healthy individuals. The CD4 subset is designated the helper/inducer subset.

The effects of histamine on the expression of antigenic determinants on T lymphocytes have been investigated by several groups. Although results have been somewhat variable, histamine appears to have some regulatory effect on T-cell surface antigens. Histamine can suppress rosetting of normal human T cells in a dose-dependent manner (5×10^{-4}-5×10^{-7} M) (71). This effect was not observed when human T cells were obtained from the blood of atopic subjects. Treatment of SRBCs with neuraminidase prior to rosetting resulted in the abolition of histamine's effect on rosette formation by normal human T cells. Inhibition of E-rosette formation of normal T cells was also observed when either histamine type I or type II receptor agonists were used in the study. The mechanisms by which activation of either histamine receptor produced this effect has not been explored.

In another study, Verhaegen et al. (72) reported the opposite effects of histamine on rosetting. They found that histamine suppressed rosetting of T cells from atopic donors, but did not affect rosetting of T cells from normal individuals. Again the effects of histamine were dose dependent (3×10^{-6}-3×10^{-7} M) and were reversed by pretreatment of human PBLs with either histamine type I or type II antagonists.

The histamine type II receptor agonist impromidine increases the number of cells expressing the Fc receptors specific for immunoglobulin G (73). This effect was reversed by the histamine type II receptor antagonist cimetidine. Birch and Polmar (73) reported that when T cells with theophylline-resistant CD2 receptors were treated with impromidine they lost their capacity to help B-cell differentiation. In a separate study these same authors (74,75) found that impromidine induced suppressor activity. Impromidine reduced the number of CD4 cells and increased the number of CD8 cells. Impromidine also increased the number of cells expressing B_2-microglobin. Therefore, histamine type II receptors play a role in the modulation of the T-cell phenotype. The biochemical events involved in these effects have not been elucidated.

VI. CONCLUSIONS

Since the discovery of histamine at the turn of the century its role as a modulator of various biologic functions has been progressively revealed. Although the role of histamine as a mediator of inflammation has been well known for some time, its role as an immunomodulator has only recently gained serious attention.

Diverse approaches have demonstrated the importance of histamine as an immune modulator. The most convincing types of data include: (a) Cells containing histamine (e.g., mast cells) are concentrated in close association with the sites of generation of the immune response (76). The precursors of these histamine-filled cells are associated with the precursors of lymphoid cells. The mucosal mast cells are dependent upon interleukin-3, a T-cell growth factor, for their proliferation and growth. (b) Release of histamine is stimulated by a number of factors key to the immune response. They include release of a lymphokine (e.g., histamine-releasing factor) and a variety of immunologic and nonimmunologic stimuli that are ubiquitous accompaniments of the immune response. (c) The receptors for histamine are nonrandomly distributed on lymphocyte subsets. Suppressor T cells can control the expression of histamine receptors on helper and cytolytic T cells. (d) Histamine influences the release of lymphokines, stimulating some and inhibiting others. (e) Histamine affects the expression of lymphocyte cell surface antigens.

The complexity of the immune response makes defining the mechanisms by which histamine regulates lymphocyte function difficult. Information concerning the role of histamine as an immune modulator is mainly derived from in vitro experiments. Recently, experiments have been done to derivatize histamine in order to make its effects lymphocyte specific. How these derivatives of histamine can eventually be tested as therapeutic immune modulators will be discussed in Chapter 6 in the second section of this book.

REFERENCES

1. Rocklin, R. E., and D. J. Beer, Histamine and immune modulation. In Advances in Internal Medicine (Stollerman, G. H., Ed.), Yearbook, Chicago, (1983), pp. 225–251.
2. Beer, D. J., and R. E. Rocklin, Histamine modulation of lymphocyte biology: Membrane receptors, signal transduction and functions, C.R.C. Crit. Rev. Immunol. 7:55–91 (1987).
3. Plaut, M., Lymphocyte hormone receptors, Ann. Rev. Immunol. 5:621–669 (1987).
4. Khan, M. M., and K. L. Melmon, Are autacoids more than theoretic modulators of immunity? Clin. Immunol. Rev. 4:1–30 (1985).
5. Melmon, K. L., and M. M. Khan, Histamine and its lymphocyte-selective derivatives as immune modulators, Trends Pharmacol. Sci. 8:437–441 (1987).
6. Melmon, K. L., R. E. Rocklin, and R. P. Rosenkranz, Autacoids as modulators of the inflammatory and immune response, Am. J. Med. 71:100–106 (1981).
7. Khan, M. M., and K. L. Melmon, Selected autacoids as modulators of lymphocyte function. In The Pharmacology of Lymphocytes (Morley, E. J., and Bray, M. A., Eds.), Springer-Verlag, Berlin Heidelberg, 363–383 (1988).
8. Razin, E., R. L. Stevens, K. F. Austen, J. P. Caulfield, A. Hein, F. T. Liu, M. Clabby, G. Nabel, H. Cantor, and S. Feidman, Cloned mast cells derived from immunized lymph node cells and from fetal liver exhibit characteristics of bone marrow derived mast cells, Immunology 52:563–575 (1984).
9. Feldbert, W., Distribution of histamine in the body. In Histamine (Wolstenhome, G. E. W., and O'Connors, C. M., Eds.), Little Brown, Boston (1956), pp. 4–13.
10. Pepys, J., Fixation of tuberculin in skin of tuberculin sensitive human subjects, Clin. Sci. 14:253-265 (1955).
11. Bourne, H. R., L. M. Lichtenstein, and K. L. Melmon, Histamine augments leukocyte adenosine 3′,5′-monophosphate and blocks antigenic histamine release, Science 173:743–745 (1971).
12. Bourne, H. R., L. M. Lichtenstein, and K. L. Melmon, Pharmacologic control of allergic histamine release *in vitro*: Evidence for an inhibitory role of 3′,5′-adenosine monophosphate in human leukocytes, J. Immunol. 108: 695–704 (1972).

13. Plaut, M., L. M. Lichtenstein, and C. S. Henney, Properties of a subpopulation of T cells bearing histamine receptor, J. Clin. Invest. 57:1051–1058 (1975).
14. Bourne, H. R., L. M. Lichtenstein, K. L. Melmon, C. S. Henney, Y. Weinstein, and G. M. Shearer, Modulation of inflammation and immunity by cyclic AMP, Science 184:19–28 (1974).
15. Melmon, K. L., H. R. Bourne, Y. Weinstein, and M. Sela, Receptors for histamine can be detected on the surface of selected leukocytes, Science 177:707–709 (1972).
16. Ballet, J. J., and E. Merler, The separation and reactivity *in vitro* of a subpopulation of human lymphocytes which bind histamine. Correlation of histamine reactivity with cellular maturation, Cell. Immunol. 24:250–269 (1976).
17. Kedar, E., and B. Bonavida, Histamine receptor bearing leukocyte (HRL): I. Detection of histamine receptor-bearing cells by rosette formation with histamine-coated erythrocytes. J. Immunol. 113:1544–1552 (1974).
18. Plaut, M., and W. Roszkowski, Lymphocyte subpopulations bearing histamine receptors. In Histamine Receptors (Yellin, T. O., Ed.), Spectrum Holliswood, New York (1979), pp. 361–385.
19. Roszkowski, W., M. Plaut, and L. M. Lichtenstein, Selective display of histamine receptors on lymphocytes, Science 195:683–685 (1977).
20. Rocklin, R. E., D. K. Greineder, B. H. Littman, and K. L. Melmon, Modulation of cellular immune function *in vitro* by histamine receptors bearing lymphocytes: Mechanism of action, Cell. Immunol. 37:162–173 (1978).
21. Garavoy, M., M. Reddish, and R. E. Rocklin, Inhibition of helper T cell function and expressionof "Ia" by histamine-induced suppressor factor, J. Immunol. 130:357–361 (1983).
22. Suzuki, S., and R. Huchet, Mechanisms of histamine induced inhibition of lymphocyte response to mitogens, Cell. Immunol. 62:396–405 (1981).
23. Lima, M., and R. E. Rocklin, Histamine modulates *in vitro* IgG production (by pokeweed mitogen-stimulated) human mononuclear cells, Cell. Immunol. 64:324–336 (1981).
24. Schwartz, A., P. W. Askenase, and R. K. Gershon, Histamine inhibition of the *in vitro* induction of cytotoxic T cell responses, Immunopharmacology 2:179–190 (1980).
25. Nair, P. M. N., and S. A. Schwartz, Effect of histamine antagonists on natural and antibody-dependent cellular cytotoxicity of human lymphocytes *in vitro*, Cell. Immunol. 81:45–60 (1983).
26. Dohlsten, M., H. O. Sjogren, and R. A. Carlsson, Histamine inhibits interferon-γ production via suppression of interleukin-2 synthesis, Cell. Immunol. 101:493–501 (1986).
27. Dohlsten, M., H. O. Sjogren, and R. A. Carlsson, Histamine acts directly on human T cells to inhibit interleukin-2 and interferon-γ production. Cell. Immunol. 101:65–74 (1987).

28. Lappin, D., and K. Whaley, Effects of histamine on monocyte complement production: Inhibition of C2 production mediated by its action on H_2 receptors, Clin. Exp. Immunol. 41:497–504 (1980).
29. Lappin, D., H. L. Moseley, and K. Whaley, Effects of histamine on monocyte complement production, Clin. Exp. Immunol. 42:515–522 (1980).
30. Busse, W. W., and J. Sosman, Histamine inhibition of neutrophil lysosomal enzyme release: An H_2 histamine receptor response, Science 194:737–738 (1976).
31. Anderson, R., A. M. Glover, and A. R. Rabson, The *in vitro* effects of histamine andmetiamide on neutrophil motility and their relationship to intracellular cyclic nucleotide levels, J. Immunol. 118:1690–1696 (1977).
32. Singh, U., and J. J. T. Owen, Studies on the maturation of thymus stem cells. The effects of catecholamines, histamine and peptide hormones on the expression of T cell alloantigen, Eur. J. Immunol. 6:59–62 (1976).
33. Anwar, A. R. E., and A. B. Kay, The ECF-A tetrapeptide and histamine selectively enhance human eosinophil complement receptors, Nature 269: 522–524 (1977).
34. Anwar, A. R. E., and A. B. Kay, Enhancement of human eosinophil complement receptors by pharmacologic mediators, J. Immunol. 131:1245–1250 (1978).
35. Arrang, J.-M., G. M. Garbag, J. C. Lancelot, J.-M. Lecomte, H. Pollard, M. Robba, W. Shunack, and J. C. Schwartz. Highly potent and selective ligands for histamine H_3-receptors. Nature 327:117–123 (1987).
36. Ishikawa, S. and N. Sperelakis. A novel class (H_3) of histamine receptors on perivascular nerve terminals. Nature 327:158–160 (1987).
37. Weinstein, Y., K. L. Melmon, H. R. Bourne, and M. Sela, Specific leukocyte receptors for small endogenous hormones: Detection by cell binding to insolubilized hormone preparations, J. Clin. Invest. 52:1349–1361 (1973).
38. Melmon, K. L., Y. Weinstein, G. M. Shearer, H. R. Bourne, and S. Bauminger, Separation of specific antibody-forming mouse cells by their adherence to insolubilized endogenous hormones, J. Clin. Invest. 53:22–30 (1974).
39. Melmon, K. L., Y. Weinstein, G. M. Shearer, and H. R. Bourne, Separation of leukocytes by their amine receptors: Subsequent immunologic functions. In Cyclic AMP, Cell Growth and the Immune Response (Braun, W., Lichtenstein, L. M., and Parker, C. W., Eds.), Springer-Verlag, New York (1974), pp. 135–146.
40. Cohen, M. G., A. J. Munro, B. N. Dracott, R. J. Ife, and M. R. Vickers, Histamine receptors of leukocytes: The binding of histamine serum albumin conjugates is nonspecific, Int. Arch. Allergy Appl. Immunol. 76:9–15 (1985).
41. Casale, T. B., S. Wescott, D. Rodbard, and M. Kaliner, Characterization of histamine H_1 receptors on human mononuclear cells, Int. J. Immunopharmacol. 7:639–645 (1985).

42. Cameron, W., K. Doyle, and R. E. Rocklin, Histamine type 1 (H_1) receptor radioligand binding studies on normal T cell subsets, B cells and monocytes, J. Immunol. 136:2116–2120 (1986).
43. Dyer, J., K. Warren, S. Merlin, D. D. Metcalf, and M. Kaliner, Measurement of plasma histamine: description of an improved method and normal values, J. Allergy Clin. Immunol. 70:82–87 (1982).
44. Kaplan, A. P., L. Gray, R. E. Schaff, Z. Horakova, and M. A. Beaver, *In vivo* studies of mediator release in cold urticaria and cholinergic urticaria, J. Allergy Clin. Immunol. 55:394–402 (1975).
45. Khan, M. M., P. Sansoni, E. G. Engleman, and K. L. Melmon, Pharmacologic effects of autacoids on subsets of T cells: Regulation of expression/function of histamine-2 receptors by a subset of suppressor cells, J. Clin. Invest. 75:1578–1583 (1985).
46. Lichtenstein, L. M. The interdependence of allergic and inflammatory processes. In: Johansson, S.G.O., Strandberg, K., Uvnas, B., eds. Molecular and biological aspects of the acute allergic reaction. New York, Plenum, 233–254 (1976).
47. Shearer, G. M., Y. Weinstein, and K. L. Melmon, Enhancement of immune response potential of mouse lymphoid cells fractionated over insolubilized conjugated histamine columns, J. Immunol. 113:597–607 (1974).
48. Sansoni, P., M. M. Khan, K. L. Melmon, and E. G. Engleman, Immunoregulatory T cells in man. Histamine-induced suppressor T cells are derived from a Leu-2^+ ($T8^+$) subpopulation distinct from that which gives rise to cytotoxic T cell, J. Clin. Invest. 75:650–656 (1985).
49. Aune, T. M., and C. W. Pierce, Mechanisms of SIRS action at the cellular and biochemical level. In Lymphocytes, Vol. 9 (Pick, E., Ed.), Academic Press, New York (1984), pp. 257–268.
50. Schnaper, H. W., C. W. Pierce, and T. M. Aune, Identification and initial characterization of concanavalin A and mitogen induced human suppressor factors: Evidence for a human equivalent of murein soluble immune response suppressor (SIRS), J. Immunol. 132:2429–2435 (1984).
51. Webb, D. R., K. Mason, G. Semenuk, T. M. Aune, and C. W. Pierce, Purification and analysis of isoforms of soluble immune response suppressor (SIRS), J. Immunol. 135:3238–3242 (1985).
52. Schnaper, H. W., and T. M. Aune, Suppression of immune responses to sheep erythrocytes by the lymphokine soluble immune response suppressor (SIRS) *in vivo*, J. Immunol. 137:863–867 (1986).
53. Schnaper, H. W., and T. M. Aune, Identification of the lymphokine soluble immune response suppressor (SIRS) in urine of nephrotic children, J. Clin. Invest. 76:341–349 (1985).
54. Schnaper, H. W., and T. M. Aune, Steroid sensitive mechanism of soluble immune response suppressor production in steroid responsive nephrotic syndrome, J. Clin. Invest. 79:257–264 (1987).
55. Schnaper, H. W., T. M. Aune, and R. K. Roby, A role for histamine type II (H_2) receptor binding in production of lymphokine, soluble immune respones suppressor (SIRS), J. Immunol. 139:1185–1190 (1987).

56. Rocklin, R. E., D. K. Greinder, and K. L. Melmon, Histamine induced suppressor factor (HSF): Further studies on the nature of the stimulus and the cell which produces it, Cell. Immunol. 44:404–415 (1979).
57. Rocklin, R. E., Histamine induced suppressor factor (HSF): Effect on migration inhibiting factor (MIF) production and proliferation, J. Immunol. 118:1734–1738 (1977).
58. Lima, M., and R. E. Rocklin, Histamine modulates *in vitro* IgG production (by pokeweed mitogen stimulated) human mononuclear cells, Cell. Immunol. 64:324–326 (1981).
59. Beer, D. J., C. A. Dinarello, L. J. Rosenwasser, and R. E. Rocklin, Human monocyte-derived soluble product(s) has an accessory function in the generation of histamine and concanavalin A-induced suppressor T cells, J. Clin. Invest. 70:393–400 (1982).
60. Beer, D. J., L. J. Rosenwasser, C. A. Dinarello, and R. E. Rocklin, Cellular interactions in the generation and expression of histamine induced suppressor activity cell, Immunology 69:101–112 (1982).
61. Rocklin, R. E., L. Kiselis, D. J. Beer, P. Rossi, F. Maggi, and J. A. Bellanti, Augmentation of prostaglandin and thromboxan production by human monocytes exposed to histamine-induced suppressor factor (HSF), Cell. Immunol. 77:92–98 (1983).
62. Rocklin, R. E., and A. Habarek-Davidson, Pharmacologic modulation *in vitro* of human histamine-induced suppressor cell activity, Int. J. Immunopharmacol. 6:179–186 (1984).
63. Nair, M. P. N., J. M. Cilik, and S. A. Schwartz, Histamine induced suppressor factor inhibition of NK cells: Reversal with interferon and interleukin-2, J. Immunol. 136:2456–2462 (1986).
64. Berman, J. S., R. G. McFadden, W. W. Cruikshank, D. M. Center, and D. J. Beer, Functional characteristics of histamine receptor-bearing mononuclear cells. II. Identification and characterization of two histamine-induced human lymphokines that inhibit lymphocyte migration, J. Immunol. 133: 1495–1504 (1984).
65. McFadden, R. G., W. W. Cruikshank, and D. M. Center, Modulation of lymphocyte migration by human lymphokines. III. Characterization of a lymphocyte migration inhibitory factor, Cell. Immunol. 85:154–167 (1984).
66. Center, D. M., and W. W. Cruikshank, Modulation of lymphocyte migration by human lymphokines. I. Identification and characterization of chemoattractant activity for lymphocytes from mitogen stimulated mononuclear cells, J. Immunol. 128:2563–2568 (1982).
67. Center, D. M., W. W. Cruikshank, J. S. Berman, and D. J. Beer, Functional characteristics of histamine receptor-bearing monoclonal cells. I. Selective production of lymphocyte chemoattractant lymphokines with histamine used as a ligand, J. Immunol. 131:1854–1859 (1983).
68. Cruikshank, W. W., and D. M. Center, Modulation of lymphocyte migration by human lymphokines. II. Purification of lymphocytic factor (LCF), J. Immunol. 128:2569–2574 (1982).

69. Khan, M. M., K. L. Melmon, C. G. Fathman, B. Hertel-Wulff, and S. Strober, The effects of autacoids on cloned murine lymphoid cells: Modulation of IL-2 secretion and the activity of natural suppressor cells, J. Immunol. 134: 4100–4106 (1985).
70. Tsien, R. Y., T. Pozzan, and T. J. Rink, T-cell mitogens cause early changes in cytoplasmic free Ca^{2+} and membrane potential in lymphocytes, Nature 295:68–71 (1982).
71. Hall, T. J., P. M. Lydyard, and J. Brostoff, Effect of histamine H_1 and H_2 agonists on E-rosette formation in normal and atopic subjects, Int. Arch. Allergy Appl. Immunol. 69:380–384 (1982).
72. Verhaegen, H., W. DeCodk, and J. DeCree, Histamine receptor-bearing peripheral T lymphocytes in patients with allergies. J. Allergy and Clinical Immunology 59:266–268 (1977).
73. Birch, R. E., and S. H. Polmar, Induction of FC gamma receptors on a subpopulation of human T lymphocytes by adenosine and impromidine an H_2 histamine agonist, Cell. Immunol. 57:455–467 (1981).
74. Birch, R. E., and S. H. Polmar, Pharmacologic modification of immunoregulatory T lymphocytes. I. Effect of adenosine, H_1 and H_2 histamine agonists upon T lymphocyte regulation of B lymphocyte differentiation *in vitro*, Clin. Exp. Immunol. 48:218–230 (1982).
75. Birch, R. E., A. K. Rosenthal, and S. H. Polmar, Pharmacological modification of immunoregulatory T lymphocytes II. Modulation of T lymphocytes cell surface characteristics, Clin. Exp. Immunol. 48:231–238 (1982).
76. Khan, M. M., D. M. Fishwild, K. L. Melmon, E. G. Engleman, and J. A. Bauer, A subset of human rosetted lymphocytes contains previously unidentified histamine. Clin. Immunol. Immunopath. 52:147–159 (1989).

3

Histamine-Induced Suppressor Cell Systems in Guinea Pigs and Humans

DENNIS J. BEER *Boston University School of Medicine, Boston, Massachusetts*

ROSS E. ROCKLIN *Boehringer Ingelheim Pharmaceuticals, Inc., Ridgefield, Connecticut, and New England Medical Center Hospital, Boston, Massachusetts*

I. INTRODUCTION

Immune responses are similar to other complex biologic processes, such as blood clotting and complement activation, in that they are modulated by a series of positive and negative regulatory signals (1). A major negative regulatory influence on the immune system is provided by suppressor T lymphocytes. Since the original observations of Gershon and Kondo (2,3), it has been documented clearly that T- and B-cell function is in part modulated by a complex interaction between effector cells and regulatory suppressor cells (4,5). Perturbations in suppressor-cell function may initiate or contribute to a variety of immunopathologic disorders (6,7).

Functionally, distinct subsets of T lymphocytes with suppressor capabilities have been defined both serologically with monoclonal antibodies directed at relatively stable cell-surface glycoproteins (8–10) and by the presence of functional histamine type II (H_2) receptors. Models of immune-induced inflammation have demonstrated that histamine induces an inhibitory signal to leukocytes that participate in inflammatory reactions. In particular, histamine interaction with histamine type II receptor–bearing lymphocytes induces the elaboration of a suppressor lymphokine that results in the dampening of both T- and B-cell function (reviewed in Ref. 11-13). Since histamine is liberated in vivo during inflammatory responses, its ability to activate suppressor cells and thereby modify the cellular phase of an inflammatory reaction places histamine into the category of an endogenous physiologic mediator, or autacoid (14). This chapter will review histamine-induced suppressor-cell systems in guinea pigs and humans.

II. HISTAMINE-INDUCED SUPPRESSOR-CELL MODULATION OF GUINEA PIG T-LYMPHOCYTE FUNCTION

Histamine initially was demonstrated to suppress in vivo and in vitro components of cellular-immune reactions in sensitized guinea pigs (15). The intradermal injection of 10^{-3} M histamine along with antigen into guinea pigs previously sensitized to orthochlorobenzoyl-bovine gammaglobulin (OCB-BGG) caused a 50% reduction on the size of the developing delayed hypersensitivity skin test reaction (Table 1). Inhibition of delayed-type skin reactivity by histamine in this model system was partially reversed by addition of the histamine type I (H_1) receptor antagonist chlorpheniramine, and was completely prevented by addition of the histamine type II receptor antagonist burimamide (Table 1) (15).

The histamine-induced suppression of cutaneous delayed hypersensitivity could be accounted for in part by its in vitro inhibitory effects on certain lym-

Table 1 Effect of Histamine on 24-Hr Delayed Hypersensitivity Skin Test

	Skin Test Reagents			
	OCB-BGG[a]	OCB-BGG + Histamine[b]	OCB-BGG + Histamine + Burimamide[b]	OCB-BGG + Histamine + Chlorpheniramine[b]
Area of DTH response[c]	28.5 ± 5.3	16.3 ± 5.4	32.9 ± 10.5	21.8 ± 6.2
% change from OCB-BGG	0	-43[d]	+15	-23

[a]Orthochlorobenzoyl-bovine gammaglobulin-immunized guinea pigs injected intradermally with 50 μg of specific antigen.
[b]Histamine and the antihistamines were used at concentrations of 10^{-3} M.
[c]The area of the delayed-type hypersensitivity response represents the radius squared in millimeters square.
[d]Different from OCB-BGG alone, $p < 0.01$.

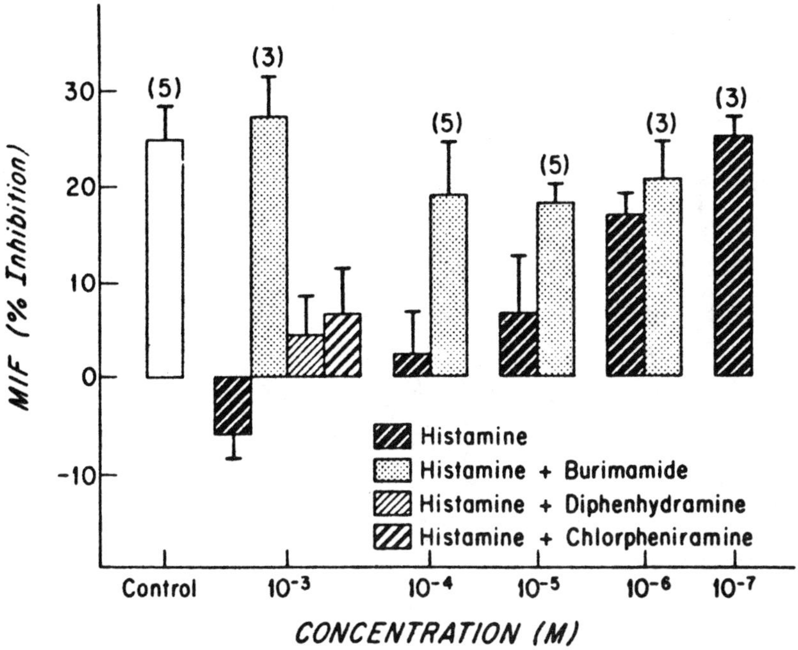

Figure 1 Effect of histamine on MIF production by OCB-BGG–immune guinea pig lymph node lymphocytes. Suppression of MIF by histamine was concentration dependent. Histamine type II receptor antagonists restored MIF production to normal.

phocyte responses, including the production of the inflammatory lymphokine macrophage migration inhibitory factor (MIF) as well as antigen-induced lymphocyte proliferation. At concentrations of 10^{-5}-10^{-3} M, histamine reversibly inhibited MIF production (Fig. 1), but did not interfere with the macrophage response to preformed MIF, nor did it interfere with antigen binding to macrophages or with macrophage presentation of antigen to lymphocytes (15,16). The in vitro proliferative response of sensitized guinea pig lymphocytes to specific antigen was inhibited by 10^{-6}-10^{-4} M histamine. The histamine-induced suppression of lymphokine production and lymphocyte proliferation was reversed by the addition of burimamide, but not by the addition of chlorpheniramine or diphenhydramine (15). Taken collectively, these studies suggested that histamine interacting with a histamine type II receptor either directly or indirectly (see below) inhibited lymphokine production and lymphocyte proliferation.

Although agents that raise intracellular levels of cyclic 3′, 5′-monophospate (AMP) have been demonstrated to inhibit guinea pig MIF production (17),

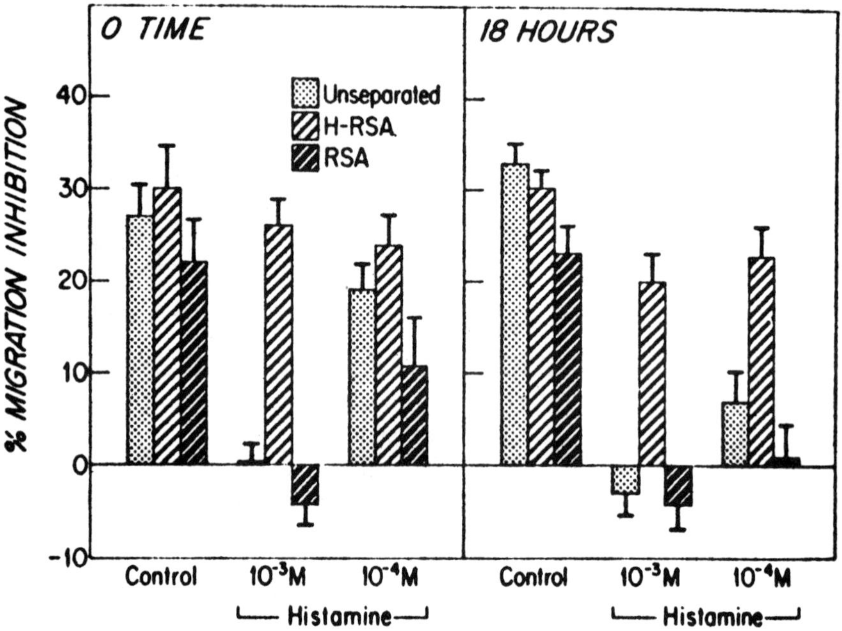

Figure 2 Immune lymph node cells were chromatographed on H-RSA and RSA columns and either tested immediately (panel A) for their sensitivity to histamine or allowed to "recover" for 18 hr (panel B) before exposing them to histamine. Cells allowed to recover for 18 hr still produced MIF in the presence of histamine, indicating that histamine receptor–bearing lymphocytes were retained on the H-RSA column and did not pass through in a desensitized state.

it was not clear from Rocklin's initial studies (15) that histamine-induced suppression of MIF production and lymphocyte proliferation was mediated via this direct mechanism. In fact, subsequent observations by Rocklin and associates (16,18,19) indicated that histamine inhibited MIF production indirectly by activating suppressor cells, which in turn regulated MIF-secreting cells. Passage of immune lymph node cells over histamine-affinity columns made of insolubilized conjugates of histamine (histamine [H] linked to rabbit serum albumin [RSA] bound to sepharose [S]) rendered the nonadherent cells insensitive to histamine; that is, these nonadherent lymph node cells when exposed to antigen in the presence of histamine made MIF and proliferated to the same extent as antigen-stimulated cells in the absence of histamine. Cells that passed through control columns (RSA or histidine methylester-RSA columns) retained their sensitivity to histamine. That cells bearing histamine receptors were actually removed by H-RSA-S columns and were not present in a histamine-unresponsive state was

Table 2 Effect of Histamine-Induced Suppressor Factor (HSF) on Guinea Pig MIF Production

Supernatant[a]	MIF Activity[b]	% Suppression[c]
Control	26 ± 1.8	0
Histamine (10^{-3} M)	1 ± 2.6	96[d]
Histamine (10^{-4} M)	6 ± 5.0	77[d]
Histamine (10^{-5} M)	16 ± 5.8	39[d]
Histamine (10^{-6} M)	31 ± 3.0	-18
Histamine (10^{-3} M) + burimamide (10^{-3} M)	25 ± 4.2	4
Histamine (10^{-3} M) + chlorpheniramine (10^{-3} M)	4 ± 4.8	84[d]

[a]Supernatants were derived from 10×10^6 lymph node cells/ml in medium TC-199 alone (control) or in the presence of various concentrations of histamine with and without histamine types I and II receptor antagonists for 24 hr at 37°C. The supernatants were harvested, dialyzed, and then used to culture sensitized lymph node cells for specific antigen-induced MIF production.
[b]Percent migration inhibition of guinea pig macrophages exposed to supernatants derived from orthochlorobenzoyl-bovine gammaglobulin (OCB-BGG)–sensitized lymph node cells incubated with OCB-BGG (100 μg/ml) (control). Except for the above control, the sensitized lymph node cells were cocultured with specific antigen plus histamine or histamine plus histamine types I and II receptor antagonist-conditioned supernatants.
[c]Percent suppression of MIF production (1 - experimental supernatant/control) × 100.
[d]Different from control, $p < 0.05$.

suggested by experiments in which cells that were not adherent to a histamine-affinity column were allowed to recover for 18 hr before antigen stimulation. In these experiments, H-RSA-S–passed cells did not regain their sensitivity to histamine and had normal antigen-induced MIF production (Fig. 2) (16).

Further studies by Rocklin (18) into the mechanism of histamine-induced suppression of cellular immune responses determined that suppressor function by cells bearing histamine type II receptors was mediated through a soluble product. It was found that lymph node cells from immune or nonimmune guinea pigs elaborated a nondialyzable factor, termed histamine-induced suppressor factor (HSF), into the culture supernatant following incubation with 10^{-5}-10^{-3} M histamine for 2 hr. When supernatants containing HSF were cocultured with antigen-pulsed sensitized lymphocytes, MIF production and lymphocyte proliferation were suppressed. Investigation into the cell source of HSF revealed that this was elaborated by lymphocytes, but not by macrophages (18). Furthermore, its production could be blocked by a histamine type II receptor antagonist (burimamide), but not by a type I receptor antagonist (chlorpheniramine) (Table 2). The inhibitory effects of HSF were reversible. If lymphocytes were

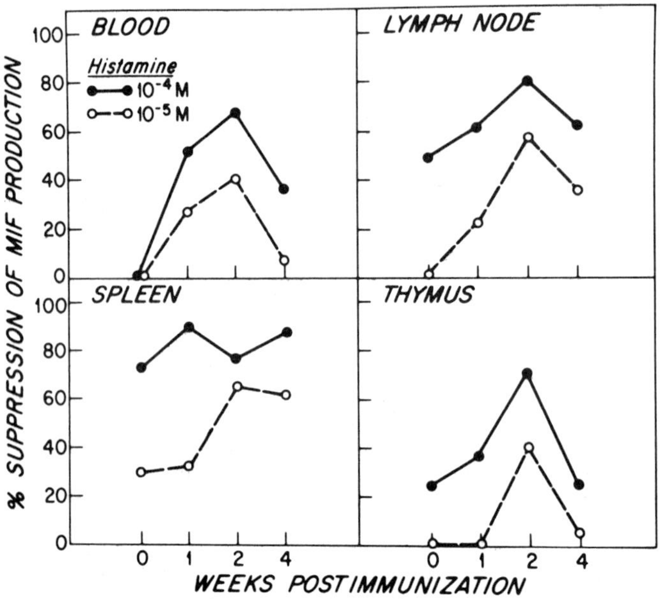

Figure 3 The source of lymphoid tissues and the kinetics of HSF-producing cells. Equal numbers of lymph node, spleen, blood, and thymus cells from nonimmune (time 0) and from guinea pigs immunized (1–4 weeks) with OCB-BGG were cultured with or without histamine (10^{-5} and 10^{-4} M) and HSF production measured. HSF production was detected in lymph node and spleen cells of nonimmune animals, but not in their blood or thymus cells. Following immunization, HSF-producing cells were found in the thymus and blood. Peak HSF activity in all tissues was detected at 2 weeks postimmunization. MIF production in the presence of control supernatants from lymph node, spleen, blood, and thymus varied from 30 to 48% inhibition of migration.

washed free of the factor after a 24-hr incubation and recultured with fresh medium and antigen, the cells were able to produce MIF. Sephadex G-100 molecular sieve chromatography of histamine-conditioned lymphocyte supernatants demonstrated that the suppressor activity eluted in a region between 23,000 and 40,000 daltons.

Rocklin and colleagues (19) addressed other aspects of guinea pig–derived HSF. Histamine-induced suppressor activity could be detected in populations of cells from spleen and lymph nodes prior to active immunization with OCB-BGG of the donor, but not in cells from the donor's blood or thymus (Fig. 3). Following immunization with antigen, increased HSF activity was detected in cells from the donor's spleen and lymph nodes. The peak response was seen 2 weeks postimmunization, a time when significant amounts of HSF were elaborated also by cells from the blood and thymus. It was found that T-cell–enriched, but not B-cell–enriched populations, made significant amounts of HSF. When lymph node cells of immunized donors were chromatographed over histamine-affinity columns the nonretained cells were unable to generate HSF. In contradistinction, cells retained on the column and subsequently eluted were able to produce HSF.

To determine further the type of histamine receptor involved in HSF production, lymph node cells from immunized guinea pigs were incubated with histamine type I (2-methylhistamine) or type II (4-methylhistamine) receptor agonists (19). Although both agonists induced the generation of HSF at high concentrations (10^{-3} M), only the histamine type II agonist stimulated production of HSF at lower concentrations (10^{-5} M). These HSF-producting lymphocytes appeared to be sensitive selectively to histamine type II receptor agonists and the induction of HSF by high concentrations of the type I agonist probably resulted from loss of type I receptor specificity with consequent activation of T-cell type II receptors.

Immediate-type hypersensitivity mediators other than histamine also were studied to determine their ability to induce suppressor factor activity from OCB-BGG–immunized guinea pig lymph node cells. Serotonin, slow-reacting substance of anaphylaxis, eosinophil chemotactic factor, and prostaglandin E_1 (PGE_1) were unable to induce suppressor factor activity in lymph node cell populations (19). Furthermore, other agents which raise intracellular cyclic AMP such as isoproterenol and cholera toxin as well as the dibutyryl form of cyclic AMP itself were unable to generate suppressor-factor activity in lymph node cells (19). Thus, histamine appeared to be unique among the mediators in inducing elaboration of a suppressor factor. These findings also suggest that the ability of histamine to induce HSF may not reside in the conventional histamine type II receptor activation pathway linked to cyclic AMP accumulation, but rather to an as yet undefined second messenger pathway.

Taken collectively, this series of observations in guinea pigs by Rocklin and associates (15,16,18,19) developed the concept that histamine released by any of various mechanisms from tissue mast cells or infiltrating basophils into the microenvironment might down regulate cellular immune reactions. The next step was to extend these observations to humans (reviewed in Refs. 11-13).

III. HISTAMINE-INDUCED SUPPRESSOR-CELL MODULATION OF HUMAN T-LYMPHOCYTE FUNCTION

Many investigators have focused on the pharmacologic effects of histamine on human lymphocyte proliferation (reviewed in Refs. 11-13). Ballet and Merler (20) reported that high concentrations of histamine inhibited the proliferative response to alloantigens induced by mixed lymphocyte culture (MLC). The influence of histamine (10^{-8}-10^{-3} M) on the proliferative response of T cells in autologous and allogeneic MLCs was analyzed further by Damle and Gupta (21). Pretreatment of responder T cells, but not stimulator non-T cells, with histamine for 24 hr resulted in a dose-dependent diminished proliferative response in both autologous and allogeneic MLCs. A minimum of 4 hr of incubation of responder T cells with histamine (10^{-4} M) was required to suppress the autologous and allogeneic MLC response. Suppression of the MLCs increased as the time of incubation with histamine approached 24 hr. Histamine-induced suppression of the MLC was prevented by the presence of an equimolar concentration of the histamine type II receptor antagonist cimetidine, but not by the presence of the type I receptor antagonist chlorpheniramine. Preincubation of responder T cells for 24 hr with either of two histamine type II receptor agonists, 4-methylhistamine and dimaprit, inhibited T-cell proliferation to the same extent as histamine in autologous and allogeneic MLCs. In contrast, preincubation of responder T cells with either of the two histamine type I receptor agonists, 2-methylhistamine and 2-pyridylethylamine, failed to inhibit the MLC-induced proliferative response. Taken together, these last sets of findings suggest that histamine inhibition of MLC-induced T-cell proliferation was mediated by histamine type II receptors.

Damle and Gupta's report (21) included data which suggested that the histamine-induced suppression of human MLC-induced T-cell proliferation was indirect and mediated by a histamine-activatable suppressor-cell system. Lymphocytes pretreated with histamine (10^{-5} and 10^{-4} M), followed by mitomycin C treatment, when cocultured with fresh autologous T cells suppressed their proliferative responses in both the autologous and allogeneic MLCs. In addition, supernatants obtained from T cells cultured with 10^{-4} M histamine for 24 hr also suppressed MLC responses by fresh autologous T cells. Combined with the studies mentioned above, these observations suggest that inhibition of MLC-induced proliferation by histamine was mediated through activation of suppressor T cells via their histamine type II receptor with subsequent elaboration of a soluble suppressor factor(s).

Histamine in a dose-dependent manner consistently inhibited the proliferative response of human lymphocytes induced by suboptimal concentrations of T-cell mitogens such as concanavalin A (Con A) and phytohemagglutinin (PHA) (reviewed in Refs. 11-13). The sensitivity to histamine-induced inhibition of T-cell proliferation was in part determined by such factors as HLA (histocompatibility leukocyte antigen) phenotype (22), and the presence or absence of an allergic diathesis (23-25). The latter will be discussed in further detail in a separate chapter.

Employing a coculture assay system initially developed to analyze the Con A-induced suppressor-cell system (26), Rocklin and Haberek-Davidson (27)

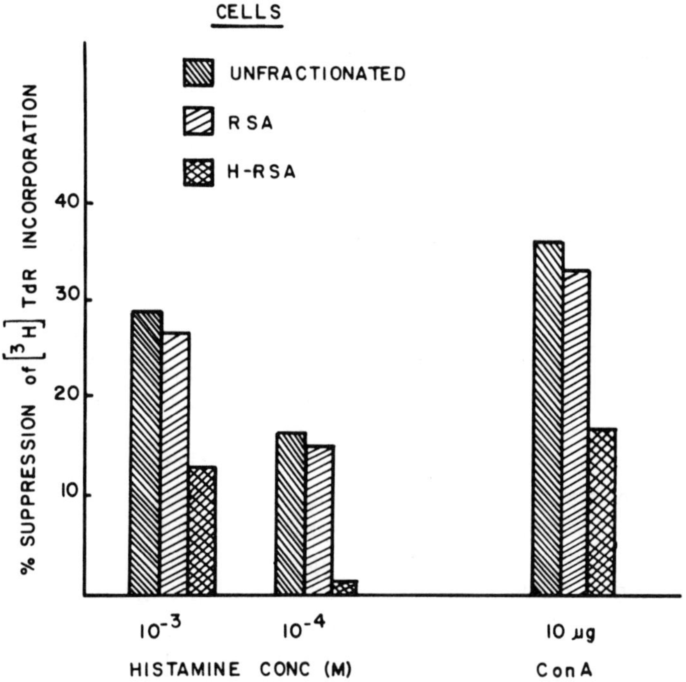

Figure 4 Chromatography of mononuclear cells on insolubilized conjugates of histamine-Sepharose. Mononuclear cells were incubated with histamine (H-RSA) or control (RSA) beads and the nonadherent cells collected. The nonretained cells were then incubated with histamine or concanavalin A (Con A) and their suppressor activity was measured. H-RSA columns (but not RSA columns) significantly depleted the histamine-responsive cells. In addition, Con A reactivity also was decreased in the suppressor cell assay.

were able to demonstrate clearly that histamine inhibition of mitogen-stimulated lymphocyte proliferation was the result of histamine activation of a suppressor T-cell bearing histamine type II receptors. In their model, aliquots of human blood mononuclear cells were cultured in vitro in the absence or presence of histamine (10^{-8}-10^{-3} M) for 24 hr, mitomycin C treated to prevent their own proliferation, washed, and then cocultured with autologous PHA-pulsed indicator cells. The results indicated that histamine in a dose-dependent fashion suppressed the PHA-induced proliferative response. A minimum of 2 hr was required to activate T cells by histamine to express suppressor function. Passage of suppressor cells over histamine-affinity columns (but not control columns) prior to their exposure to histamine depleted the nonadherent T cells of histamine-activatable cells (Fig. 4). An additional finding was that Con A-inducible suppressor cells also adhered to these histamine-affinity columns. The activation of these suppressor cells was mimicked by histamine type II, but not type I, receptor agonists and was blocked by type II, but not type I, receptor antagonists.

Employing the coculture method for generation and expression of histamine-induced T-cell suppressor activity, Rocklin and associates (28) were able to detect a soluble suppressor factor that was elaborated in vitro by human lymphocytes in response to histamine (histamine-induced suppressor factor, HSF). The human suppressor T cells induced to produce HSF were shown to be included in the suppressor/cytotoxic subset (as defined by the presence of receptors for the Fc portion of immunoglobulin G [IgG] and their staining with the monoclonal antibodies directed against the OKT8 and Leu 2 epitopes) (21,29, 30). Using a murine monoclonal antibody, designated 9.3, which previously had been shown to distinguish precursors of cytotoxic T cells (9.3^+) from precursors of antigen-specific suppressor T cells (9.3^-), Sansoni et al. (30) demonstrated that the histamine-induced suppressor T cell was phenotypically Leu 2^+, 9.3^-.

Human HSF has been characterized by enzyme treatment, sensitivity to reduction and alkylation, molecular sieve chromatography, and polyacrylamide gel electrophoresis (31). It was found to have a wide pH stability (pH 3-10), to be sensitive to temperatures more than 80°C, and to have the properties of a glycoprotein by virtue of its sensitivity to chymotrypsin, trypsin, sodium periodate, and neuraminidase. Human HSF did not appear to have a serine group(s) in its active site, since its biologic activity remained intact after treatment with an irreversible serine esterase inhibitor. Furthermore, HSF did not appear to have inter- or intramolecular disulfide bridges because treatment with denaturing and/ or reducing agents followed by alkylation did not alter its suppressor activity. Electrophoresis of HSF in polyacrylamide gels at pH 8.7 under nonreducing conditions revealed two regions of suppressor activity: one migrating with albumin and the other anodal to albumin (acidic glycoproteins). Molecular sieve chromatography revealed an apparent molecular weight for HSF of 25,000–40,000. Furthermore, gel filtration of supernatants generated by stimulating human blood mononuclear cells with dimaprit (but not 2-pyridylethylamine), Con A, or specific antigen resulted in similar elution profiles with regard to inhibition of lymphocyte proliferation; that is, the 25–40 kDa fractions of supernatants generated by each ligand suppressed lymphocyte proliferation to a similar degree. These findings provide indirect evidence that T cells, triggered by antigen-specific or nonspecific stimuli, elaborate physicochemically similar suppressor molecules capable of modulating T-cell function.

The effect of various metabolic inhibitors on the generation of suppressor cells was investigated in the coculture system (32). Human blood mononuclear cells were stimulated with histamine for 24 hr in the presence or absence of metabolic inhibitors, washed, and cocultured with lectin-stimulated autologous mononuclear cells. The generation of histamine-induced suppressor T cells was demonstrated to require active cellular metabolism, since inhibition of transcription (actinomycin D), translation (puromycin or cycloheximide), oxidative phosphorylation (sodium azide), and glycolysis (2-deoxyglucose) all significantly reduced histamine induction of suppressor activity. Inhibitors or cytoskeletal function such as cytochalasin B and colchicine also markedly reduced histamine generation of suppressor activity. There was no apparent requirement for deoxyribonucleic acid (DNA) synthesis in the histamine induction of suppressor cells, since treatment of the cells with mitomycin C (50 μg/ml) had no effect on suppression.

Employing the coculture assay and techniques for fractionation of blood mononuclear cells, the requirement of the macrophage/monocyte in the activation and expression of histamine-responsive human suppressor T cells was explored (33-35). Histamine activation of human suppressor T cells required the presence of monocytes. Monocyte-depleted T-lymphocyte populations containing less than 2% monocytes were unable to be activated by histamine to express suppressor activity. If, during the generation phase of the coculture assay, the T-cell population was reconstituted with 5-10% autologous monocytes in the form of glass-adherent cells, exposure to histamine resulted in suppressor activity (34).

The requirement for intact monocytes in the activation process could be bypassed by suspending the nonadherent T-cell population in supernatants derived from allogeneic monocytes stimulated with heat-killed *Staphylococcus albus* (34,35). These crude monocyte-derived supernatants contained leukocyte pyrogen (LP) and lymphocyte-activating factor (LAF) activities. Sequential separation of the crude monocyte supernatants using gel filtration (Fig. 5) immunoadsorption, and isoelectric focusing demonstrated that only those fractions containing both LP and LAF activities were capable of reconstituting histamine-induced nonadherent T-lymphocyte suppressor activity. By itself, LP/LAF (interleukin-1) did not activate T-suppressor cells nonspecifically, but rather served as an accessory factor that was required for the generation of histamine-induced suppressor T cells (Fig. 6) (35).

Additionally, further investigation has demonstrated the requirement of monocytes in the effector stage of histamine-induced suppressor activity (34,36, 37). The role of monocytes in the effector phase of suppression was analyzed using T-cell populations cultured in the presence of dialyzed monocyte supernatant factors in both the generator and effector stages of the coculture assay. Despite the presence of monocyte supernatant, depletion of monocytes from both the suppressor (generation phase) and indicator (effector phase) populations resulted in a marked reduction in the expression of histamine-induced sup-

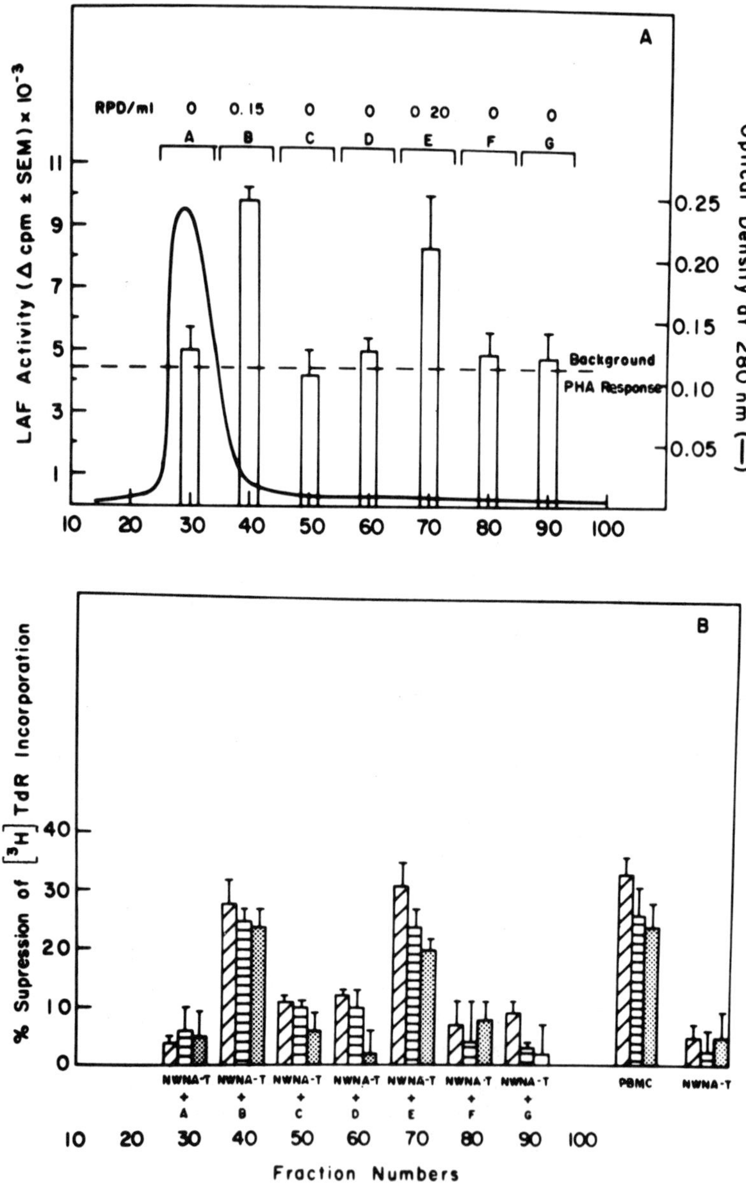

Figure 5 Sephadex G-50 gel filtration of crude monocyte supernatant showed coincident peaks (~ 40 and 15 kDa) of pyrogenicity, lymphocyte-activating factor activity (panel A), and the ability to reconstitute histamine and Con A–induced suppressor activity of the nylon wool nonadherent T-cell population (panel B). ▨ , 1 mM histamine; ▤ , 0.1 mM histamine; ▩ 20 μg/ml Con A

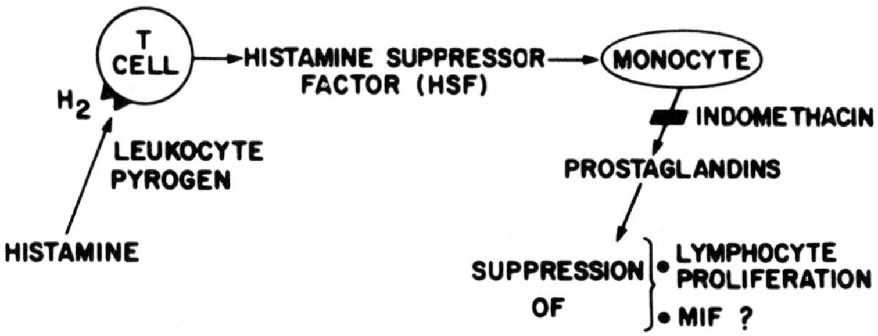

Figure 6 A proposed model of the in vivo monocyte-lymphocyte interactions required for the expression of histamine-induced suppression. Histamine, in the presence of monocytes or their secretory products, activated a subpopulation of T lymphocytes to elaborate soluble substances capable of stimulating mononuclear phagocytes to synthesize prostaglandins that subsequently suppressed mitogen-stimulated lymphocyte proliferation.

pressor activity. Thus, unlike the generation phase of suppressor-cell activation where a nondialyzable monocyte-derived factor could partially replace or augment the function of intact monocytes, the effector phase appeared to require for full expression of histamine-induced suppressor activity the presence of monocytes or a factor not present in the dialyzed partially purified monocyte supernatants.

The addition of indomethacin (1 μg/ml) at the time of coculture (effector phase) when monocytes were present in the indicator phase population abrogated histamine-induced suppression (34,37). In contrast, indomethacin had no effect during the generation phase of suppressor-cell activation. Moreover, addition of exogenous 10^{-8} and 10^{-7} M PGE_2 (a known inhibitor of T-cell proliferation) (36) to mononuclear cell cultures reconstituted histamine-induced suppressor activity in the presence of indomethacin. Taken collectively, these observations suggested that monocytes or prostanoids derived from monocytes were required for full expression of histamine-induced suppressor-cell activity (Fig. 6).

The necessary relationship between histamine-induced suppressor T cells and monocytes was strengthened further by investigations demonstrating the ability of HSF-containing supernatants to increase prostanoid production from monocytes (37). Monocytes, but not lymphocytes, incubated with supernatants containing HSF activity increased their production of prostaglandins E_2 and $F_2\alpha$, and thromboxane B_2 by 169, 53, and 49%, respectively. When suppressor supernatants were generated with histamine or dimaprit and separated by molecular sieve chromatography, the elution profiles for the factor(s) inducing suppression of lymphocyte proliferation (25–40 kDa) and augmenting PGE_2 pro-

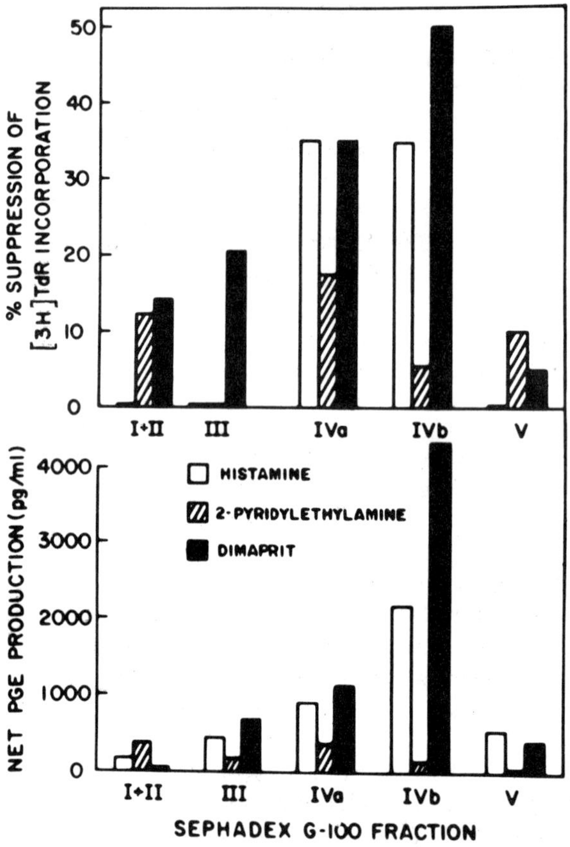

Figure 7 Serum-free HSF was generated with histamine (or a histamine type I or type II receptor agonist) and chromatographed by gel filtration on Sephadex G-100. The fractions were assayed in parallel for [^{3}H] thymidine incorporation and augmentation of PGE_2 production. Both histamine and dimaprit (but not 2-pyridylethylamine) generated supernatants that inhibited proliferation (fractions 4a and 4b; 25–40 kDa) and augmented PGE_2 production (fraction 4b; 25 kDa).

duction (25 kDa) overlapped, but were not identical (Fig. 7). Collectively, these data suggest that HSF-mediated inhibition of lymphocyte proliferation may occur at least in part through the augmented production of prostaglandins and/or thromboxanes by monocytes.

Unlike the extensive investigations into histamine-induced suppression of human lymphocyte proliferation, there is far less known about the effects of histamine on human lymphokine secretion. Studies by Dohlsten et al. (38,39) demonstrated that histamine, via interaction with a histamine type II receptor, directly suppressed CD4 (helper/inducer) production of interleukin-2 and interferon-γ. This direct inhibition of CD4 lymphokine production was independent of the presence or absence of CD8 (suppressor/cytotoxic) cells.

Rigal et al. (40) demonstrated that in vitro elaboration of human leukocyte migration inhibitory factor (LIF) was decreased by the addition of histamine. This histamine-induced suppression of LIF production was secondary to a soluble mediator with an apparent molecular weight between 10 and 50 kDa that was elaborated by human T cells stimulated with histamine. No other studies address the effects of histamine-induced human suppressor factors on lymphokine production.

Natural killer (NK) and cytotoxic lymphocytes possess an important but poorly understood capacity to destroy tumor cells both in vitro and in vivo. Nair and Schwartz (41) showed that human blood lymphocytes precultured with histamine for 24 hr demonstrated a significant decrease in their NK and antibody-dependent cellular cytotoxic activities, and when combined in coculture with autologous cytotoxic lymphocytes suppressed the NK activity of these effector cells. In a subsequent study, Nair et al. demonstrated that culture supernatants of lymphocytes stimulated with 10^{-8}–10^{-3} M histamine contained a soluble suppressor factor (histamine-induced soluble suppressor factor [HISSF]) that significantly inhibited the NK function of allogeneic lymphocytes. The NK activity suppressive effect of HISSF was dose dependent. By itself, HISSF was not cytotoxic and produced its suppressive effect on a mixed lymphocyte population and on NK-enriched large granular lymphocytes (LGLs). Production of HISSF was specifically blocked by the histamine type II receptor antagonist cimetidine, but not by the type I receptor antagonist clemastine fumurate. Although HISSF inhibited the cytotoxicity of LGLs, LGLs themselves did not produce HISSF. Inhibition of NK activity by HISSF was reversed completely by treating effector lymphocytes with interferon-α for a short period or culturing them with interleukin-2 for 36 hr.

Preliminary characterization of HISSF by ultrafiltration indicated an apparent molecular weight greater than 20 kDa. However, it is unclear whether HISSF is similar or identical to HSF, or instead is a structurally and functionally distinct lymphokine. The final answer to the relationship of HISSF and HSF awaits further physicochemical and functional characterization of the two molecules.

IV. HISTAMINE-INDUCED SUPPRESSOR-CELL MODULATION OF HUMAN B-LYMPHOCYTE FUNCTION

A number of studies (reviewed in Refs. 11-13) in humans have demonstrated that histamine receptor-bearing cells exert a regulatory influence on immuno-

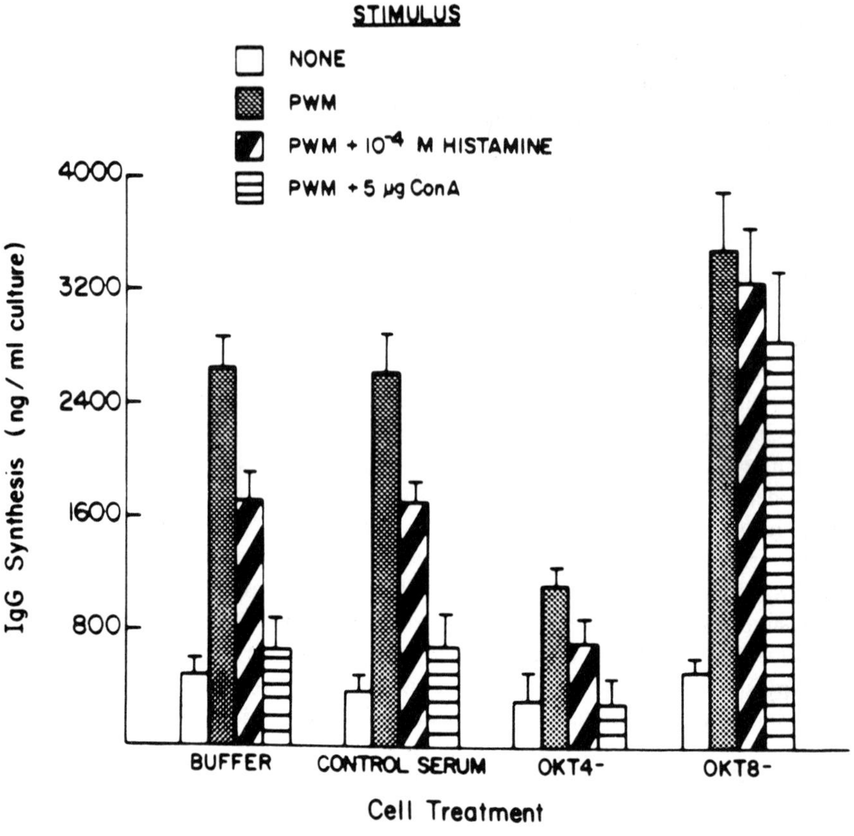

Figure 8 Treatment of histamine- and concanavalin A (Con A)–induced suppressor cells with monoclonal antibodies directed against T-cell subsets. T-enriched cells were incubated in buffer alone, buffer + complement, OKT4 antiserum + complement, or OKT8 antiserum + complement, washed, and then incubated with or without histamine or Con A for 24 hr. After incubation, the remaining cells ($OKT4^-$ or $OKT8^-$) were cocultured with autologous E-rosette-negative cells that were then stimulated by pokeweed mitogen. Histamine- and Con A–induced suppressor cells were contained within the $OKT8^+$ cell population.

globulin production. The majority of these studies pointed out that the major effect of histamine in down regulating immunoglobulin production was mediated through T-cell suppressor mechanisms.

In an in vitro model of immunoglobulin production by human blood mononuclear cells using pokeweed mitogen as a stimulant, histamine in a dose-dependent manner was shown to significantly suppress production of IgG (measured by double antibody radioimmunoassay) (43). Kinetic experiments indicated that the effect of histamine was not due to direct toxicity because the suppression was only seen if histamine was added within 72 hr following the addition of mitogen, but not thereafter.

In order to characterize the histamine-responsive suppressor cell in this model system, a coculture technique was employed. Human blood mononuclear cells were either separated into E-rosette-positive (T cell–enriched) or E-rosette–negative (T cell–depleted, B cell–enriched) populations and irradiated or treated with monoclonal antibodies directed against the CD4 or CD8 membrane glycoproteins plus complement. These cells were then stimulated with histamine or Con A for 24 hr. These potential suppressor cell populations were cocultured with pokeweed mitogen-stimulated autologous E-rosette–negative cells, and IgG production was measured. The histamine- and Con A–responsive suppressor cell was contained within the T cell–enriched population and was identified by reactivity with OKT8 antisera, but not OKT4 antisera (Fig. 8) (43). Efforts to discern histamine receptor specificity led to confusing results in the above study. It was found that suppression of IgG production occurred with histamine types I and II receptor agonists. Attempts to reverse the histamine-induced suppression using selective histamine types I and II receptor antagonists revealed that diphenhydramine, but not cimetidine, reversed the histamine-induced suppression of IgG production. These data suggested that T cells bearing both functional histamine types I and II receptors may be involved in the regulation of IgG production.

A study by Hebert et al. (44) measured the effects of histamine-induced suppressor activity on pokeweed mitogen-generated IgG synthesis in vitro as measured by a modified reverse hemolytic plaque assay. Addition of autologous or allogeneic histamine-stimulated suppressor T cells at the end of a 7-day culture caused a significant suppression of the IgG response. On the other hand, addition of suppressor cells at the beginning of the culture did not suppress the synthesis of IgG. These observations suggested that the histamine-induced suppressor cells did not act by blocking the proliferation of B cells or B-cell precursors, but rather they acted by inhibiting the synthesis or release of IgG by mature B cells.

The latter results demonstrating that histamine-induced suppressor activity affects only the late phase of antibody production appears contradictory to the study of Lima and Rocklin (43) which demonstrated an effect of histamine-induced suppressor activity in the early phases of antibody production. These discrepancies may be related more to differences in experimental design rather than to actual disparate data. A subsequent study (45), described below, further clarified the kinetics of histamine-induced suppression of humoral responses.

Table 3 Histamine-Induced Suppressor Activity Inhibition of DR Antigen Expression on MLC-Activated T Lymphocytes

			MLC-activated T lymphocytes[a]	
Cell	HLA phenotype	Antigens	Control supernatant (%)	HISA[b] (undiluted) (%)
1	A1, B8, DR3			
	(homozygous)	Ia	62	18
		DR3	51	21
		DR1	2	2
		(Neg. control)		
2	A1, A2, B12, B35			
	DR1, DR7	Ia	50	28
		DR1	48	20
		DR7	50	23
		DR3	2	2
		(Neg. control)		

[a]T lymphocytes were activated in one-way MLC by incubating 2×10^6 irradiated blood lymphocytes from HLA-mismatched individuals for 6 days in RPMI 1640-enriched media at 37°C, 5% CO_2 atmosphere. Cells recovered from triplicate wells were washed and examined for antigen expression by indirect immunofluorescence.
[b]Histamine-induced suppressor activity.

Employing a model of polyclonal B-cell activation induced during a primary MLC, the effect of T cell-derived histamine-induced suppressor activity (HISA) on the humoral immune response was examined (45). The addition of HISA on day 0 to MLC-induced plaques (measured by a protein A plaque assay) resulted in a reduction in the mean number of IgG, IgM, and IgA PFC by 60–80%. The histamine-induced lymphokine was active at a titer of 1/1000 and suppressed all the isotypes equally well. Experiments were then carried out to determine whether the factor was acting on T cells initially being activated to become helper cells, or whether the factor affected the function of activated T helper cells. If HISA was present only during the helper T-cell generation phase, or only at the time of coculture, the subsequent total plaque-forming B-cell response was inhibited by up to 80%. This indicated that the histamine-induced factor inhibited both the activation of helper T cells and their effector function.

It is known that activated T cells express Ia/DR antigens. Another way to evaluate the effect of HISA on helper T-cell function was to determine its effect

Table 4 Inhibition of MLC-Derived Helper Factor–Induced Plaque–Forming Cell Response by Histamine-Induced Suppressor Activity

	IgG (PFC/10^6)	Percent inhibition[c]	IgM (PFC/10^6)	Percent inhibition[c]
B cells + control supernatant (sup.)	25		50	
B cells + MLC (sup.)	1400–1500[a]		1000–1100[a]	
B cells + sup. 50% + HISA[b] 12.5%		27–32		27–31
B cells + sup. 50% + HISA 25%		47–50		38–42
B cells + sup. 50% + HISA 37.5%		47–50		40–43
B cells + sup. 50% + HISA 50%		71–73		43–46

[a]Range of IgG and IgM PFC produced in four separate experiments. Nylon column–purified B lymphocytes were cultured for 6 days in 50% derived helper factor supernatant and 50% control media.

[b]Histamine-induced suppressor activity.

[c]Concentration (%) of HISA (undiluted) after replacing portion of control media. Range of percent inhibition in four experiments are shown.

on the expression of DR antigens. As shown in Table 3, DR antigens were normally detected on 50–60% of activated T cells generated by day 6 of an MLC. The presence of detectable DR antigens on the surface of activated T cells was reproducibly reduced by half by HISA. Whether the factor was restricted in its action to the CD4+, Ia+ helper T cell, or whether other T-cell subsets might also be affected was not determined.

Another aspect of these studies (45) involved the direct effect of HISA on B-cell function. Allogeneic-effect helper factors, i.e., lymphokines which are known to provide help for B cells, were employed. Increasing concentrations of HISA led to a significant inhibition of the PFC response to preformed helper factors (Table 4). To achieve a 50% reduction in B-cell responses to helper factors required at least half-strength HISA. A similar reduction in primary MLC-generated PFC responses was achieved with significantly lower concentrations (1/1000 dilution) of HISA. These findings suggested that in the sequence of cellular interactions required for antibody production the phase of T-cell activation may be more sensitive to the inhibitory effects of HISA than the subsequent phase of B-cell activation. Taken together, the data suggested that a histamine-induced lymphokine inhibited polyclonal B-cell activation by interfering with the generation and effector function of helper T cells as well as the B-cell response to preformed helper factors. Since HISA also inhibited the expression of DR antigens on activated T cells, this may serve to limit cooperation between T and B cells and help explain the inhibitory effects of HISA on immunoglobulin production.

Soluble immune response suppressor (SIRS) is an immunosuppressive protein which inhibits antibody production and tumor cell division in vitro (46) and plaque-forming cell and delayed-type hypersensitivity responses in vivo (47). Initially defined as a murine T-cell product induced by Con A or interferon (46, 48), more recent work (49) has identified human SIRS with antigenic, functional, and physical similarities to the murine analog. Because histamine had been reported to activate suppressor cells, Schnaper et al. (50) investigated the potential role for histamine in SIRS production. Human mononuclear cells incubated for 1 hr with 10^{-4} or 10^{-5} M histamine released a suppressive substance (as measured by inhibition of an in vitro polyclonal IgM plaque-forming cell assay) into culture supernatants that was physically, functionally, and antigenically similar to previously described human SIRS. The T-lymphocyte subset activated by histamine to produce SIRS was contained within the CD8, but not the CD4, population of cells. Cimetidine and ranitidine, two structurally distinct histamine type II receptor antagonists, inhibited histamine-induced CD8 cell elaboration of SIRS. Of further interest, activation of lymphocytes to produce SIRS by Con A or interferon also was blocked by cimetidine or ranitidine. This observation raised the possibility that histamine release induced by Con A or interferon from basophils contaminating the lymphocyte cultures may be the final mechanism for SIRS production. Alternatively, the data were consistent with the possibility that the histamine type II receptor antagonists prevent either binding of Con A or interferon to the appropriate receptors, or triggering of suppressor cell activity once the ligand has bound to the receptor. The precise role of histamine type II receptor binding in SIRS production and the relationship of the previously described histamine-induced suppressor activities, HSF and HISSF, to the SIRS pathway remain to be defined.

V. CONCLUSIONS

Although the role of histamine as a mediator of immediate-type hypersensitivity responses has been known since the early part of this century, its role as an immunomodulator has become increasingly apparent over the past 20 years. In this chapter describing histamine-induced suppressor-cell systems, we reviewed the in vitro observations originating in animal studies and progressing to humans, which promote the concept of histamine serving as a negative-feedback regulator of lymphocyte function. In vivo, release of histamine from tissue mast cells and basophils may be induced by a number of different mechanisms (51-53). Once released, histamine, via interaction with histamine type II receptors on a subset of CD8 lymphocytes, may activate the suppressor limb of an inflammatory reaction and dampen the response by decreasing production or release of inflammation-promoting lymphokines and inhibiting lymphocyte proliferation.

In keeping with the concept of an immune response being a complex series of events modulated by both negative and positive influences, it should come as no surprise that the above described role of histamine as an inhibitor of the immune response has a proinflammatory counterpart. In addition to inducing a series of lymphokines which suppress immune reactions, histamine also induces from a different T-cell subset a series of lymphokines which promote or amplify immune responses. These histamine-induced lymphokines are discussed elsewhere in this book. In the final analysis, the extent and character of an immune response in vivo represents the balance among all the local factors which contribute to its occurrence.

ACKNOWLEDGMENTS

This work was supported by U.S. Public Health Service Grants HL-32802 and AI-16362.

We thank Randi White and Sharon Davignon for their expert assistance in the preparation of this manuscript.

REFERENCES

1. Cantor, H., and R. K. Gershon, Immunological circuits: Cellular composition, Fed. Proc. 38:2058-2064 (1979).
2. Gershon, R. K., and K. Kondo, Antigenic competition between heterologous erythrocytes. I. Thymic dependency, J. Immunol. 106:1524-1531 (1971).
3. Gershon, R. K., and K. Kondo, Antigenic competition between heterologous erythrocytes. II. Effect of passive antibody administration, J. Immunol. 106:1532-1539 (1971).
4. Fauci, A. S., and R. E. Ballieux, Antibody Production in Man: *In Vitro* Synthesis and Clinical Implication, Academic Press, New York, (1979).
5. Broder, S., Cellular regulation of immune function, J. Allergy Clin. Immunol. 65:239-241 (1980).
6. Waldmann, T. A., and S. Broder, Suppressor cells in the regulation of the immune response. In Progress in Clinical Immunology, vol. 3 (Schwartz, R. S., Ed.), Grune & Stratton, New York (1977), pp. 155-199.
7. Reinherz, E. L., A. Rubinstein, R. S. Geha, A. J. Stelkaus, F. S. Rosen, and S. F. Schlossman, Abnormalities in immunoregulatory T cells in disorders of immune function, N. Engl. J. Med. 301:1018-1022 (1979).

8. Reinherz, E. L., P. C. Kung, G. Goldstein, and S. F. Schlossman, Separation of functional subsets of human T cells by a monoclonal antibody, Proc. Natl. Acad. Sci. U.S.A. 76:4061–4065 (1979).
9. Reinherz, E. L., P. C. Kung, G. Goldstein, and S. F. Schlossman, A monoclonal antibody reactive with the human cytotoxic/suppressor T cell subset previously defined by a heteroantiserum termed TH_2, J. Immunol. 124: 1301-1307 (1980).
10. Reinherz, E. L., P. C. Kung, G. Goldstein, R. H. Levey, and S. F. Schlossman, Discrete stages of intrathymic differentiation: Analysis of normal thymocytes and leukemic lymphoblasts of T-cell lineage, Proc. Natl. Acad. Sci. U.S.A. 77:1588–1592 (1980).
11. Plaut, M., and L. S. Lichtenstein, Histamine and immune responses. In Pharmacology of Histamine Receptors (Ganellin, C. R., and Parsons, M. G., Eds.), John Wright, London (1982), pp. 392–435.
12. Beer, D. J., S. M. Matloff, and R. E. Rocklin, The influence of histamine on immune and inflammatory responses. In Advances in Immunology, vol. 35 (Kunkel, H. G., and Dixon, F. J., Eds.), Academic Press, Orlando, Florida (1984), pp. 209-268.
13. Beer, D. J., and R. E. Rocklin, Histamine modulation of lymphocyte biology: Membrane receptors, signal transduction and functions. In CRC Critical Reviews in Immunology, vol. 7 (Atassi, M. Z., Ed.), CRC Press, Orlando, Florida (1987), pp. 55–91.
14. Melmon, K. L., R. E. Rocklin, and R. P. Rosenkranz, Autacoids as modulators of the inflammatory and immune response, Am. J. Med. 71:100–106 (1981).
15. Rocklin, R. E., Modulation of cellular-immune responses in vivo and in vitro by histamine receptor-bearing lymphocytes, J. Clin. Invest. 57:1051–1058 (1976).
16. Rocklin, R. E., D. Greineder, B. H. Littman, and K. L. Melmon, Modulation of cellular immune function in vitro by histamine receptor-bearing lymphocytes: Mechanism of action, Cell. Immunol. 37:162–173 (1978).
17. Pick, E., Soluble lymphocytic mediators. I. Inhibition of macrophage migration inhibitory factor production by drugs, Immunology 26:649–658 (1974).
18. Rocklin, R. E., Histamine-induced suppressor factor (HSF): Effect on migration inhibitory factor (MIF) production and proliferation, J. Immunol. 118:1934–1938 (1977).
19. Rocklin, R. E., D. K. Greineder, and K. L. Melmon, Histamine-induced suppressor factor (HSF): Further studies on the nature of the stimulus and the cell which produces it, Cell. Immunol. 44:404–415 (1979).
20. Ballet, J. J., and E. Merler, The separation and reactivity in vitro of a subpopulation of human lymphocytes which bind histamine. Correlation of histamine reactivity with cellular maturation, Cell. Immunol. 24:250–269 (1976).
21. Damle, N. K., and S. Gupta, Autologous mixed lymphocyte reaction in man. II. Histamine-induced suppression of the autologous mixed lympho-

cyte reaction by T-cell subsets defined with monoclonal antibodies. J. Clin. Immunol. 1:241–249 (1981).
22. Staszak, C., J.S. Goodwin, G. M. Troup, D. R. Pahtak, and R. C. Williams, Decreased sensitivity to prostaglandin and histamine in lymphocytes from normal HLA-B12 individuals: A possible role in autoimmunity, J. Immunol. 125:181–185 (1980).
23. Stannegard, I. L., and O. Stannegard, Increased sensitivity of lymphocytes from atopic individuals to histamine-induced suppression, Scand. J. Immunol. 6:1225–1231 (1977).
24. Martinez, J. D., J. Santos, D. J. Stechschulte, and N. I. Abdou, Nonspecific suppressor cell function in atopic subjects, J. Allergy Clin. Immunol. 64: 485–490 (1979).
25. Beer, D. J., M. E. Osband, R. P. McCaffrey, N. A. Soter, and R. E. Rocklin, Abnormal histamine-induced suppressor-cell function in atopic subjects, N. Engl. J. Med. 306:454–458 (1982).
26. Shou, L., S. A. Schwartz, and R. A. Good, Suppressor cell activity after concanavalin A treatment of lymphocytes from normal donors, J. Exp. Med. 113:1100–1110 (1976).
27. Rocklin, R. E., and A. Haberek-Davidson, Histamine activates suppressor cells *in vitro* using a co-culture technique, J. Clin. Immunol. 1:73–79 (1981).
28. Rocklin, R. E., B. Sherry, and H. Dolben, Production and assay of histamine-induced suppressor factor (HSF) by human lymphocytes, Afr. J. Clin. Exp. Immunol. 3:199–208 (1981).
29. Rocklin, R. E., J. Breard, S. Gupta, R. A. Good, and K. L. Melmon, Characterization of the human blood lymphocytes that produce a histamine-induced suppressor factor, Cell. Immunol. 51:226–237 (1980).
30. Sansoni, P., E. D. Silverman, M. M. Khan, K. L. Melmon, and E. G. Engleman, Immunoregulatory T cells in man: Histamine-induced suppressor T cells are derived from a Leu2+ (T8+) subpopulation distinct from that which gives rise to cytotoxic T cells, J. Clin. Invest. 75:650–656 (1985).
31. Rocklin, R. E., A. Blidy, and M. Kamal, Physicochemical characterization of human histamine-induced suppressor factor (HSF), Cell. Immunol. 76: 243–252 (1983).
32. Rocklin, R. E., and A. Haberek-Davidson, Pharmacologic modulation *in vitro* of human histamine-induced suppressor cell activity, Int. J. Immunopharmacol. 6:179–186 (1984).
33. Hebert, J., R. Beaudoin, M. Aubin, and M. Fontaine, The regulatory effect of histamine on the immune response: Characterization of the cells involved, Cell. Immunol. 54:49–57 (1980).
34. Beer, D. J., L. J. Rosenwasser, C. A. Dinarello, and R. E. Rocklin, Cellular interactions in the generation and expression of histamine-induced suppressor activity, Cell. Immunol. 69:101–112 (1982).
35. Beer, D. J., C. A. Dinarello, L. J. Rosenwasser, and R. E. Rocklin, Human monocyte-derived soluble product(s) has an accessory function in the generation of histamine and concanavalin A-induced suppressor T cells, J. Clin. Invest. 70:393–400 (1982).

36. Staszak, C., and J. S. Goodwin, Is prostaglandin a mediator for the inhibitory action of histamine, hydrocortisone, and isoproterenol, Cell. Immunol. 54:351-361 (1980).
37. Rocklin, R. E., I. Kiselis, D. J. Beer, P. Rossi, F. Maggi, and J. Bellanti, Augmentation of prostaglandin and thromboxane production *in vitro* by monocytes exposed to histamine-induced suppressor factor (HSF), Cell. Immunol. 77:92-98 (1983).
38. Dohlsten, M., H. O. Sjogren, and R. Carlsson, Histamine inhibits interferon-gamma production via suppression of interleukin-2 synthesis, Cell. Immunol. 101:493-501 (1986).
39. Dohlsten, M., H. O. Sjogren, and R. Carlsson, Histamine acts directly on human T cells to inhibit interleukin-2 and interferon-gamma production, Cell. Immunol. 109:65-74 (1987).
40. Rigal, D., J. C. Monier, and G. Souweine, The effect of histamine on leukocyte migration test in man. I. Demonstration of a LIF production inhibitor (LIF-PI), Cell. Immunol. 46:360-372 (1979).
41. Nair, M. P. N., and S. A. Schwartz, Effect of histamine and histamine antagonists on natural and antibody-dependent cellular cytotoxicity of human lymphocytes *in vitro*, Cell. Immunol. 81:45-60 (1983).
42. Nair, M. P. N., J. M. Cilik, and S. A. Schwartz, Histamine-induced suppressor factor inhibition of NK cells: Reversal with interferon and interleukin 2, J. Immunol. 136:2456-2462 (1986).
43. Lima, M., and R. E. Rocklin, Histamine modulates *in vitro* IgG production by pokeweed mitogen-stimulated human mononuclear cells, Cell. Immunol. 64:324-336 (1981).
44. Hebert, J., R. Beaudoin, M. Fontaine, and G. Fradet, The regulatory effect of histamine on immune responses. II. Effect on the *in vitro* IgG synthesis, Cell. Immunol. 58:366-371 (1981).
45. Garovoy, M. R., M. A. Reddish, and R. E. Rocklin, Histamine-induced suppressor factor (HSF): Inhibition of helper T cell generation and function. J. Immunol. 130:357-361 (1983).
46. Aune, T. M., and C. W. Pierce, Mechanism of SIRS actions at the cellular and biochemical level. In Lymphokines, vol. 9 (Pick, E., Ed.), Academic Press, New York (1984), pp. 257.
47. Schnaper, H. W., and T. M. Aune, Suppression of immune response to sheep erythrocytes by the lymphokine soluble immune response suppressor (SIRS) *in vivo*, J. Immunol. 137:863-867 (1986).
48. Webb, D. R., K. Mason, G. Semenuk, T. M. Aune, and C. W. Pierce, Purification and analysis of the isoforms of soluble immune response suppressor (SIRS), J. Immunol. 135:3238-3242 (1985).
49. Schnaper, H. W., C. W. Pierce, and T. M. Aune, Identification and initial characterization of concanavalin A- and interferon-induced human suppressor factors: Evidence for a human equivalent of murine soluble immune response suppressor (SIRS), J. Immunol. 132:2429-2435 (1984).

50. H. W. Schnaper, T. M. Aune, and R. K. Roby, A role for histamine type II (H-2) receptor binding in production of the lymphokine, soluble immune response suppressor (SIRS), J. Immunol. 139:1185–1190 (1987).
51. Dvorak, A. M., M. C. Mihm, Jr., and H. F. Dvorak, Morphology of delayed-type hypersensitivity reactions in man. II. Ultrastructural alterations affecting the microvasculature and the tissue mast cells, Lab. Invest. 34:179–191 (1976).
52. Thueson, D. O., L. S. Speck, M. A. Lett-Brown, and J. A. Grant, Histamine-releasing activity (HRA). I. Production by mitogen- or antigen-stimulated human mononuclear cells, J. Immunol. 123:626–632 (1979).
53. Dy, M., and B. Lebel, Skin allografts generate an enhanced production of histamine and histamine-producing cell-stimulating factor (HCSF) by spleen cells in response to mitogens, J. Immunol. 130:2343–2347 (1983).

4

Histamine in the Immunoregulation of Cellular Cytotoxicity

STANLEY A. SCHWARTZ and MADHAVAN P. N. NAIR *University of Michigan, Ann Arbor, Michigan*

I. INTRODUCTION

Histamine is a well-recognized soluble mediator of inflammation; its range of target tissues includes the vasculature, smooth muscles, and exocrine glands. Regarding the latter, histamine, a potent gastric secretagogue, can stimulate the production of copious amounts of gastric juice containing hydrochloric acid and pepsin. Two classes of physiological histamine receptors have been identified, designated histamine type I (H_1) and type II (H_2) receptors. Histamine type I receptors are associated with bronchoconstriction and contraction of gastrointestinal smooth muscle, whereas gastric secretion involves activation of type II receptors. Some effects, such as decrease in vascular tone, involve activation of both histamine types I and II receptors.

Histamine and a variety of other mediators of inflammation are present in the cytoplasmic granules of mast cells and basophils. These cells also possess membrane receptors for the Fc portion of immunoglobulin E (IgE). When antigens (or more specifically, allergens) bind to two or more cell-bound IgE secretion involves activation of type II receptors. Some effects, such as decrease in vascular tone, involve activation of both histamine types I and II receptors.

molecules, cytoplasmic degranulation occurs with a resultant liberation of free histamine and subsequent manifestation of allergic symptoms. As atopy is so widespread, numerous pharmacologic antagonists of histamine type I receptors have been produced for clinical use. Recently, several histamine type II receptor antagonists have also been developed and are finding extensive application in the treatment of duodenal and gastric ulcers.

II. CELL-MEDIATED CYTOTOXICITY

Leukocyte-mediated cytotoxic activities appear to be a significant host defense mechanism. Cellular cytotoxicity may require genetic identity between the target and effector cells, as manifested by cytotoxic T lymphocytes (CTLs), or it may be completely independent of histocompatibility restrictions, as exemplified by natural killer (NK) and antibody dependent cellular cytotoxic (ADCC) cells. Cytotoxic T lymphocytes also require prior exposure to target cell antigens to become activated, whereas NK and ADCC effector cells do not need this "education" process and can lyse target cells de novo.

Lymphocytes mediating NK-cell activity have been proposed as a first-line host response to malignant and virus-infected cells. Natural killer cells are operationally defined on the basis of their in vitro functional activities. When allogeneic human peripheral blood lymphocytes (PBLs) from healthy donors are mixed with the K562 cell line derived from a patient with erythroleukemia, the NK cells present within the PBLs spontaneously kill the tumor target cells. The microcytotoxicity assay for NK-cell activity has been generally standardized in most laboratories to consist of the admixture of effector cells, either PBL- or NK-enriched subpopulations, with ^{51}Cr-radiolabeled K562 target cells at effector-to-target cell ratios ranging approximately between 100:1 to 10:1. Cytotoxicity is proportional to and measured by the release of ^{51}Cr into the media from lysed tumor target cells after a 4-hr culture period.

The isolation of relatively pure populations of NK cells has not yet been accomplished. However, isopycnic fractionation of PBLs by centrifugation over discontinuous gradients of colloidal silica (Percoll, Pharmacia Fine Chemicals, Piscataway, New Jersey) has yielded subpopulations greatly enriched for NK-cell activities. Phenotypic characterization of NK cell–enriched preparations has shown that they are large granular lymphocytes (LGLs), approximately 8-10 μ in diameter, with cytoplasm containing azurophilic granules.

Considerable controversy surrounds the hematopoietic origin of NK cells as they bear markers for both monocytes and T-lymphocyte lineages (1). Because of the granular appearance of the cytoplasm of NK cells, several workers have raised the question of whether they are related to basophils or mast cells. To examine this issue, Rosenthal and colleagues (2) cloned three different NK-cell lines possessing granular cytoplasm, which were then analyzed for intracellular histaminase-sensitive histamine as well as high-affinity surface Fc receptors for IgE. None of the clones were found to possess either cytoplasmic histamine or IgE membrane receptors, thus failing to support a mast cell or basophil lineage for NK cells. In animal studies, a murine basophilic mast cell line and a rat basophilic leukemic cell line manifested cytotoxic activities, but were unable to kill specific NK targets (3). While a cloned human NK cell line was noted to resemble basophils by ultrastructural analysis and even expressed IgE receptors, the clone was unable to synthesize histamine (4). This wide spectrum of phenotypic and functional characteristics of various NK-cell clones is consistent with the current impression that NK cells are a heterogeneous subpopulation of lymphocytes.

III. REGULATION OF CELLULAR CYTOTOXICITY

Lymphocytes have long been recognized to possess a wide variety of specific receptors for biologically active substances. Early recognition of the inhibitory effect of histamine on the activities of CTLs can be attributed to Schayer (5). It was suggested that the inhibition of CTLs by histamine was due to decreased induction rather than suppression of their effector functions (6). However, Plaut and collaborators (7) demonstrated that specific activation of histamine type II receptors resulted in increased intracellular cyclic adenosine monophosphate (cAMP) levels in effector cells with concomitant inhibition of cytolysis. Other investigators have shown that histamine can also inhibit a variety of lymphocyte functions, including blast transformation, B-cell differentiation, and lymphokine production (for a review, see Ref. 8). Later studies indicated that the immunosuppressive activities of histamine were mediated through suppressor lymphocytes bearing histamine type II receptors (9). Surface marker analysis of these histamine-induced suppressor cells demonstrated that they are a unique subpopulation of T cells which express the $CD8^+$ antigen (10). Rocklin and his colleagues have previously identified and characterized a soluble mediator produced by histamine-activated suppressor cells, which they called histamine-induced suppressor factor, or HSF (11). Like histamine-induced suppressor cells, HSF can inhibit a wide variety of lymphocyte functions, including proliferative responses to antigens and lymphokine and antibody production.

In addition to their immune surveillance functions, NK cells have also been shown to regulate various immunologic activities (12-15). Consequently, it is reasonable to expect that NK and ADCC activities are also under immunologic control. We have previously reported that preculture of lymphocytes with or without concanavalin A can inhibit various in vitro immunologic functions through the activation of suppressor T cells (16). In the absence of added lectin, suppressor-cell induction by in vitro culture appears to be the result of an autologous mixed lymphocyte reaction (17). Culture-activated suppressor cells secrete a soluble suppressor factor (SSF) with a wide range of inhibitory activities, including suppression of (1) T-lymphocyte proliferative responses (18), (2) polyclonal B-cell activation (18), (3) myeloid colony formation in soft agar (unpublished observations), and (4) NK and ADCC functions (19).

Besides histamine, several pharmacologic agents can increase suppressor-cell activities, including amphotericin B (20) and corticosteroids (21). It has been shown that the histamine types I and II receptor antagonists, clemastine fumarate and cimetidine respectively, inhibit the NK and ADCC activities of human lymphocytes in vitro when added directly to the cell culture, and this inhibition could be partially reversed by histamine (22-25). Although complete reversal was not achieved with the histamine concentrations used, perhaps increased histamine concentrations would restore cytotoxic activities to original control levels. When lymphocytes were cultured with histamine for 24 hr, not only were their own NK and ADCC activities decreased, but these histamine-treated cells were also capable of suppressing the cytotoxic activities of fresh autologous effector cells in coculture experiments (25). Thus, histamine not only directly inhibits cytotoxicity, but it can also activate suppressor cells which can inhibit cytotoxic functions. It appears then that lymphocytes with histamine receptors may have dual roles in both mediating and regulating NK and ADCC functions.

IV. ACTIVATION OF SUPPRESSOR CELLS

Suppressor cells are essential to the control of various immunologic functions. When histamine-treated lymphocytes capable of suppressing NK and ADCC activities were examined for their surface marker phenotypes, it was noted that the relative proportion of $CD8^+$ cells increased after culture with histamine, whereas the percentage of $CD3^+$ and $CD4^+$ lymphocytes remained unchanged (25). This suggests that histamine-induced $CD8^+$ cells are either recruited from an undefined precursor pool or from $CD3^+$ and $CD4^+$ subpopulations. Alternatively, histamine-activated lymphocytes may exhibit a complex phenotype with coexpression of all three surface markers. Multiparameter analysis by flow cytometry may resolve this question.

In contrast to the effects of histamine on purified lymphocytes, when histamine was added directly to total peripheral blood mononuclear leukocytes containing approximately 15% monocytes, NK cytotoxicity was increased significantly (26). Enhancement of NK activity was also manifested by dimaprit, a specific histamine type 2 receptor agonist. However, when adherent cells were removed from the cultures, NK enhancement by histamine was completely eliminated. Monocytes are capable of suppressing NK activities through the elaboration of soluble factors. Monocytes and neutrophils were found to produce soluble factors which could modulate the cytotoxic activities of NK cells (27). Coculture of NK cells with autologous granulocytes or their diffusates across a Millipore filter resulted in augmented cytotoxicity, whereas reciprocal experiments with monocytes or their diffusates resulted in decreased killing of targets. While these effects were not due to interferon in the case of the granulocyte diffusates, nor to prostaglandins or lysozyme released by monocytes, rigorouse characterization of the specific moieties had not yet been accomplished. Histamine type II receptor blockers, such as cimetidine and ranitidine, could prevent histamine-induced enhancement of NK activity in the presence of monocytes, but were ineffective in adherent cell–depleted cultures (28). By contrast, however, both clemastine, a specific histamine type II receptor antagonist, and an isomer of clemastine with a low affinity for the type I receptor suppressed NK cytotoxicity. The authors concluded that this latter effect was thus independent of histamine receptor activation. Like histamine, serotonin could increase the NK activity of total human mononuclear cells, but enhancement was not additive when histamine also was present (29). From the above observations one might speculate that the paradoxical effects of histamine are possibly operating through different histamine type II receptors on monocytes and lymphocytes, but there is no evidence that the type II receptor is heterogeneous. However, activation of the same receptor on different leukocyte subpopulations can have different physiologic effects. Thus, binding of histamine by monocytes inhibits their ability to suppress NK activity, whereas histamine can activate suppressor T lymphocytes, which can then down regulate NK cell functions.

Earlier studies showed that histamine can directly down regulate CTL activities by binding to type II receptors on effector cells (6,7). Histamine appears to suppress CTL effector responses by stimulating an increase in intracellular cAMP levels. When murine CTLs were initially precultured alone without added drugs and subsequently treated with cAMP-enhancing agents such as histamine, the cells failed to produce increased levels of intracellular cAMP and became refractory to histamine-mediated suppression of cytotoxicity (30). This is similar to the observations described above in which preculture of human lymphocytes can induce suppressor cells capable of inhibiting NK and ADCC activities (17). It is possible that both situations involve activation of autologous mixed lymphocyte reactions. It is unlikely, however, that any appreciable histamine release occurs during the autologous mixed lymphocyte reaction to result in down regulation of CTL activity by histamine receptor desensitization. Prior incubation of cloned cytotoxic T lymphocytes with histamine results in their desensitization to subsequent histamine-induced enhancement of intracellular cAMP production (31). The effect appeared to be mediated by stimulation of a histamine type II receptor. By contrast, it was recently reported that cloned T cells activated with interleukin (IL-2) showed increased affinity and responsiveness to histamine type II receptor agonists capable of stimulating cAMP production (32). One can speculate on the basis of the disparity between different culture effects on cAMP activation by histamine. Perhaps as observed by Zhang and coworkers (33), various subpopulations of cytotoxic T cells respond differentially to cAMP-modulating substances such as histamine. The apparent paradox may also be explained by the observation that although both cytotoxic and suppressor T lymphocytes bear the CD8 surface antigen, they are two distinct subpopulations with differential responses to histamine (9). A similar differential response to histamine has been reported with regard to chemoattractant lymphokine production (34). $CD4^{+}$ and $CD8^{+}$ lymphocyte subsets secrete two biochemically different lymphokines which manifest similar lymphocyte migration inhibition activity. Kinetic influences may also underlie the differential immunoregulatory effects of histamine. Thus, when histamine was injected into experimental animals during the late phase of CTL activation it stimulated the response (35). This was paralleled in vitro by enhancement of IL-2 production by concanavalin A–activated splenocytes when histamine or histamine plus histaminase was added to the culture, suggesting that CTL augmentation is mediated by oxidized histamine via increased IL-2 production.

Further evidence for apparent opposing effects of histamine on lymphocytes exists. Histamine could either inhibit or stimulate IL-2 production by T helper cells depending upon the presence or absence of antigen, respectively (36). These activities, however, were unaffected by cimetidine.

In an extensive analysis of a large group of congener derivatives and conjugates of histamine, it was noted that a unique subset of suppressor cells, natural suppressor cells (NSs), possess both histamine type I and II receptors which could be differentially activated (37). Such observations may subsequently form a basis for a rational pharmacology of histamine derivatives specifically expressing immunomodulatory activities without coincident manifestations of adverse side effects.

While several investigators have described direct actions of histamine on CTL activity, recent studies suggest that histamine-induced inhibition of CTL responses may also involve the activation of suppressor mechanisms (38). Suppression could be reversed with IL-2 containing culture supernates and by the specific histamine type II antagonists, cimetidine and mifentidine, and not by ranitidine or type I antagonists.

In our earlier report (25) we noted an unusual phenomenon: Both clemastine fumarate and cimetidine, a histamine type I and type II histamine receptor blocker, respectively, could inhibit the NK and ADCC activities of lymphocytes as well as partially purified NK effector cells in a dose-dependent manner. This inhibition of cytotoxicity was observed at several effector-to-target

Table 1 Suppression of NK Activity of Lymphocytes by HISSF Derived from T3+ and T3− Lymphocyte Cultures[a]

Source of HISSF	% Cytotoxicity[b] (K562)	% Suppression[c]
Mock HISSF (T3+ cells)[d]	52.5	
HISSF (T3+ cells)[e]	30.3	42.2
Mock HISSF (T3− cells)[f]	54.7	
HISSF (T3− cells)[g]	50.6	7.4

[a]1 × 10^6 allogeneic PBLs were incubated for 40 hr with either mock HISSF or HISSF (20% v/v) prepared from T3+ or T3− lymphocytes separated by panning technique, washed, and tested for their cytotoxicity against K562 target cells.
[b]Percent cytotoxicity was calculated at a 50:1 effector to target cell ratio.
[c]Percent suppression was calculated on the basis of cytotoxicity observed with lymphocytes treated with mock HISSF.
[d]Supernates prepared from T3+ lymphocytes cultured without added histamine.
[e]Supernates prepared from T3− lymphocytes precultured with 10^{-3} M histamine.
[f]Supernates prepared from T3− lymphocytes cultured for 24 hr without added histamine.
[g]Supernates prepared from T3− lymphocytes, precultured with 10^{-3} M histamine for 24 hr. All culture supernatants were dialysed, sterilized, and used.

cell ratios and could be reversed by histamine. Unlike the observations of Hellstrand and Hermodsson (26,29) above, this effect was not dependent upon the presence or absence of monocytes, and was specifically due to inhibition of target binding by effector lymphocytes. While we did not observe any decrease in cytotoxicity when a wide range of histamine was added to NK cultures, Hall and coworkers (39) found that high doses (~ 10^{-4} M) of histamine as well as specific histamine type I and type II histamine receptor agonists could induce a slight inhibition of NK-cell cytotoxicity. We further noted that preculture of lymphocytes for 24 hr with histamine caused a significant decrease in their NK and ADCC activities with a concomitant increase in the proportion of CD8+ cells. Coculture experiments revealed that this immunoregulatory activity was due to the activation of suppressor cells capable of inhibiting cytotoxic activities.

Subsequently, we reported that histamine-activated suppressor cells produced a soluble factor which alone inhibited NK and ADCC activities (40). This histamine-induced soluble suppressor factor (HISSF) is produced by T lymphocytes and is equally effective against autologous and allogeneic NK effector cells (Table 1). We have also prepared a monoclonal antibody (IgM) against HISSF which is capable of abrogating its suppressive activities (Fig. 1). Production of this factor could be blocked by the histamine type II antagonist, cimetidine, but

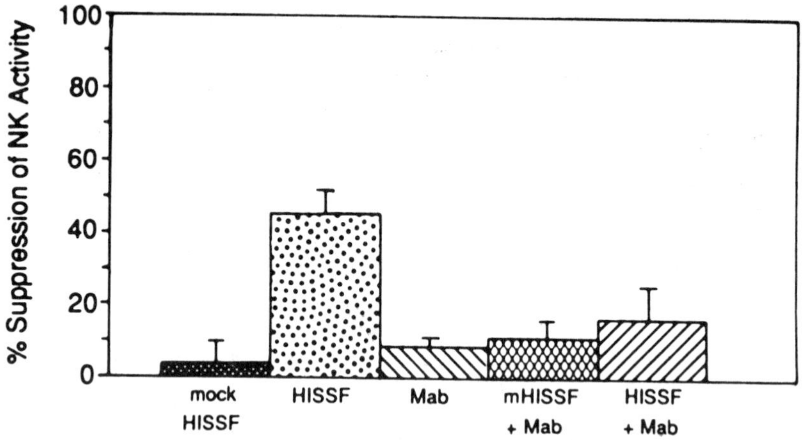

Figure 1 Lymphocytes (1×10^6) were cultured for 48 hr in media alone or containing 20% mock HISSF or 20% HISSF with and without added monoclonal antibody (Mab) prepared against HISSF. NK activity was determined in a 4 hr ^{51}Cr-release assay using K562 target cells at an effector to target ratio of 50:1. While HISSF produced significant suppression of NK activity, this effect could be reversed by adding Mab.

not by clemastine fumarate, a type I blocker. Of particular interest was the ability of the biologic modifier substances, interleukin-2 and interferon-α, to completely reverse the inhibition of cytotoxicity mediated by HISSF. Purified HISSF may have immunopharmacologic potential in the management of certain diseases associated with suppressor cell dysfunctions. Conversely, the capacity of biological response modifiers to reverse HISSF-induced inhibition may be of therapeutic benefit in certain diseases associated with increased circulating histamine. Whether HISSF is identical to the histamine-induced suppressor factor, HSF, described by Rocklin and colleagues (41) remains to be determined; our recently developed monoclonal antibody to HISSF will be useful in the comparison of HSF and HISSF.

V. CLINICAL SIGNIFICANCE

Recognition of the role of the histamine type II receptor in the activation of suppressor T cells formed the basis for the therapeutic use of the type II antagonist, cimetidine, in the treatment of various disorders manifesting secondary immunosuppression. Several conditions associated with increased number or activity of suppressor cells have been found to be responsive to histamine type

II antagonist treatment, including malignant, immunodeficiency, and autoimmune diseases. As previously noted, cellular cytotoxic activities are important host defense mechanisms against neoplasms. Using a tumor-bearing mouse model, Gifford et al. showed that treatment with cimetidine prolongs expression of active tumor immunity (42). Concomitant in vitro experiments demonstrated that this effect was probably due to inhibition of tumor-associated suppressor cells which down regulate cell-mediated cytotoxicity.

Although histamine may indirectly decrease the host's immune responses to malignancies by increasing suppressor-cell activities, histamine may also have a direct inhibitory effect on tumor cells. In a tumor-bearing mouse model, Burtin et al. (43) noted an inverse correlation between tumor incidence and tissue histamine levels. As tissue histamine seems to be a function of the presence of mast cells, tumor incidence and metastasis were also inversely correlated with tissue mast cell numbers.

A major adverse side effect of most treatment regimens for cancer is immunosuppression. Ironically, several different malignancies also seem to induce secondary immunodeficiency via activation of the host's endogenous suppressor monocytes/macrophages and lymphocytes. Regarding the former, prostaglandins have been identified as their probable mediators of immunosuppression. This has led to the use of prostaglandin synthetase inhibitors (e.g., indomethacin) in several clinical conditions. Histamine type II receptor blockers have also found their way into the therapeutic armamentorium against cancer. Allen and coworkers (44) observed that patients with B-cell chronic lymphocytic leukemia showed depressed to absent NK activity in their peripheral blood. When these patients were treated with an oral regimen of 1.2 gm of cimetidine daily for 3 weeks, their NK activities increased significantly. Interestingly, the NK activity of PBLs from normal donors decreased after 2 weeks of cimetidine administration, but returned to pretreatment levels by the third week. Malignant melanoma patients treated with a combination of recombinant human interferon-α and cimetidine showed evidence of tumor regression presumably in part through inhibition of suppressor cell activity (45). Subsequent in vitro studies demonstrated that cimetidine could stimulate the NK and ADCC activities of peripheral lymphocytes from melanoma patients and some patients with metastatic colorectal cancer (46). Moreover, cimetidine could augment interferon-induced enhancement of both NK- and K-cell cytotoxicities, suggesting that cimetidine and interferon activate a different mechanism. These observations support the therapeutic application of a combination of potential immunomodulators in the treatment of various malignancies associated with immunodepression.

Activity of the NK cell was found to be diminished in patients with severe atopic eczema (47). In view of the several observations above, it is not unreasonable to presume that this might be secondary to increased circulating histamine levels. However NK-cell activity from these patients was still sensitive to further inhibition by histamine and the depressed NK activity was associated with reduced numbers of circulating NK cells. While no specific pathogenic mechanism for this effect was elucidated, perhaps increased circulating histamine levels prevented recruitment of active NK cells from precursors.

Suppressor cells have been considered as one mechanism for the induction and maintenance of immunologic tolerance, consequently preventing autoimmune reactions. Indeed it has been demonstrated that suppressor-cell activity is depressed in patients with various autoimmune disorders such as systemic lupus erythematosus and juvenile rheumatoid arthritis (48-51). Chronic active hepatitis is a condition whose pathogenesis may be due to autoimmune mechanisms. Patients with chronic active hepatitis were studied for the presence of circulating suppressor/cytotoxic T cells with membrane receptors for histamine (52). In comparison to normal volunteers and control subjects with metabolic or vascular liver disease, chronic active hepatitis patients had fewer circulating histamine receptor-bearing suppressor/cytotoxic T cells. Those patients who were hepatitis B surface antigen negative had even lower numbers of histamine receptor-bearing suppressor/cytotoxic T cells than patients who were hepatitis B surface antigen positive. Moreover, there was an inverse correlation between serum immunoglobulin levels and numbers of histamine receptor-positive cells. Thus, with a decrease in suppressor cells, increased immunoglobulin synthesis could occur.

Studies of patients with systemic sclerosis also demonstrated decreased cytotoxic functions of peripheral blood monocytes (52). Suppressed monocyte ADCC correlated inversely with cellular cAMP levels. Treatment of patients' cells with histamine stimulated cAMP production comparable to normals; however, in these studies ADCC activity was not determined after histamine treatment.

Multiple sclerosis (MS) is another critical condition in which cellular cytotoxic activities may be modulated by histamine. Merrill and Mohlstrom (54) developed a model system wherein primary cultures of oligodendrocytes served as targets of ADCC effector cells from MS patients and controls. While MS patients' ADCC responses to oligodendrocyte targets were depressed compared to controls, addition of cimetidine significantly enhanced cytotoxicity. The authors suggested that endogenous histamine production and type II receptor binding could be responsible for the suppressive effect. In such a situation, histamine may be serving to protect the host against progression of an autoimmune process.

VI. CONCLUSIONS

It has been our intention to document the very wide spectrum of immunoregulatory activities mediated by histamine, with particular emphasis on cellular cytotoxic functions. Like other biologic systems, histamine can mediate differential reactions which can even be mutually antagonistic. Overall, however, histamine appears to manifest a wide spectrum of activities that down regulate various immune functions either directly or through the activation of suppressor cells. The availability of numerous histamine receptor antagonists provides us with the potential for unique new therapies directed at a range of disorders associated with immunologic dysfunction. Chemical derivatives of histamine itself, devoid of adverse effects but possessing immunoregulatory activities, may eventually be developed and find ready pharmacologic application. We have progressed significantly from the time, not so long ago, when histamine was soley recognized as a noxious component of allergic reactions to the present recognition of its important role in the complex immunologic network.

REFERENCES

1. Ritz, J., R. E. Schmidt, J. Michon, T. Hercend, and S. F. Schlossman, Characterization of functional surface structures on human natural killer cells, Adv. Immunol. 42:181–211 (1988).
2. Rosenthal, K. L., T. Ishizaka, D. Befus, G. Dennert, H. Hengartner, and J. Bienenstock, Expression of IgE receptors and histamine in cloned natural killer cell lines, J. Immunol. 133:642–646 (1984).
3. Okuno, T., Y. Takagaki, D. H. Pluznik, and J. Djeu, Natural cytotoxic (NC) cell activity in basophilic cells: Release of NC-specific cytotoxic factor by IgE receptor triggering, J. Immunol. 136:4652–6568 (1986).
4. Galli, S. J., A. M. Dvorak, T. Ishizaka, G. Nabel, H. Der Simonian, H. Cantor, and H. F. Dvorak, A cloned cell with NK function resembles basophils by ultrastructure and expresses IgE receptors, Nature 298:288–290 (1982).
5. Schayer, R. W., Induced synthesis of histamine, microcirculatory regulation and the mechanism of action of the adrenal glucocorticoid hormones, Prog. Allergy 7:187–212 (1963).
6. Schwartz, A., P. W. Askenase, and R. K. Gershon, Histamine inhibition of the in vitro induction of cytotoxic T-cell responses, Immunopharmacology 2:179–190 (1980).
7. Plaut, M., L. Lichtenstein, E. Gillespie and C. S. Henney, Studies on the mechanism of lymphocyte mediated cytolysis. IV. Specificity of the histamine receptor on effector T cells. J. Immunol. 111:389–394 (1973).
8. Beer, D. J., and R. E. Rocklin, Histamine modulation of lymphocyte biology: Membrane receptors, signal transduction and functions, CRC Crit. Rev. Immunol. 7:55–91 (1987).
9. Rocklin, R. E., Modulation of cellular immune responses in vivo and in vitro by histamine receptor-bearing lymphocytes, J. Clin. Invest. 57:1051–1058 (1976).
10. Sansoni, P., E. D. Silverman, M. M. Khan, M. L. Melmon, and E. G. Engleman, Immunoregulatory T cells in man. Histamine induced suppressor T cells are derived from a Leu 2^+ ($T8^+$) subpopulation distinct from that which gives rise to cytotoxic T cells. J. Clin. Invest. 75:650–656 (1985).

11. Rocklin, R. E., Histamine-induced suppressor factor (HSF): Effect on migration inhibitory factor (MIF) production and proliferation, J. Immunol. 118:1734–1738 (1977).
12. Cudkowicz, G., and P. S. Hochman, Do natural killer cells engage in regulated reactions against self to ensure homeostasis? Immunol. Rev. 44:13–41 (1979).
13. Kumagai, K., R. Suzuki, S. Suzuki, and S. Arai, Immunoregulatory effects of NK cells. In Mechanisms of Cytotoxicity by NK Cells (Herberman, R. B., and Callewaert, D. M., Eds.), Academic Press, Orlando, Florida (1985), pp. 489–498.
14. Robles, C. P., P. Pereira, P. Wortley, and S. B. Pollack, Regulation of the B cell response by NK cells. In Mechanisms of Cytotoxicity by NK Cells (Herberman, R. B., and Callewaert, D. H., Eds.), Academic Press, Orlando, Florida (1985), pp. 499–506.
15. Targan, S., J. Brieva, W. Newman, and R. Stevens, Is the NK lytic process involved in the mechanism of NK suppression of antibody producing cells, J. Immunol. 134:666–669 (1985).
16. Shou, L., S. A. Schwartz, and R. A. Good, Suppressor cell activity after concanavalin A treatment of lymphocytes from normal donors, J. Exp. Med. 143:1100–1110 (1976).
17. Nair, M. P. N., and S. A. Schwartz, Suppression of natural killer activity and antibody-dependent cellular cytotoxicity by cultured human lymphocytes, J. Immunol. 126:2221–2229 (1981).
18. Shou, L., S. A. Schwartz, R. A. Good, R. Peng, and C. L. Chen, A human soluble suppressor factor affecting lymphocyte responses in vitro, Proc. Natl. Acad. Sci. U.S.A. 77:6096–6100 (1980).
19. Nair, M. P. N., and S. A. Schwartz, Suppression of human natural and antibody-dependent cytotoxicity by soluble factors from unstimulated normal lymphocytes, J. Immunol. 129:2511–2518 (1982).
20. Nair, M. P. N., and S. A. Schwartz, Immunomodulatory effects of amphotericin-B on cellular cytotoxicity of normal human lymphocytes, Cell. Immunol. 70:287–300 (1982).
21. Nair, M. P.N., and S. A. Schwartz, Immunomodulatory effects of corticosteroids on natural killer and antibody-dependent cellular cytotoxic activities of human lymphocytes, J. Immunol. 132:2876–2882 (1984).
22. Lang, I., K. Torok, P. Gergely, K. Nekam, and G. Y. Petranyi, Effect of histamine receptor blocking on human antibody-dependent cell-mediated cytotoxicity, Scand. J. Immunol. 13:361–366 (1981).
23. Lang, I., P. Gergely, and G. Y. Petranyi, Effect of histamine-receptor blocking on human spontaneous lymphocytes mediated cytotoxicity, Scand. J. Immunol. 14:573–576 (1981).
24. Ruiz-Arguelles, A., K. B. Seroogy, and R. E. Ritis, Jr., In vitro effect of cimetidine on human cell-mediated cytotoxicity. I. Inhibition of natural killer cell activity, Cell Immunol. 69:1–12 (1982).
25. Nair, M. P. N., and S. A. Schwartz, Effect of histamine and histamine antagonists on natural and antibody-dependent cellular cytotoxicity of human lymphocytes in vitro, Cell. Immunol. 81:45–60 (1983).

26. Hellstrand, K., and S. Hermodsson, Histamine H2-receptor-mediated regulation of human natural killer cell activity, J. Immunol. 137:656–660 (1986).
27. Yang, I., and D. Zucker-Franklin, Modulation of natural killer (NK) cells by autologous neutrophils and monocytes, Cell. Immunol. 86:171–182 (1984).
28. Hellstrand, K., and S. Hermodsson, Differential effects of histamine receptor antagonists on human natural killer cell activity, Int. Arch. Allergy Appl. Immunol. 84:247–255 (1987).
29. Hellstrand, K., and S. Hermodsson, Role of serotonin in the regulation of human natural killer cell cytotoxicity, J. Immunol. 139:869–875 (1987).
30. Plaut, M., G. Marone, and E. Gillespie, The role of cyclic AMP in modulating cytotoxic lymphocytes. II. Sequential changes during culture in responsiveness of cytotoxic lymphocytes to cyclic AMP-active agents. J. Immunol. 131:2945–2952 (1983).
31. Schreurs, J., M. O. Dailey, and H. Schulman, Pharmacological characterization of histamine H2 receptors on clonal cytolytic T lymphocytes. Evidence for histamine-induced desensitization, Biochem. Pharmacol. 33:3375–3382 (1984).
32. Dailey, M. O., J. Schreurs, and H. Schulman, Hormone receptors on cloned T lymphocytes. Increased responsiveness to histamine, prostaglandins, and beta-adrenergic agents as a late stage event in T cell activation, J. Immunol. 140:2931–2936 (1988).
33. Zhang, Y. H., N. K. Mak, K. N. Leung, and N. H. Hunt, Modulation of T cells by cyclic AMP in murine influenza virus infection. I. In vitro inhibition of cytotoxic T lymphocytes by exogenous cyclic AMP analogues and by agents which increase intracellular cyclic AMP concentrations, Immunopharmacology 13:37–45 (1987).
34. Berman, J. S., W. W. Cruikshank, D. M. Center, A. C. Theodore, and D. J. Beer, Chemoattractant lymphokines specific for the helper/inducer T-lymphocyte subset, Cell. Immunol. 95:105–112 (1985).
35. Droge, W., H. Schmidt, S. Nick, and B. Sonsky, Histamine augments interleukin-2 production and the activation of cytotoxic T lymphocytes, Immunopharmacology 11:1–6 (1986).
36. Khan, M. M., K. L. Melmon, G. C. Fathman, B. Hertel-Wulff, and S. Strober, The effects of autocoids on cloned murine lymphoid cells: Modulation of IL2 secretion and the activity of natural suppressor cells, J. Immunol. 134: 4100–4106 (1985).
37. Khan, M. M., D. Marr-Leisy, M. S. Verlander, M. R. Bristow, S. Strober, M. Goodman, and K. L. Melmon, The effects of derivatives of histamine on natural suppressor cells, J. Immunol. 137:308–314 (1986).
38. French, S., M. Walker, B. Susskind, and R. Faanes, Modulation of in vitro cellular immune responses by histamine agonists or antagonists in murine species, Arzneimittelforschung 35:390–394 (1985).
39. Hall, T. J., S. H. Chen, J. Brostoff, and P. M. Lydyard, Modulation of human natural killer cell activity by pharmacological mediators, Clin. Exp. Immunol. 54:493–500 (1983).

40. Nair, M. P. N., J. M. Cilik, and S. A. Schwartz, Histamine-induced suppressor factor inhibition of NK cells: Reversal with interferon and interleukin 2, J. Immunol. 136:2456–2462 (1986).
41. Rocklin, R. E., A. Blidy, and M. Kamal, Physicochemical characterization of human histamine-induced suppressor factor, Cell. Immunol. 76:243–252 (1983).
42. Gifford, R. R. M., B. V. Voss, J. R. Schmidtke, and R. M. Ferguson, Histamine type-2 receptor antagonist immune modulation. I. Increased cell-mediated cytotoxicity in normal and in down-regulated systems, Surgery 103:184–192 (1988).
43. Burtin, C., C. Ponvert, A. Fray, P. Scheinmann, G. Lespinats, B. Loridon, P. Canu, and J. Paupe, Inverse correlation between tumor incidence and tissue histamine levels in W/WV, WV/+, and +/+ mice, J. Natl. Cancer Inst. 74:671–674 (1985).
44. Allen, J. I., H. J. Spyropoulos, B. Grant, J. C. Eagon, and N. E. Kay, Cimetidine modulates natural killer cell function of patients with chronic lymphocytic leukemia, J. Lab. Clin. Med. 109:396–401 (1987).
45. Flodgren, P., S. Borgstrom, P. E. Jonsson, C. Lindstrom, and H. O. Sjogren, Metastatic malignant melanoma: Regression induced by combined treatment with interferon HuIFN-x (Le) and cimetidine, Int. J. Cancer 32: 657–665 (1983).
46. Flodgren, P., and H. O. Sjogren, Influence in vitro on NK and K cell activities with and without simultaneous exposure to interferon, Cancer Immunol. Immunopathol. 19:28–34 (1985).
47. Hall, T. J., R. Rycraft, and J. Brostoff, Decreased natural killer cell activity in atopic eczema, Immunology 56:337–344 (1985).
48. Sagawa, A., and N. I. Abdou, Suppressor cell dysfunction in systemic lupus erythematosus, cells involved and in vitro correction, J. Clin. Invest. 62:789-796 (1978).
49. Sakane, T., A. D. Steinberg, and I. Green, Studies of immune functions of patients with systemic lupus erythematosus. I. Dysfunction of suppressor T-cell activity related to impaired generation of rather than response to, suppressor cells, Arthritis Rheum. 21:657–664 (1978).
50. Kaufman, D. B., and E. Bostwick, Defective suppressor T-cell activity in systemic lupus erythematosus. Clin. Immunol. Immunopathol. 13:9–18 (1979).
51. Strelkauskas, A. J., R. T. Callery, J. McDowell, Y. Borel, and S. F. Schlossman, Direct evidence for loss of human suppressor cells during active autoimmune disease, Proc. Natl. Acad. Sci. U.S.A. 75:5150–5154 (1978).
52. Colombo, M., M. G. Rumi, L. Roffi, and E. Del-Ninno, Decrease in suppressor/cytotoxic T-cells with histamine receptors in patients with chronic active hepatitis, Liver 4:201–207 (1984).
53. Herlin, T., J. Eggert, K. Kragballe, and H. Zachariae, Abnormal monocyte cytotoxicity and cyclic-AMP levels in systemic sclerosis, Arch. Dermatol. Res. 276:279–282 (1984).

54. Merrill, J. E., and C. Mohlstrom, Regulation of antibody-dependent cellular cytotoxicity in multiple sclerosis by central nervous system hormones, Int. Arch. Allergy Appl. Immunol. 82:195–201 (1987).

5

Histamine-Induced Human Lymphocyte Chemoattractant Lymphokines: Mechanisms for the Amplification of Cell-Mediated Immune Responses

DENNIS J. BEER, WILLIAM W. CRUIKSHANK, JEFFREY S. BERMAN, JOHN BERNARDO, ARTHUR C. THEODORE, and DAVID M. CENTER
Boston University School of Medicine, Boston, Massachusetts

I. INTRODUCTION

Delayed-type or cellular hypersensitivity responses initiated by activated lymphocytes are characterized by a mononuclear cell infiltrate consisting of macrophages and lymphocytes, the majority of which are not specifically sensitized for the antigen eliciting the reaction (1). The cellular content of this form of immune response is dependent upon increased vascular permeability permitting the egress of circulating cells, the elaboration of cell type-specific chemoattractant factors, and local cellular activation and proliferation.

Because basophils and mast cells have been noted in delayed-type hypersensitivity tissue reactions (2-6), and because histamine, the major vasoactive amine contained within human metachromatic cells, can be released into the microenvironment during these inflammatory responses via immunoglobulin E (IgE)-independent mechanisms (2,3,7-10), our laboratory has been investigating in vitro histamine modulation of human lymphocyte accumulation. Histamine directly may augment the development of lymphocyte infiltration by causing gaps between endothelial cells of the postcapillary venule and allowing circulating lymphocytes to migrate into extravascular tissue spaces. Beyond this, our laboratory has foucsed on histamine-induced human lymphokines which function as chemoattractants and activators of resting human T cells. This chapter will detail the identification, physicochemical characterization and basic biology of these histamine-induced lymphokines, and put our observations into the context of an amplification schema for T cell–dependent immune responses.

II. IDENTIFICATION AND PHYSICOCHEMICAL CHARACTERIZATION

Several studies (11–13) have identified and characterized three histamine-induced human lymphokines which influence nonactivated lymphocyte migration (Table 1). Utilizing a modified Boyden chamber assay to assess lymphocyte migration, Center et al. (11) identified chemoattractant activity for rat splenic and human blood T lymphocytes from histamine-conditioned human mononuclear cell supernatants. Neutrophil or monocyte chemoattractant activity was not detected in these supernatants, nor was histamine itself chemoattractant for T lymphocytes. Production of T-cell chemoattractant activity was seen over a histamine concentration range between 10^{-7} and 10^{-4} M, with peak activity induced at 10^{-4} M histamine (12). A histamine time-course experiment revealed induction of T-cell chemoattractant activity within 4 hr of mononuclear cell culture (12). The histamine dose response and time course for production of lymphocyte chemoattractant activity is similar to that reported by Rocklin and Haberek-Davidson (14) for the production of the other well-described histamine-induced lymphokine, histamine-induced suppressor factor (HSF).

As illustrated in Figure 1, Sephadex G-100 molecular sieve chromatography of histamine-conditioned mononuclear cell supernatants demonstrated that the lymphotactic activity was eluted at a region between bovine serum albumin and ovalbumin corresponding to an apparent molecular weight of 56,000 (11,12). Analysis of molecular size by sodum dodecyl sulfate-polyacrylamide gel electrophoresis (SDS-PAGE) revealed that the 56,000 molecular weight lymphocyte chemoattractant factor (LCF) was a tetramer of a 14,000 molecular weight species (15,16). This lymphocyte chemoattractant was a cationic molecule as determined by its elution pattern from a Sephadex QAE anion exchange matrix with a single isoelectric point of 9.1 (11). The biologic activity of LCF was stable to heating at 56°C for 30 min, but sensitive to the effects of neuraminidase and trypsin (see Table 1) (11).

Further characterization of the chemoattractant activity of this lymphokine by checkerboard analysis (17) showed it to be predominantly chemokinetic and not chemotactic in nature (11). That is to say, it enhanced the random (nondirected) migration of T cells, and its effects were independent of any concentration gradient across the target cell surface. As will be discussed below,

Table 1 Physicochemical and Functional Characteristics of Histamine-Induced Lymphocyte Chemoattractant Lymphokines

Lymphokine	Cell of origin	Physicochemical characteristics	Biologic activities
Lymphocyte chemoattractant factor (LCF)	H_2 receptor–bearing CD8 (suppressor/cytotoxic) T cells	MW 56,000 (tetramer of 14,000); cationic sialoprotein with a pI of 9.1	Selective chemokinetic activity for CD4 cells; Selective induction of IL-2 receptors and HLA-DR on CD4 cells
Lymphocyte migration inhibitory factor 35K ($LyMIF_{35K}$)	H_1 receptor-bearing CD4 (helper/inducer) T cells	MW 30–40,000; cationic sialoprotein with a pI of 8.5	Noncytotoxic inhibitor of CD4 lymphocyte migration
Lymphocyte migration inhibitory factor 75K ($LyMIF_{75K}$)	H_1 receptor–bearing CD4 (helper/inducer) T cells	MW 70-80,000; cationic protein with a pI of 7.5	Noncytotoxic inhibitor of T-lymphocyte migration

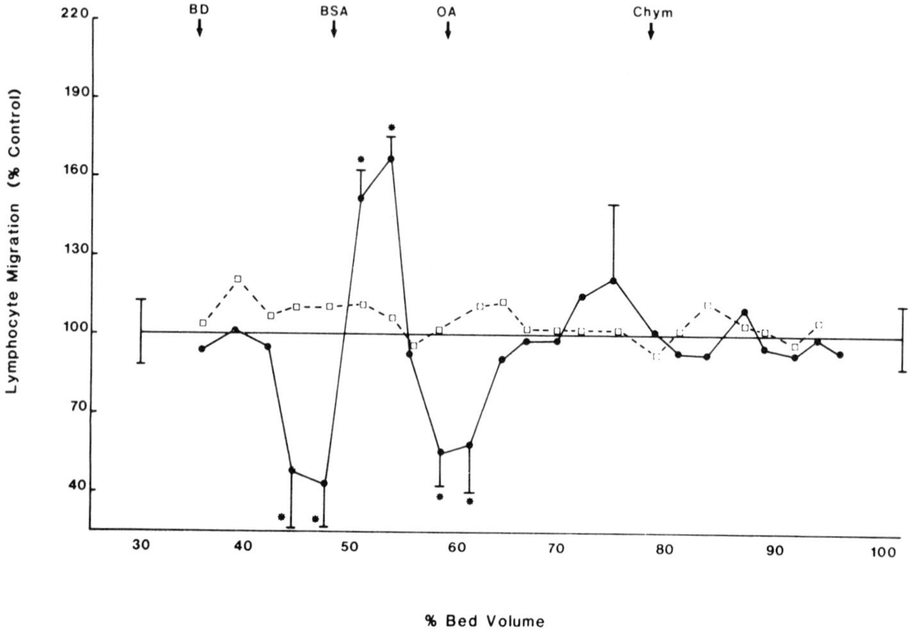

Figure 1 Representative Sephadex G-100 chromatogram of a mononuclear cell supernatant generated in the presence (●– – –●) or absence (□– – –□) of histamine (10^{-4} M). T-lymphocyte migration is expressed on the ordinate as percent of buffer control migration (designated 100%). *denotes migration that was different from control ($p < 0.01$).

from a biologic perspective, the chemokinetic activity of this factor, though capable of attracting T cells to an inflammatory site, is not alone capable of immobilizing cells at an inflammatory focus.

The physicochemical characterization of LCF separates it from HSF which has been characterized as two species of acidic glycoproteins with molecular weights between 25,000 and 40,000 (18). In addition, partially purified LCF (molecular sieve and anion exchange chromatography) did not possess suppressor activity as assessed by inhibition of mitogen-induced lymphocyte proliferation (11).

In the course of purifying LCF from histamine-stimulated human mononuclear cells, Sephadex G-100 molecular sieve chromatography also demonstrated the presence of two simultaneously generated noncytotoxic inhibitors of T-lymphocyte migration (see Fig. 1) (11,12). These two lymphocyte migration-inhibitory factors (LyMIFs) were distinct from LCF and were cationic

Table 2 LYMIF$_{35K}$ Inhibition of LCF-Stimulated Migration

Test sample		T lymphocyte migration[a]
LyMIF$_{35K}$	10 μl	72 ± 3.9[b]
	50 μl	43 ± 4.2[b]
	100 μl	36 ± 2.0[b]
LyMIF$_{35K}$	10 μl + LCF 100 μl	55 ± 3.0[a,b]
	50 μl + LCF 100 μl	42 ± 4.6[a,b]
	100 μl + LCF 100 μl	29 ± 3.1[a,b]
	LCF 100 μl alone	165 ± 6.6[b]

[a]Data expressed as a percentage ± SEM of control migration.
[b]Different from control, $p < 0.05$
[c]Different from the effect of LCF alone, $p < 0.05$.

proteins with apparent molecular weights of 70,000–80,000 (LyMIF$_{75K}$) and 30,000–40,000 (LyMIF$_{35K}$) (12). LyMIF$_{35K}$ was characterized as a glycoprotein with an isoelectric point of 8.5, whose biologic activity was restricted to T cells, and was susceptible to neuraminidase treatment and heat inactivation, but was not destroyed by trypsin (12). Trypsin treatment of the parent LyMIF$_{35K}$ protein resulted in a 22,000- to 25,000-dalton protein which retained T-cell migration inhibitory activity (19). LyMIF$_{75K}$ had an isoelectric point of 7.5, and its biologic activity was susceptible to degradation by trypsin, but was not sensitive to neuraminidase treatment or heating (see Table 1) (12). These physicochemical characteristics suggested that these histamine-induced lymphokines were distinct from one another and different from previously described migration-inhibitory factors for other leukocyte types. Similar to LCF, these lymphocyte migration inhibitory lymphokines did not possess suppressor activity (12).

In addition to demonstrating LyMIF$_{35K}$ inhibition of random T cell migration, McFadden et al. (19) documented the effect of LyMIF$_{35K}$ on stimulated migration. As shown in Table 2, a partially purified preparation of LCF enhanced lymphocyte migration to 165% of control. In a similar manner to the inhibition of random motion, three concentrations of LyMIF$_{35K}$ inhibited the LCF-induced migratory responses in a dose-dependent fashion. This suggested that the mechanism of action of LyMIF$_{35K}$ was independent of the stimulatory process.

The mechanism of LyMIF$_{35K}$ inhibition of lymphocyte migration may be related to its ability to alter the adhesiveness of lymphocytes. McFadden et al. (19) adapted a nylon wool column assay (20) and demonstrated that LyMIF$_{35K}$ increased the adherence of a preselected relatively nonadherent T lymphocyte population in direct proportion to its inhibitory effect on cell migration (Fig. 2).

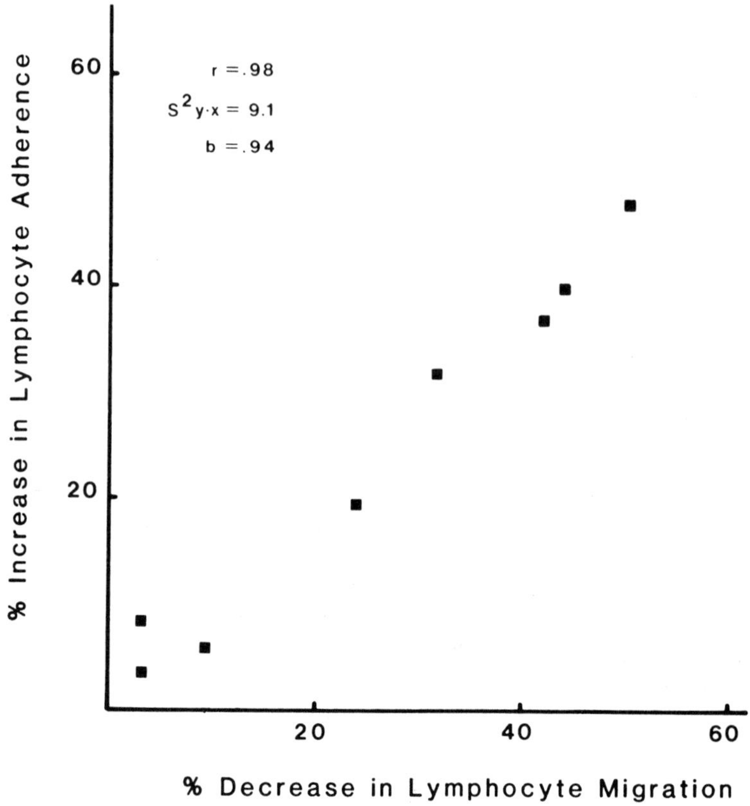

Figure 2 The effect of various preparations of $LyMIF_{35K}$ on T-lymphocyte adherence. The percentage decrease in lymphocyte migration of each $LyMIF_{35K}$ sample is compared to the percentage increase of lymphocytes that adhered to nylon wool columns. Samples of $LyMIF_{35K}$ in the lower left of the graph were formerly active in their capacity to inhibit migration, but had lost this activity after prolonged storage or heat treatment.

The finding of simultaneous generation of T cell–specific chemokinetic and immobilizing lymphokines is consistent with the pattern and proposed mechanism of accumulation of other leukocyte types at sites of activated lymphocytes (21). Thus, monocytes (22) and polymorphonuclear leukocytes (23) are attracted by chemoattractant lymphokines and then immobilized by MIF (24) and LIF (25), respectively. The stimulation of lymphocyte migration with low concentrations of LCF and inhibition of lymphocyte migration with higher concentration of LyMIFs is consistent with the postulated mechanism in vivo where distant cells must necessarily first sense low levels of lymphokines. When these cells migrate closer to sites of lymphocyte activation, thereby experiencing higher concentrations of lymphokines, immobilization of these leukocytes could occur.

III. CELL OF ORIGIN

Although T lymphocytes constitute a heterogeneous population of cells, numerous observations (26-28) have demonstrated a linkage between T-cell phenotype, as defined by the presence of certain membrane macromolecules, and T-cell function, as defined by in vitro assay systems. The results of studies (11-13, 16) defining the T cell of origin of the histamine-induced lymphocyte chemoattractant lymphokines further support the association between lymphocyte phenotype and lymphocyte function.

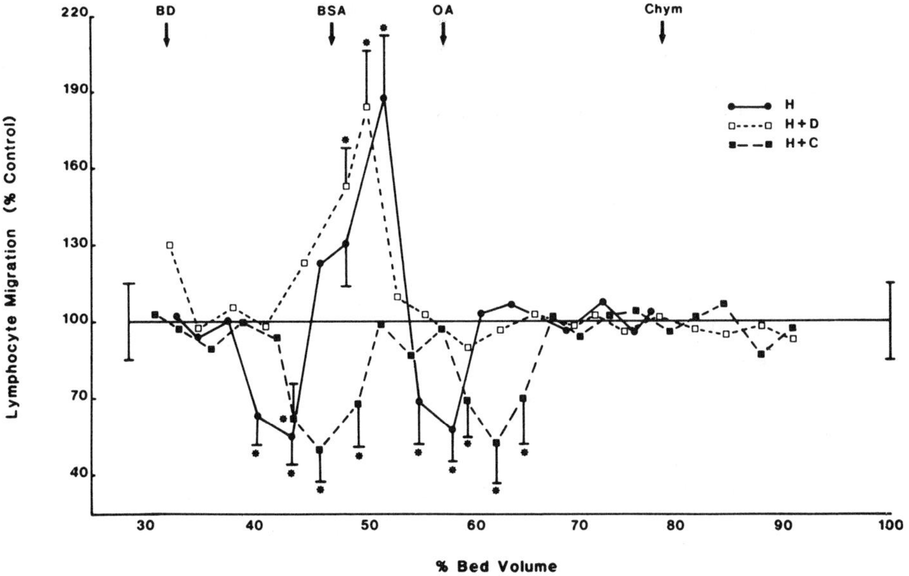

Figure 3 Representative Sephadex G-100 chromotograms of mononuclear cell supernatants generated in the presence of histamine (10^{-4} M) (●——●), histamine plus cimetidine (10^{-6} M) (■ – – – ■), or histamine plus diphenhydramine (10^{-5} M) (□ – – – □). T-lymphocyte migration is expressed on the ordinate as percent of buffer control migration (designated 100%). *Denotes migration that was different from control ($p < 0.01$).

Table 3 Representation of the Migratory Responses of T-Lymphocytes to Partially Purified Histamine and Con A–Induced Supernatants from Human Lymphocytes Fractionated on Histamine Affinity Matrices

	Lymphokine activities		
Stimulant	LCF_{56K}[a]	$LyMIF_{35K}$[a]	$LyMIF_{75K}$[a]
Unfractionated			
histamine (10^{-4} M)	+	+	+
Con A (10 μg/ml)[b]	+	+	+
H-EACA-Sepharose[c]			
histamine	–	–	–
Con A[b]	–	–	–
EACA Sepharose[d]			
histamine	+	+	+
Con A[b]	+	+	+

[a]Data are expressed as presence (+) or absence (–) of expected lymphokine activities in chromatography fractions of appropriate molecular weights.
[b]Crude Con A–induced (but no histamine–induced) supernatants from unfractionated lymphocytes and from lymphocytes nonadherent to either a control or histamine affinity column all possessed significant monocyte chemoattractant activity.
[c]Histamine affinity matrix: histamine-epsilon-aminocaproic acid Sepharose.
[d]Control column: epsilon-aminocaproic acid Sepharose.

Fractionation via differential adherence properties of blood mononuclear cells demonstrated that LCF and LyMIF production was restricted to the nylon wool nonadherent T-lymphocyte population (11–13). As shown in Figure 3, Sephadex G-100 gel filtration of supernatants generated from mononuclear cells incubated with histamine plus cimetidine (a histamine type II [H_2] receptor antagonist) resulted in selective production of $LyMIF_{35K}$ and $LyMIF_{75K}$; no LCF was produced (11,12). In contrast, cells incubated with histamine and diphenhydramine (a histamine type I [H_1] receptor antagonist) produced LCF, whereas no $LyMIF_{35K}$ or $LyMIF_{75K}$ were detected (12). Cells incubated with either histamine antagonist alone did not generate LCF or LyMIF activity. Collectively, these data suggested that LCF was the product of histamine type II receptor–bearing T lymphocytes, and that both $LyMIF_{35K}$ and $LyMIF_{75K}$ were products of histamine type I receptor–bearing T lymphocytes (11,12) (see Table 1).

Previous studies (15,19,29) have described concanavalin A (Con A)-induced lymphocyte chemoattractant and migration inhibitory lymphokines which were physicochemically and functionally identical to those induced by histamine. A subsequent investigation (11) assessed the ability of a lymphocyte

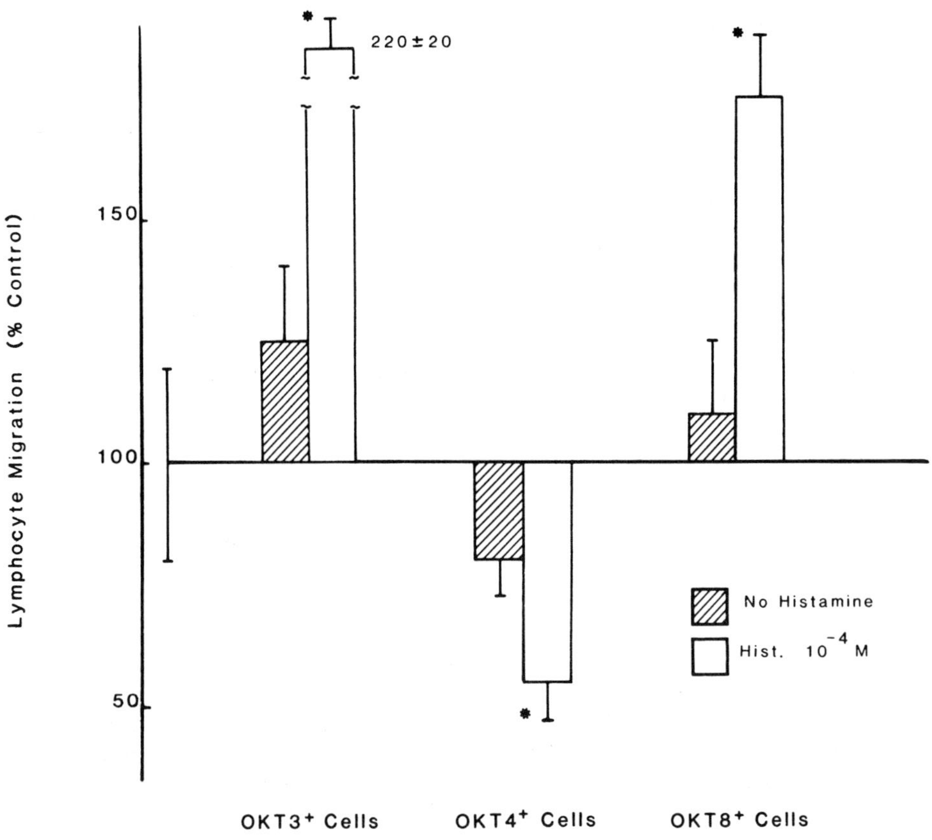

Figure 4 The effect of crude lymphocyte supernatants on T-lymphocyte migration. Human T cells or purified T-lymphocyte subsets were incubated either with or without histamine (10^{-4} M) for 24 hr. The harvested supernatants were then assayed for their ability to alter lymphocyte migration in a modified Boyden chamber assay. Lymphocyte migration is expressed on the ordinate as percent of buffer control migration (designated 100%). *Denotes migration that was different from control ($p < 0.01$).

population depleted of histamine receptor-bearing cells to generate these lymphokines in response to histamine or Con A. Cells nonadherent to a histamine affinity matrix (histamine-EACA-Sepharose) and stimulated with each ligand did not produce LCF or either of the LyMIFs, whereas supernatants generated in parallel from histamine or Con A stimulation of unfractionated or control column (EACA-Sepharose)-passed lymphocytes contained all three lymphokines

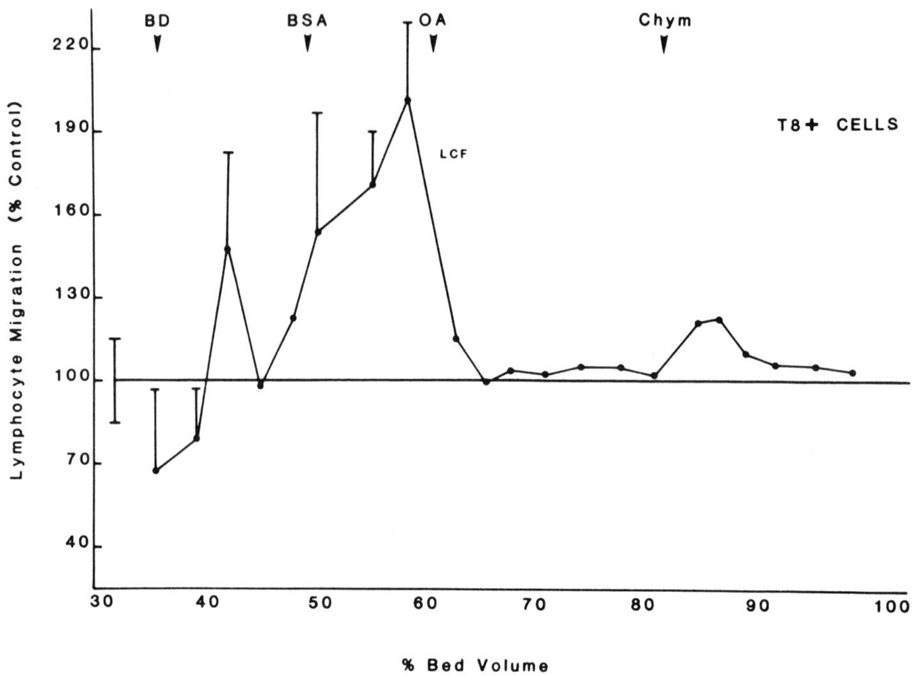

Figure 5 Representative Sephadex G-100 chromatogram of a CD8 lymphocyte supernatant generated in the presence of histamine (10^{-4} M). T-lymphocyte migration is expressed on the ordinate as percent of buffer control migration (designated 100%). *Denotes migration that was different from control ($P < 0.01$).

(Table 3). Interestingly, cells nonadherent to a histamine-affinity matrix produced significant monocyte chemoattractant activity following activation with Con A (but not histamine). These data, taken together with the histamine antagonist-blocking studies, suggested that all LCF production in response to either histamine or the polyclonal lymphocyte activator Con A can be attributed to histamine type II receptor-bearing lymphocytes, and that all LyMIF production, regardless of stimulus, can be attributed to histamine type I receptor-bearing lymphocytes. The cell of origin of these lymphokines appeared independent of the activating ligand (histamine or Con A). Data demonstrating that Con A induction of T-cell chemoattractants was not inhibitable by either cimetidine or diphenhydramine suggested that Con A did not stimulate cells to produce these lymphokines through direct activation of histamine receptors or through the release of histamine from contaminating basophils (12).

A subsequent study (13) further defined the human T cell of origin of these chemoattractant lymphokines (see Table 1). Nylon wood nonadherent human T-cell populations were enriched for CD4 (helper/inducer) and CD8 (suppressor/cytotoxic) lymphocyte subsets by negative selection and were then incubated with histamine. As shown in Figure 4, supernatants derived from histamine-stimulated unfractionated T cells and CD8 cells significantly enhanced T-lymphocyte migration, whereas supernatants derived from histamine stimulated CD4 cells significantly inhibited T-cell migration. When supernatant derived from CD8 lymphocytes was fractionated by molecular sieve chromatography, LCF activity was observed, but LyMIF activity was not (Fig. 5). Along these same lines, experiments performed by Van Epps and colleagues (30) demonstrated a mitogen-induced human T-cell chemoattractant with physicochemical characteristics similar to those of histamine-induced LCF whose production also was restricted to human CD8 lymphocytes. In regard to migration inhibitory activity, when supernatant derived from CD4 lymphocytes cells was similarly fractionated, both $LyMIF_{75K}$ and $LyMIF_{35K}$ were noted, but LCF was absent (Fig. 6). In conjunction with the histamine receptor data presented above, it appeared that LCF production was limited to histamine type II receptor-bearing lymphocytes of the CD8 phenotype and that $LyMIF_{75K}$ and $LyMIF_{35K}$ production was limited to histamine type I receptor-bearing lymphocytes of the CD4 phenotype (see Table 1).

As discussed elsewhere in this book, histamine can induce T cells to elaborate a suppressor factor (HSF) capable of inhibiting lymphocyte proliferative responses to mitogens (14,31) or alloantigens (32) and the production of lymphokines (33). As is the case with human T cells elaborating LCF, histamine-induced human suppressor cells have been shown to be included in the histamine type II receptor-bearing CD8 subset of T cells (32,34). The question that arises is whether these two distinct lymphokines were derived from the same cell. Recent observations suggested that HSF and LCF are derived from two distinct cell populations contained within the histamine type II receptor-bearing CD8 lymphocyte subset. Work from several laboratories (35,36) has demonstrated that lymphocytes from atopic individuals compared to those from normal subjects generated less suppressor activity upon stimulation with histamine. In a preliminary study, Hollingsworth et al. (37) analyzed the generation of histamine-induced suppressor and lymphocyte chemoattractant activities in normal and atopic subjects. Histamine-induced suppressor activity was reduced in atopics compared to that in normal controls, whereas lymphocyte chemoattractant activity was equivalent between the two groups. These data suggested that HSF and LCF were elaborated by two different histamine type II receptor-bearing CD8 cell types or, alternatively, the same cell could produce both lymphokines and the defect in atopics represents an abnormality of specific protein

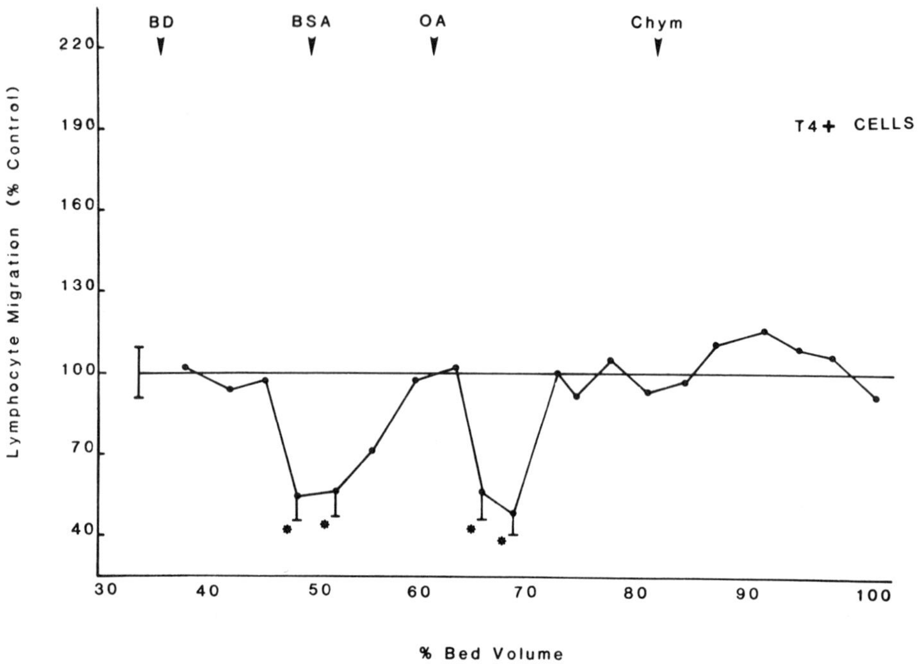

Figure 6 Representative Sephadex G-100 chromatogram of a CD4 lymphocyte supernatant generated in the presence of histamine (10^{-4} M). T-lymphocyte migration is expressed on the ordinate as percent of buffer control migration (designated 100%). *Denotes migration that was different from control ($P < 0.01$).

synthesis or release. In support of the former was the finding that certain human T-cell hybridomas (fusion products of PHA-stimulated human T cells and cells from the human CEM lymphoma line) constitutively produced either suppressor activity or T-lymphocyte chemoattractant activity, but never both activities (16).

Finally, Damle et al. (38) have shown that the human CD8 T-cell population can be divided further with a murine monoclonal antibody, designated 9.3, into subpopulations that include precursors of antigen-specific cytotoxic (Leu 2^+, 9.3^+) and suppressor (Leu 2^+, 9.3^-) cells. Sansoni et al. (34) separated human CD8 lymphocytes with this monoclonal antibody and each subset was incubated with histamine prior to determining their ability to suppress PHA-induced T-cell proliferation and pokeweed mitogen–induced B-cell differentiation. The results indicated that the lymphocyte population containing precursors of antigen-specific suppressor cells (Leu 2^+, 9.3^-), but not precursors of antigen-specific cytotoxic cells (Leu 2^+, 9.3^+), included all histamine-inducible suppressor cells. These data suggested that the human CD8 cell population was in fact both phenotypically and functionally heterogeneous, and that the distinct suppressor and T-cell chemoattractant lymphokines could arise from distinct cells within the histamine type II receptor-bearing CD8 lymphocyte subset. It remains to be seen whether LCF is derived from the cytotoxic (Leu 2^+, 9.3^+) subset.

IV. TARGET CELL SPECIFICITY

Berman et al. (13) defined the target cell specificity of the three histamine-induced chemoattractant lymphokines. Partially purified (Sephadex G-100 followed by QAE anion exchange column chromatography) LCF, $LyMIF_{75K}$, and $LyMIF_{35K}$ were assayed for their ability to alter the migration of T-cell subsets. As shown in Table 4, LCF stimulated the migration of CD4 lymphocytes, but not that of CD8 lymphocytes. Similarly, $LyMIF_{35K}$ selectively inhibited the random migration of CD4 cell, but not that of CD8 lymphocytes (Table 4). $LyMIF_{75K}$ inhibited equally the random migration of both T-cell subsets. Along these same lines, the mitogen-induced T-cell chemoattractant described by Van Epps et al. (30) was selective for the CD4 lymphocyte subset. The selective action of LCF and $LyMIF_{35K}$ on CD4 cells provides a possible mechanism by which histamine might promote the formation of a predominantly CD4 T-lymphocytic cellular inflammatory infiltrate. For instance, in sarcoidosis of the lung, a disease process characterized by selective recruitment of CD4 lymphocytes to the lung (39), it is tempting to hypothesize that production of LCF and $LyMIF_{35K}$ in the early stages of sarcoidosis could account for the accumulation of T helper/inducer lymphocytes which then participate in the pathogenesis of the disease (40,41).

Table 4 Target Cell Specificity of the Chemoattractant Lymphokines

	Chemoattractant		
Target cell	LCF	$LyMIF_{35K}$	$LyMIF_{75K}$
CD3	163 ± 4[a,b]	55 ± 5[b]	56 ± 6[b]
CD4	161 ± 3[b]	53 ± 6[b]	60 ± 5[b]
CD8	95 ± 6	102 ± 6	60 ± 4[b]

[a]Data expressed as percentage ± SEM of control migration.
[b]Different from control, $p < 0.05$.

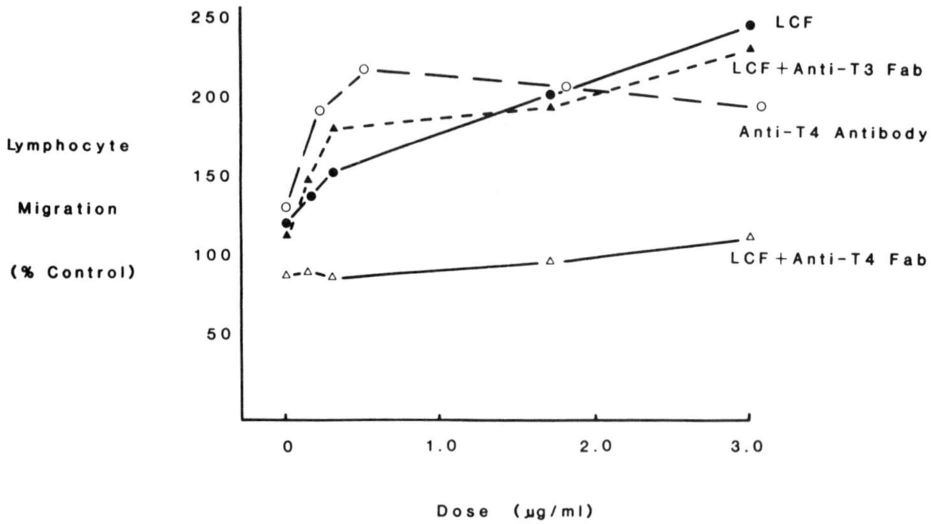

Figure 7 Inhibition of LCF-induced migration of CD4 lymphocytes by anti-CD4 Fab fragments. A representative dose response curve of CD4 cells stimulated with varying doses of LCF. Lymphocyte migration is expressed on the ordinate as percent of buffer control migration (designated 100%). LCF-induced significant ($p < 0.01$) migration at all concentrations greater than 0.3 μg/ml.

V. INTERACTION OF LYMPHOCYTE CHEMOATTRACTANT FACTOR AND CELL SURFACE MEMBRANE CD4

The findings that LCF acted solely on CD4 cells and that cells induced by LCF to migrate could be in the nonactivated state (G_0 phase of the cell cycle) suggested that the receptor for LCF must be unique to the CD4 cell population and that it must be present on the cell surface in the resting state. In a recent series of experiments, Cruikshank et al. (42) have provided data which strongly suggested that LCF elicited its effects via interaction with the CD4 cell surface glycoprotein.

Anti-CD4 antibody was able to induce a migratory response in CD4, but not CD8, lymphocytes that was qualitatively (i.e., chemokinetic) and quantitatively similar to that seen with LCF. Additionally, neither anti-CD8 antibody nor monovalent anti-CD4 Fab fragments induced a migratory response in CD4 lymphocytes. However, anti-CD4 Fab fragments could inhibit the T-cell migratory response to divalent anti-CD4. These findings suggested that the CD4 antigen could be involved in signaling of lymphocyte migration. These investigators (41) next determined if the monovalent Fab fragments from either anti-CD4 or

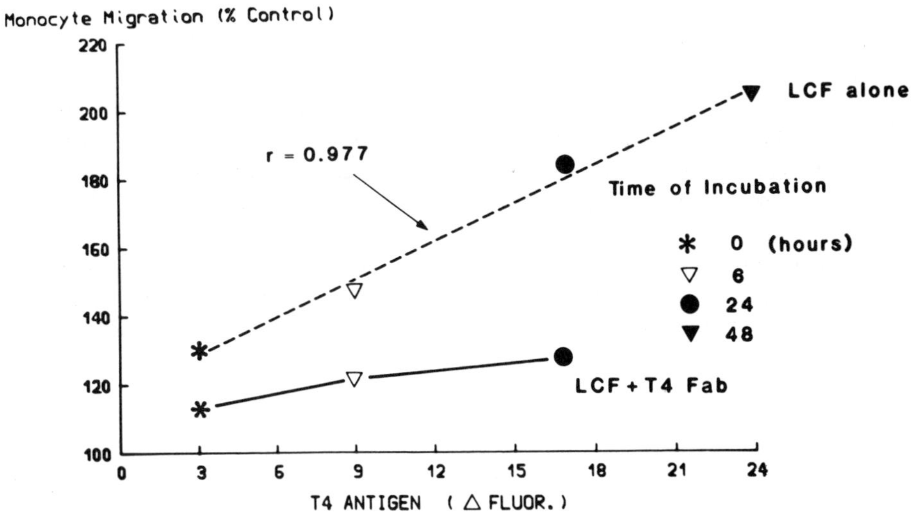

Figure 8 Correlation of monocyte migration induced by LCF with expression of CD4 antigen. Freshly isolated blood monocytes were incubated for 0, 6, 24, or 48 hr. At each time point, cells were harvested and half were stained with fluorescently labeled anti-CD4 antibody and half were assayed for LCF-induced migration. The increase in fluorescence along the axis represents an increase in CD4 antigen expression compared with cells stained with fluorescently labeled irrelevant antibody. Monocyte migration is expressed on the ordinate as percent of buffer control migration (designated 100%).

anti-CD3 antibodies could effect LCF-induced migration. As shown in Figure 7, anti-CD4 Fab fragments, but not anti-CD3 fragments, blocked the LCF-induced T-cell migratory response. Taken together with the previous observation that divalent anti-CD4 induced a chemokinetic T-cell response, these latter findings were consistent with two possibilities. Either anti-CD4 Fab fragments were inhibiting the effect of LCF by sterically inhibiting LCF binding to cell surface CD4 or anti-CD4 Fab fragments binding to the cell generated a negative intracellular signal that precluded an LCF-induced migratory response. The finding that anti CD3-induced T-cell migration was unaffected by coincubation with anti-CD4 Fab fragments strongly suggested that anti-CD4 Fab fragments do not elicit a negative signal but rather blocked the action of LCF by sterically inhibiting the binding of the ligand to the cell surface.

To further define the relationship between LCF and the CD4 membrane glycoprotein, Cruikshank et al. (42) analyzed the interaction of LCF with CD4-bearing monocytes which are devoid of cell surface CD3. CD4 antigen, identical to that expressed by lymphocytes, had been noted to be present in low amounts on freshly isolated monocytes (43,44). As mentioned previously, the migratory response of freshly isolated monocytes to LCF was not statistically significant. However, as monocytes were incubated with 10% fetal bovine serum in vitro for 6-48 hr, the LCF-induced chemoattractant response became increasingly more apparent (Fig. 8). Most interestingly, the extent of chemoattractant response of monocyte migration was completely blocked by coincubation with anti-CD4 Fab on the monocyte cell surface. At all levels of CD4 expression, LCF-induced monocyte migratin was completely blocked by coincubation with anti-CD4 Fab fragments (Fig. 8). The migratory response to LCF was unaffected by coincubation with anti-CD3 or anti-CD8 Fab fragments or with antibody to gamma inter-

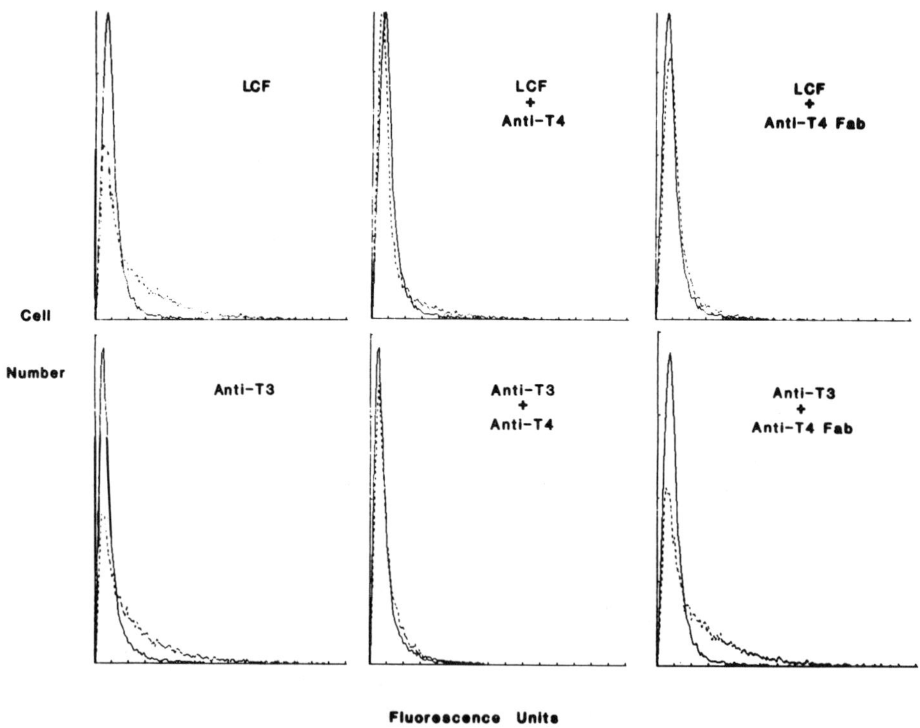

Figure 9 Representative FACS analysis of CD4 lymphocyte expression of IL-2 receptors induced by LCF and anti-CD3 antibody. The solid lines represent background staining with rhodamine-labeled monoclonal anti-Tac of T cells incubated in media for 24 hr. The dashed lines represent staining of T cells incubated with either LCF or anti-CD3 antibody for 24 hr. In certain experiments, anti-CD4 or monovalent anti-CD4 Fab fragments were added to the cultures.

feron. Taken collectively, these functional data relating LCF activity and CD4 antigen expression strongly support the concept that the CD4 cell surface glycoprotein is the receptor for LCF. Final proof of this association will come from ligand (LCF)–receptor (CD4) binding studies.

VI. LYMPHOCYTE CHEMOATTRACTANT FACTOR ACTIVATION OF CD4 CELLS

Several cellular growth factors have been reported to have chemoattractant properties (39,45–53). The association of motile responses with cell activation has been described for lymphocytes of the B-cell lineage (51,52). The progression type growth factors interleukin-2 (49) and insulin (53) have been shown to induce chemotactic responses in activated (G_1) lymphocytes. Interleukin-1, a cytokine capable fo initiating activation in resting (G_0) lymphocytes, has been reported to induce migration in resting lymphocytes (50). Since LCF was chemoattractant for resting T cells, Cruikshank et al. (42) assessed its ability to drive resting lymphocytes into the G_1 phase (defined as the up regulation on the cell surface of the interleukin-2 receptor (Tac) and HLA-DR antigen [54–56]). As shown in Figure 9, lymphocytes incubated with either LCF or divalent anti-CD3 antibody (57,58) demonstrated an increase in IL-2 receptor expression. Tac expression was noticeable by 18 hr and increased further from 24–30 hr of incubation. Lymphocyte chemoattractant factor induced Tac expression to

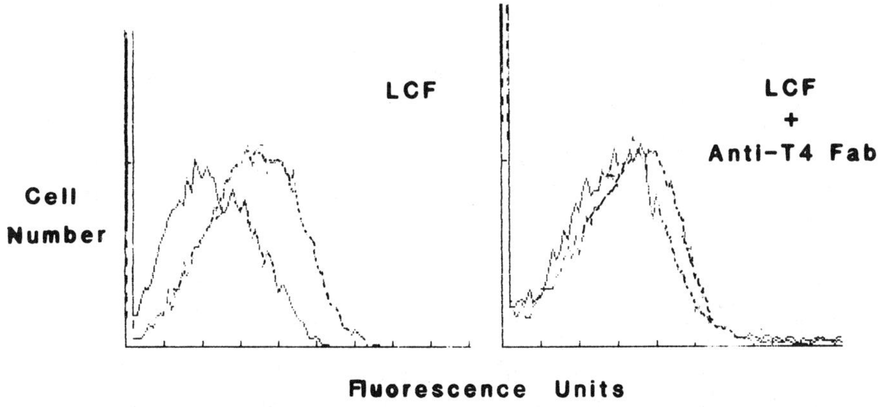

Figure 10 Representative FACS analysis of CD4 lymphocyte expression of HLA-DR antigen induced by LCF. In these experiments, CD4 cells were incubated for 24 hr with (dashed lines) or without (solid lines) LCF in the presence (right panel) or absence (left panel) of monovalent anti-CD4 Fab fragments.

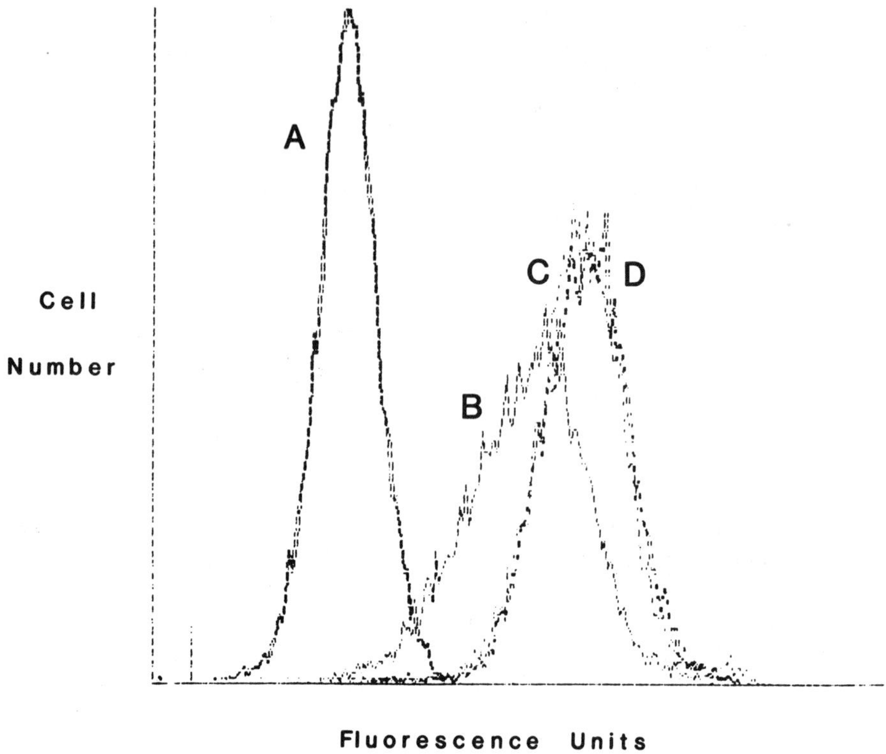

Figure 11 Representative FACS analysis of monocyte expression of HLA-DR antigen induced by LCF and gamma interferon. Fluorescently labeled anti-HLA-DR antigen was used to determine the amount of HLA-DR present on monocytes after incubation under control conditions (B); in the presence of LCF (C); or in the presence of 500 U gamma interferon (D). To determine the extent to which HLA-DR antigens are present under control conditions, untreated monocytes were stained with a fluorescently labeled irrelevant antibody, anti-CD3.

approximately the same degree as that elicited by divalent anti-CD3 antibody. The effect of LCF was unchanged by coincubation with monovalent anti-CD3 Fab fragments; however, Fab fragments of anti-CD4 antibody completely blocked the LCF induction of IL-2 receptor expression. Anti-CD4 antibody Fab fragments did not block anti-CD3 induction of Tac expression. Of note was the fact that divalent anti-CD4 antibody alone did not increase Tac expression and when cells were coincubated with anti-CD4 and either LCF or anti-CD3, Tac expression was blocked. This latter observation was in keeping with previous work (59) reporting that anti-CD4 generated a signal that blocks anti-CD3 antibody-induced cell activation. Taken together with the effects of mono- and divalent anti-CD4 on LCF-induced migration, these findings further supported the concept that cell surface CD4 was the receptor for LCF. In addition, it appeared that LCF, through interaction with CD4 had a role as a growth factor, and that LCF-induced signals resulting in cell migration and cell activation may not be identical.

As shown in Figure 10, in addition to inducing IL-2 receptor expression on CD4 lymphocytes, LCF induced a significant increase in their HLA-DR antigen expression (42). The up regulation of HLA-DR antigen expression per cell and the time course of its expression was similar to that seen for IL-2 receptor expression. As was observed with Tac staining, monovalent Fab fragment of anti-CD4 antibody (but not those of anti-CD3 antibody) were able to block LCF-induced HLA-DR cell surface expression.

Despite LCF activation of CD4 lymphocytes, LCF alone in long-term culture was unable to induce [^{3}H] thymidine incorporation, a marker of S phase, or deoxyribonucleic acid (DNA) synthesis (11). As IL-2 is essential for lymphocytes to progress from the G_1 phase into S phase and eventual proliferation (60), this suggested that LCF does not induce the production of IL-2 in CD4 T cells. This in fact has proven to be the case (Cruikshank, W. W., personal communication). Thus, LCF has the characteristics of a competence-type growth factor for CD4 lymphocytes allowing them to progress into early G_1, but unable to drive them completely through G_1 into S phase.

Since the expression of CD4 on monocytes increased as the cells were kept in culture, and since LCF induced a chemoattractant response in CD4 monocytes, Cruikshank et al. (42) determined whether LCF could cause monocyte activation as assessed by HLA-DR antigen expression. As shown in Figure 11, similar to its effect on CD4 lymphocytes, LCF induced an up regulation of HLA-DR on monocytes. The magnitude of the response was comparable to that seen for gamma interferon (61). The up regulation of cell surface HLA-DR on monocytes was blocked by coincubation with anti-CD4 Fab fragments, but not by coincubation with anti-gamma interferon antibody. These experiments provided further proof that LCF, via interaction with cell surface CD4, could result in cell activation. Implicit in both the lymphocyte and monocyte studies was the fact that the CD4 antigen can function as a growth factor receptor.

VII. CONCLUSIONS

The importance of histamine in inflammatory reactions has been appreciated ever since it was shown by Dale and Laidlaw (62) that the effects of histamine mimic those occurring during anaphylaxis; and by Bovet and Staub (63) that antihistamines could reduce the manifestations of anaphylaxis. Experimental observations in the last 2 decades have expanded upon the traditional view of histamine as the primary effector molecule in immediate-type hypersensitivity responses (reviewed in Refs. 64–66). It has become increasingly apparent that histamine and other endogenous mediators such as prostaglandins and beta-mimetic catecholamines—termed autacoids by Melmon et al. (67)—may be part of the microenvironmental physiologic process that regulates many inflammatory processes. Although the bulk of recent investigations have shown that histamine, via interaction with histamine type II receptors on various leukocyte populations, directly or indirectly induces an inhibitory signal to leukocytes which participate in inflammatory reactions, the work detailed above describing histamine-induced lymphocyte chemoattractant lymphokines provides a mechanism for histamine amplification of a lymphocyte-predominant inflammatory response.

The biology of such a system provides a model for the pathogenesis of CD4 lymphocytic infiltration into tissue (39,47). Histamine-containing cells (basophils and mast cells) have been shown to degranulate at sites of cellular immune responses (2,3,7–10). From the known amount of histamine contained in these cells, it can be estimated that histamine concentrations as high as 10^{-3} M may persist for short intervals in the microenvironment of such an immune reaction. Subsequently, the microenvironmental concentration of histamine probably falls to 10^{-4}–10^{-5} M, and eventually lower, owing to diffusion and the action of catabolic enzymes (62). By causing gaps between endothelial cells in the microcirculation, histamine directly may augment the diapedesis of lymphocytes into the tissue space. Moreover, histamine induces the production of cytokines which attract and immobilize CD4 lymphocytes at the inflammatory focus. One of these cytokines, LCF, by inducing IL-2 receptor expression, primes the cells for eventual proliferation. Lymphocyte chemoattractant factor also activates the responding lymphocytes to express HLA-DR antigen, which promotes other inflammatory responses requiring intimate cell contact. This cascade of histamine-induced effects involving CD4 lymphocyte chemoattraction and activation provides a mechanism that amplifies a signal originating from the small percentage of antigen-specific or sensitized lymphocytes present at the site of inflammation. In vivo, an amplification schema such as this occurs in concert with the effects of other cytokines and cell interactions. The net result of these various pathways determines the character and the extent of an immune-mediated inflammatory response.

ACKNOWLEDGMENTS

This work was supported by U.S. Public Health Service Grants HL 32802, HL29544, HL 19707, and a Career Investigator Award from the American Lung Association.

We thank Lisa A. Cooke for her expert assistance in the preparation of this manuscript.

REFERENCES

1. McClusky, R. T., B. Benacerraf, and J. W. McCluskey, Studies on the specificity of the cellular infiltrate in delayed hypersensitivity reactions. J. Immunol. 90:466–477 (1963).
2. Dvorak, A. M., M. C. Mihm, and H. F. Dvorak, Degranulation of basophilic leukocytes in allergic contact dermatitis reactions in man, J. Immunol. 116: 687–695 (1976).
3. Dvorak, A. M., M. C. Mihm, Jr., and H. F. Dvorak, Morphology of delayed-type hypersensitivity reactions in man, II. Ultrastructural alterations affecting the microvasculature and the tissue mast cells. Lab. Invest. 34:179–191 (1976).
4. Askenase, P. W., Role of basophils, mast cells, and vasoamines in hypersensitivity reactions with a delayed time course, Prog. Allergy 23:199–320 (1977).
5. Askenase, P. W., R. Debernardo, D. Tauben, and M. Kashgarian, Cutaneous basophil anaphylaxis. Immediate vasopermeability increases and anaphylactic degranulation of basophils at delayed hypersensitivity reactions challenged with additional antigen, Immunology 35:741–755 (1978).
6. Askenase, P. W., S. Bursztajn, M. D., Gerhson, and R. K. Gershon, T cell dependent mast cell degranulation and release of serotonin in murine delayed-type hypersensitivity, J. Exp. Med. 152:1358–1374 (1980).
7. Thueson, D. O., L. S. Speck, M. A. Lett-Brown, and J. A. Grant, Histamine-releasing activity (HRA). I. Production by mitogen- or antigen-stimulated human mononuclear cells, J. Immunol. 123:626–632 (1979).
8. Thueson, D. O., L. S. Speck, M. A. Lett-Brown, and J. A. Grant, Histamine-releasing activity (HRA). II. Interaction with basophils and physicochemical characterization, J. Immunol. 123:633–639 (1979).
9. Dy, M., and B. Lebel, Skin allografts generate an enhanced production of histamine and histamine-producing cell-stimulating factor (HCSF) by spleen cells in response to T cell mitogens, J. Immunol. 130:2343–2347 (1983).
10. Ezeamuzie, I. C., and E. S. K. Assem, Histamine releasing lymphokine: Preliminary evidence of membrane receptors on basophils, Agents and Actions 17:131–137 (1985).
11. Center, D. M., W. W. Cruikshank, J. S. Berman, and D. J. Beer, Functional characteristics of histamine receptor-bearing mononuclear cells: I. Selective production of lymphocyte chemoattractant lymphokines with histamine used as a ligand, J. Immunol. 131:1854–1859 (1983).
12. Berman, J. S., R. G. McFadden, W. W. Cruikshank, D. M. Center, and D. J. Beer, Functional characteristics of histamine receptor-bearing mononuclear cells: II. Identification and characterization of two histamine-induced

human lymphokines that inhibit lymphocyte migration. J. Immunol. 133: 1495–1504 (1984).
13. Berman, J. S., W. W. Cruikshank, D. M. Center, A. C. Theodore, and D. J. Beer, Chemoattractant lymphokines specific for the helper/inducer T lymphocyte subset, Cell. Immunol. 95:105–112 (1985).
14. Rocklin, R. E., and A. Haberek-Davidson, Histamine activates suppressor cells *in vitro* using a co-culture technique, J. Clin. Immunol. 1:73–79 (1981).
15. Cruikshank, W., and D. M. Center, Modulation of lymphocyte migration by human lymphokines: II. Purification of a lymphotactic factor, J. Immunol. 128:2569–2574 (1982).
16. Theodore, A. C., D. M. Center, W. W. Cruikshank, and D. J. Beer, A human T-T cell hybridoma-derived lymphocyte chemoattractant factor, Cell. Immunol. 98:411–421 (1986).
17. Zigmond, S. H., and J. G. Hirsch, Leukocyte locomotion and chemotaxis. New methods of evaluation and demonstration of cell-derived chemotactic factors, J. Exp. Med. 137:387–410 (1973).
18. Rocklin, R. E., A. Blidy, and M. Kamal, Physicochemical characterization of human histamine-induced suppressor factor (HSF), Cell. Immunol. 76: 243–252 (1983).
19. McFadden, R. G., W. W. Cruikshank, and D. M. Center, Modulation of lymphocyte migration by human lymphokines: III. Characterization of a lymphocyte migration inhibitory factor ($LyMIF_{35K}$), Cell. Immunol. 85:154–167 (1984).
20. Julius, M. H., G. Simpson, and L. A. Herzenberg, A rapid method for the isolation of functional thymus-derived murine lymphocytes, Eur. J. Immunol. 3:645–649 (1973).
21. Altman, L. C., Chemotactic lymphokines: A review. In Leukocyte Chemotaxis (Gallin, J., and Quie, P., Eds.), Raven Press, New York (1978), pp. 267–287.
22. Ward, P. A., H. G. Remold, and J. R. David, Leukotactic factor produced by sensitized lymphocytes, Science 163:1079–1081 (1969).
23. Ward, P. A., and A. Volkman, The elaboration of leukotactic mediators during the interaction between parenteral-type lymphocytes and F_1 hybrid cells, J. Immunol. 115:1394–1399 (1975).
24. David, J. R., S. Al-Askari, H. S. Lawrence, and L. Thomas, Delayed hypersensitivity in vitro: I. The specificity of inhibition of cell migration by antigens, J. Immunol. 93:264–273 (1964).
25. Rocklin, R. E., Partial characterization of leukocyte inhibitory factor by Concanavalin A-stimulated human lymphocytes (LIF_{ConA}), J. Immunol. 114:1161–1165 (1975).
26. Reinherz, E. L., E. L. Kung, G. Goldstein, and S. F. Schlossman, Separation of functional subsets of human T cells by a monoclonal antibody, Proc. Natl. Acad, Sci, U.S.A. 76:4061–4065 (1979).
27. Reinherz, E. L., and S. F. Schlossman, The differentiation and function of human T lymphocytes, Cell 19:821–827 (1980).

28. Romain, P. L., and S. F. Schlossman, Human T cell subsets. Functional heterogeneity and surface recognition structures, J. Clin. Invest. 74:1559-1565 (1984).
29. Center, D. M., and W. Cruikshank, Modulation of lymphocyte migration by human lymphokines: I. Identification and characterization of chemoattractant activity for lymphocytes from mitogen stimulated mononuclear cells. J. Immunol. 128:2563–2568 (1982).
30. Van Epps, D. E., D. A. Durant, and J. W. Potter, Migration of human helper/inducer T cells in response to supernatants from Con A-stimulated suppressor/cytotoxic T cells, J. Immunol. 131:697–700 (1983).
31. Rocklin, R. E., J. Breard, S. Gupta, R. A. Good, and K. L. Melmon, Characterization of the human blood lymphocytes that produce a histamine-induced suppressor factor, Cell. Immunol. 51:226–237 (1980).
32. Damle, N. K., and S. Gupta, Autologous mixed lymphocyte reaction in man. II. Histamine-induced suppression of the autologous mixed lymphocyte reaction by T-cell subsets defined with monoclonal antibodies, J. Clin. Immunol. 1:241-249 (1981).
33. Rigal, D., J. C. Monier, and G. Souweine, The effect of histamine on leukocyte migration test in man. I. Demonstration of a LIF production inhibitor (LIF-PI) Cell. Immunol. 46:360–372 (1979).
34. Sansoni, P., E. D. Silverman, M. M. Khan, K. L. Melmon, and E. G. Engleman, Immunoregulatory T cells in man: Histamine-induced suppressor T cells are derived from a Leu 2^+ ($T8^+$) subpopulation distinct from that which gives rise to cytotoxic T cells, J. Clin. Invest, 75:650–656 (1985).
35. Martinez, J. D., J. Santos, D. J. Stechshulte, and N. I. Abdou, Nonspecific suppressor cell function in atopic subjects, J. Allergy and Clin. Immunol. 64:485–490 (1979).
36. Beer, D. J., M. E. Osband, R. P. McCaffrey, N. A. Soter, and R. E. Rocklin, Abnormal histamine-induced suppressor cell function in atopic individuals, N. Engl. J. Med. 306:454–458 (1982).
37. Hollingsworth, H. M., H. Kornfeld, A. C. Theodore, D. M. Center, L. J. Rosenwasser, and D. J. Beer, Functional studies in atopic subjects provide evidence for further subfractionation of the histamine type-2 receptor-bearing human lymphocyte population (Abstract), Am. Rev. Resp. Dis. 129:A8 (1984).
38. Damle, N. K., N. Mohagheghpour, J. A. Hansen, and E. G. Engleman, Alloantigen-specific cytotoxic and suppressor T lymphocytes are derived from phenotypically distinct precursors, J. Immunol. 131:2296–2300 (1983).
39. Hunninghake, G. W., and R. G. Crystal, Pulmonary sarcoidosis: A disorder mediated by excess helper T-lymphocyte activity at sites of disease activity, N. Engl. J. Med. 305:429–434 (1981).
40. Hunninghake, G. W., J. E. Gadek, R. C. Young, O. Kawanami, V. J. Ferrans, and R. G. Crystal, Maintenance of granuloma formation in pulmonary sarco idosis by T lymphocytes within the lung, N. Engl. J. Med. 302:594-598 (1980).

41. Wahl, S. M., L. M. Wahl, and J. S. McCarthy, Lymphocyte-mediated activation of fibroblast proliferation and collagen production, J. Immunol. 121: 942–946 (1978).
42. Cruikshank, W. W., J. S. Berman, A. C. Theodore, J. Bernardo, and D. M. Center, Lymphokine activation of $T4^+$ T lymphocytes and monocytes, J. Immunol. 138:3817–3823 (1987).
43. Stewart, S. J., J. Fujimoto, and R. Levy, Human T lymphocytes and monocytes bear the same Leu-3 (T4) antigen, J. Immunol. 136:3773–3778 (1986).
44. Crocker, P. R., W. A. Jeffries, S. J. Clark, L. P. Chung, and S. Gordon, Species heterogeneity in macrophage expression of the CD4 antigen, J. Exp. Med. 166:613–618 (1987).
45. Devel, T. F., R. M. Senior, J. S. Huang, and G. L. Griffin, Chemotaxis of monocytes and neutrophils to platelet-derived growth factor, J. Clin. Invest. 69:1046–1049 (1982).
46. Seppa, H., G. Grotendorst, E. Seppa, E. Schiffmann, and G. R. Martin, Platelet-derived growth factor is chemotactic for fibroblasts, J. Cell. Biol. 92:584–588 (1982).
47. Van Voorhis, W. C., G. Kaplan, E. N. Sarno, M. A. Horwitz, R. M. Steinman, and W. R. Lewis, The cutaneous infiltrate of leprosy: Cellular characteristics and the predominant T-cell phenotype, N. Engl. J. Med. 307:1593–1597 (1982).
48. Panitch, H. S., and G. S. Francis, T lymphocyte subsets in cerebrospinal fluid in multiple sclerosis, N. Engl. J. Med. 307:560–561 (1982).
49. Kornfeld, H., J. S. Berman, D. J. Beer, and D. M. Center, Induction of human T lymphocyte motility by interleukin 2, J. Immunol. 134:3887–3890 (1985).
50. Miossec, P., C. Yu, and M. Ziff, Lymphocyte chemotactic activity of human interleukin 1, J. Immunol. 133:2007–2011 (1984).
51. Ransom, J. T., D. L. Digiusto, and J. C. Cambier, Single cell analysis of calcium mobilization in anti-immunoglobulin-stimulated B lymphocytes, J. Immunol. 136:54–57 (1986).
52. Ransom, J. T., and J. C. Cambier, B cell activation III. Independent and synergistic effects of mobilized calcium and diacylglycerol on membrane potential and Ia expression, J. Immunol. 136:66–72 (1986).
53. Berman, J. S., and D. M. Center, Chemotactic activity of porcine insulin for human T lymphocytes in vitro. J. Immunol. 138:2100–2103 (1987).
54. Krensky, A. M., and C. Clayberger, Diagnostic and therapeutic implications of T cell surface antigens, Transplantation 39:339–348 (1985).
55. Uchiyama, T. S., S. Broder, and T. A. Waldmann, A monoclonal antibody (anti-Tac) reactive with activated and functionally mature human T cells. I. Production of anti-Tac monoclonal antibody and distribution of Tac (+) cells, J. Immunol. 126:1393–1397 (1981).
56. Evans, R. L., T. J. Faldetta, R. E. Humphreys, D. M. Pratt, E. J. Yunis, and S. F. Schlossman, Peripheral human T cells sensitized in mixed lymphocyte

culture synthesize and express Ia-like antigens, J. Exp. Med. 148:1440–1445 (1978).
57. Weiss, A., R. Wiskocil, and J. Stobo, The role of T3 surface molecules in the events occurring at a pre-translation level, J. Immunol. 133:123–128 (1984).
58. Imboden, J. B., and J. D. Stobo, Transmembrane signalling by the T cell antigen receptor: Perturbation of the T3-antigen receptor complex generate inositol phosphates and releases calcium ions from intracellular stores, J. Exp. Med. 161:446–456 (1985).
59. Bank, I., and L. Chess, Perturbation of the T4 molecule transmits a negative signal to T cells, J. Exp. Med. 162:1294–1303 (1985).
60. Cotner, T., J. M. Williams, L. Christenson, H. M. Shapiro, T. B. Strom, and J. L. Strominger, Simultaneous flow cytometric analysis of human T cell activation, antigen expression, and DNA content, J. Exp. Med. 157:461–472 (1983).
61. Koeffler, H. P., J. Ranyard, L. Yelton, R. Billing, and R. Bohman, Gamma-interferon induces expression of the HLA-D antigens on normal and leukemic human myeloid cells, Proc. Natl. Acad. Sci. U.S.A. 81:4080–4084 (1984).
62. Dale, H. H., and P. P. Laidlaw, Histamine shock, J. Physiol. Lond. 52:355–390 (1919).
63. Bovet, D., and A.-M. Staub, Action protectrice des ethers phenoliques au cours de l'intoxication histaminque, C.R. Soc. Bio. (Paris) 125:547–549 (1937).
64. Plaut, M., and L. M. Lichtenstein, Histamine and immune responses. In Pharmacology of Histamine Receptors (Ganellin, C. R., and Parsons, M. E., Eds.), Wright-PSG, Bristol, England, (1982), pp. 392–435.
65. Beer, D. J., S. M. Matloff, and R. E. Rocklin, The influence of histamine on immune and inflammatory responses. In Advances in Immunology, vol. 35 (Kunkel, H. G., and Dixon, F. J., Eds.), Academic Press, Orlando, Florida (1984), pp. 206–268.
66. Beer, D. J., and R. E. Rocklin, Histamine modulation of lymphocyte biology: Membrane receptors, signal transduction, and functions. In Critical Reviews in Immunology, vol. 7 (Atassi, M. Z., Ed.) CRC Press, Boca Raton, Florida (1987), pp. 55–91.
67. Melmon, K. L., R. E. Rocklin, and R. P. Rosenkranz, Aucacoids as modulators of the inflammatory and immune response, Am. J. Med. 71:100–105 (1981).
68. Askenase, P. W., A. Schwartz, J. N. Siegel, and R. K. Gershon, Role of histamine in the regulation of cell-mediated immunity, Int. Arch Allergy Appl. Immunol. 66:225–233 (1981).

6

Histamine Regulation of Granulocyte Function

JULIE B. SEDGWICK and WILLIAM W. BUSSE *University of Wisconsin Medical School, Madison, Wisconsin*

I. INTRODUCTION

Like other leukocytes, the granulocyte has membrane-bound receptors for histamine (1-4). Studies over the past decade have shown that these receptors are an important link in regulation of this cell's activity and function in host defense and inflammation. Furthermore, information gained by study of granulocyte histamine receptors indicate that histamine, like other autacoids, often performs a paradoxical, or dualistic, role in determining granulocyte participation in inflammation.

Histamine is found preformed attached to intracellular granules of mast cells and basophils, and is released by a number of different mechanisms: antigen and surface-bound immunoglobulin E (IgE) molecules, complement anaphylatoxin particles (C3a and C5a), and nonimmunologic factors. Histamine's initial role in the inflammatory response can be viewed as a "gate keeper," as it increases vascular permeability to form channels which facilitate granulocyte trafficking from the circulation into tissues where they can participate in the inflammatory response. However, for every "turn-on" mechanism of tissue injury, forces of homeostasis provide their own regulatory activity. Histamine's action on granulocyte function is no exception to this general rule. As histamine combines with specific receptors on granulocytes, this cell's inflammatory activity is modulated. This chapter will review the available evidence which shows that activation of histamine granulocyte receptors is an important link to the host's efforts to establish homeostasis and to retain a balance between forces which either propagate or curb cellular injury.

II. NEUTROPHILS

Neutrophil participation in host defense and inflammation represents an integration of a number of key steps: chemotaxis, adherence, activation, and release of intracellular constituents. Many factors can act to initiate and then regulate neutrophil function in these processes. Histamine is one such factor and possesses both phlogistic and antiphlogistic properties. The balance, or lack of balance, between such opposing activities may determine the eventual outcome of the host response.

Histamine's contribution to tissue injury assumes an important but complex role, as indicated by an ability to modulate neutrophil chemotaxis, adherence, and lysosomal enzyme release. The eventual effect of histamine on neutrophils, and other granulocytes, is dependent upon activation of its specific membrane receptors. However, the degree and manner to which granulocytes respond to histamine activation is often complex and dependent not only on the specific receptor activated histamine type I (H_1) or type II (H_2), but the conditions under which this occurs. Experiments to establish the role of histamine in the inflammatory process have provided valuable information on the regulation of neutrophil function (Table 1).

A. Chemotaxis and Chemokinesis

1. In vitro

Histamine is not by itself chemotactic for neutrophils, but rather modulates chemotactic and chemokinetic responses to other stimuli (5). When neutrophil chemotaxis to bacterial products was evaluated with modified Boyden chambers, histamine diminished this activity in a dose-dependent fashion (6). Neutrophil levels of cyclic adenosine monophosphate (cAMP) increased following exposure to histamine, and histamine inhibition of chemotaxis was blocked by the histamine type II receptor antagonist burimamide. From these observations, it was concluded that histamine combines with the type II receptor of the neutrophil to activate adenylate cyclase and generate cAMP, which then serves as second messenger to signal suppression of neutrophil-directed movement.

To further clarify the regulatory role of histamine and its receptors in the modulation of neutrophil chemotaxis and chemokinesis (stimulated random

Table 1 Effect of Histamine on Neutrophil Function

Function	Stimulus	Effect	Receptor		
			H_1	H_2	non-H_1, non-H_2
cAMP	Histamine	↑		+	
Chemotaxis	Histamine	0			
	Casein, LPS	↓		+	
	fMLP				+?
	Zymosan, endotoxin	↓		+	
Chemokinesis	Histamine	0			
	fMLP	↑		+?	
Adherence	Histamine	↓		+	
BG release	Histamine	0			
	Zymosan	↓		+	+
	fMLP	↓			
Histaminase	IAA	↓			
Collegenase	Histamine	↑	+	+	
O_2^-	Histamine	0			
	Agg IgG	↓	+?	+	
	fMLP	↓	+?	+	
	PMS	0			
	Cal	0			
CL	fMLP	↓		+	

motility), Anderson et al. (2) used the leading front method of Zigmond and Hirsch (7), in which casein and bacterial lipopolysaccharide were chemotactic factors. The following observations were made. Histamine (1×10^{-6} M) inhibited true chemotaxis; that is, chemotaxis minus the effect of chemokinesis. Neutrophil chemotaxis was not affected by either the histamine type II receptor antagonist metiamide or the type I antagonist diphenhydramine in the absence of any other signal. However, only the type II histamine antagonist blocked histamine's inhibition of neutrophil chemotaxis to casein and bacterial lipopolysaccharide. Anderson's data suggest that type II histamine receptors participate in regulating neutrophil chemotaxis when evaluated by this method and to these stimuli.

To determine the mechanism by which histamine may regulate neutrophil motility, intracellular levels cAMP and cyclic guanosine monophosphate (cGMP) were measured following drug treatment (2). The neutrophil levels of cAMP increased during incubation with histamine, whereas no change in cGMP was observed. Further, isoproterenol and prostaglandin E_1 (PGE_1), which increase intracellular cAMP, or the dibutyryl derivative of cAMP, increased neutrophil random migration but inhibited chemotaxis to support the hypothesis that histamine modulates neutrophil motility via cAMP changes.

Histamine has also been found to suppress neutrophil chemotaxis to n-formyl-methionyl-leucyl-phenylalanine (fMLP) (8). Interestingly, neutrophils with the highest degree of unstimulated migration were the most sensitive to histamine suppression. Further, both histamine types I and II agonists inhibited chemotactic activity, but only the type II antagonist cimetidine blocked the effect of histamine or histamine agonists on neutrophil chemotaxis to fMLP. When the chemotactic peptide fMLP was used as the stimulus for chemokinesis, low concentrations of histamine, 3×10^{-9}-1×10^{-8} M, enhanced this activity (8). However, higher concentrations of histamine, $\geq 3 \times 10^{-7}$ M, suppressed chemokinesis. Although detected at much lower histamine concentrations, these results are similar to the findings of Anderson et al. (2), in which the histamine effect on chemokinesis was dose dependent. Therefore, the effect of histamine on cell movement must be examined in relationship to both random and directed movement, the stimulus for cell migration, and the concentration of modifier.

At present, most studies would agree with the earlier findings by Hill et al. (6), which showed that histamine modulation of neutrophil motility appears to be mediated through an interaction with histamine type II receptors to increase intracellular cAMP. In contrast, Seligman and coworkers (8) have proposed the presence of a single histamine receptor on neutrophils which is sensitive to both histamine types I and II agonists, but is blocked only by type II antagonists. Thus histamine could inhibit chemotaxis and enhance chemokinesis by three possible mechanisms: (1) histamine has multiple, independent effects of neutrophil motility via type II receptors; (2) neutrophils have a single histamine receptor which has a lower affinity for type II agonists than type I agonists, and is blocked only by type II antagonists; or (3) histamine's effects on neutrophil production of oxidative metabolites could disrupt regulation of the chemoattractant gradient through gneration of the MPO/H_2O_2/halide system (see below).

Knowledge that histamine modulates neutrophil chemotaxis may have direct clinical relevance. In atopic dermatitis, many patient have defective neutrophil function, an increased susceptibility to infections, and elevated levels of circulating histamine. Furthermore, neutrophil chemotaxis is markedly reduced during flares of atopic dermatitis, a time when many patients have concurrent skin infections. To explain the propensity of atopic dermatitis patients for infections, it is hypothesized that high concentrations of circulating histamine suppress neutrophil function, particularly chemotaxis, and thereby increase the patient's susceptibility to infection (9). The observation that cimetidine blocks histamine-induced inhibition of true chemotaxis has caused at least one group of investigators (10) to speculate that the use of histamine type II antagonists (particularly cimetidine) may block histamine suppression of neutrophil function and thereby promote normal granulocyte host defense. Such recommendations are only speculative at present.

As discussed above, it has been postulated that abnormalities in leukocyte chemotaxis in patients with atopic dermatitis occur as a consequence of in vivo exposure to high levels of histamine. To evaluate this possibility, leukocyte suspensions were obtained from atopic pateints and then incubated with selected antigen to release basophil histamine (11). Following this reaction, neutrophils were isolated and chemotaxis to opsonized zymosan or endotoxin was measured. Leukocytes isolated following exposure to antigen, and presumably higher concentrations of histamine, had decreased chemotaxis; these observations suggest that neutrophil movement was affected by basophil secretion of histamine. However, other factors can modify neutrophil function and may be generated during leukocyte incubation with antigen. When neutrophils from either normal or atopic subjects were incubated with histamine, chemotaxis was reduced in a dose-dependent fashion; histamine's effect was blocked by the type II antagonist cimetidine, but not promethazine, a type I blocker. Moreover, inhibition of chemotaxis by histamine was more apparent in cells from patients with atopic disease. From these observations, it was concluded that leukocytes from atopic patients are particularly "sensitive" to histamine, and that this may arise as a consequence of previous in vivo exposure to histamine. However, the changes in chemotaxis may also arise because the cells have already been partially suppressed from previous exposure to histamine, a likely possibility when the skin disease is very active.

2. In Vivo

The in vivo implications of these in vitro studies would predict diminished accumulation of neutrophils at sites of inflammation, reduced clearance of bacteria, and greater possibility for infection when histamine concentrations are increased. Increased circulating concentrations of histamine would arise following antigen activation of IgE-sensitized mast cells and basophils; histamine could then activate histamine type II receptors to suppress neutrophil chemotactic activity. In rats, Hirasawa and coworkers (12) found that local administration of histamine inhibited neutrophil infiltration, whereas cimetidine, but not the type I antagonist pyrilamine, enhanced neutrophil accumulation.

However, the effect of histamine on neutrophil motility in vivo is likely to be more complex than stated above. Although histamine directly inhibits neutrophil chemotaxis by action on membrane-bound histamine type II receptors, it may also inhibit cell movement through a separate interaction with mononuclear cells (13). Histamine stimulates mononuclear cells to secrete a soluble product which can then block release of leukocyte migration inhibitor factor (LIF); if this factor is not present, neutrophils will migrate from sites of inflammation. Therefore, the net in vivo effect of histamine on neutrophil chemotaxis inhibits neutrophil migration, via type II receptor activation, and (2) conversely "uncheck" this cell's movement by suppressing the secretion of monocyte factors.

B. Adherence

For leukocytes to participate in inflammatory reactions, chemotaxis, diapedesis, and eventually cell adherence must occur. Histamine also suppresses neutrophil adherence (14). Attempts to evaluate the effect of histamine on adherence found that leukocytes from normal and atopic subjects adhere similarly to nylon fibers. When normal leukocytes were incubated with high concentrations (1×10^{-5}-1×10^{-3} M) of histamine, cell adherence to nylon fibers was reduced, an action blocked by the histamine type II antagonist, metiamide. When, however, leukocytes from atopic subjects were similarly evaluated, histamine was less effective in inhibiting cell adherence. These findings indicate diminished histamine type II receptor function on leukocytes from atopic subjects, and suggest this occurs from generation of histamine in the allergic reactions in these patients and receptor down regulation.

The mechanism by which histamine inhibits neutrophil adherence may be related to the formation of ligand-receptor domains at adherence sites (15). Using a fluorescence-histamine probe, histamine receptors appeared as randomly distributed clusters on stationary neutrophils. With exposure to a chemotactic gradient (fMLP), the fluorescent complexes redistributed to pseudopods or to the lamellipodium and uropod which are responsible for neutrophil adherence. If there is previous accumulation of histamine-receptor complexes at these sites, membrane components needed to participate in cell adhesion may be excluded from functioning in this process. Moreover, accumulation of histamine receptors at the leading edge of migrating neutrophils may enhance cell sensitivity to further modulation from extracellular mediators, including histamine. Alternatively, decreased adherence may occur through generation of second messengers, such as cAMP, which in turn alter leukocyte adherence. The consequence of all these histamine effects will be reduced cell adherence.

C. Modulation of Lysosomal Enzyme Release

1. β-Glucuronidase

Like catecholamines and prostaglandins of the E series, histamine increases intracellular concentrations of neutrophil cAMP and inhibits β-glucuronidase (βG) release to zymosan (16). The concentrations of histamine, 1×10^{-8}-1×10^{-5} M, which inhibit βG release, are also the doses which reduce chemotaxis. Histamine regulation of βG release occurs through activation of type II receptors. The histamine type II dimaprit, but not the type I agonist 2-(2-pyramidal)ethylamine, also blocks lysosomal enzyme release (18). Furthermore, the histamine type II receptor antagonist metiamide blocks histamine modulation of βG release, whereas the type I antagonist chlorpheniramine has no effect. In contrast, Marone and coworkers (19) did not find that histamine increased cAMP or reduced βG release in neutrophils stimulated by opsonized zymosan; however, the experimental design in this study was different from previous studies and this may account for the discrepancy.

Although most investigators agree that histamine's effect on neutrophil βG release is mediated by the type II receptor, observations by Vickers et al. (20) do not totally support this concept. In their studies, histamine caused dose-dependent inhibition of βG release to opsonized zymosan. The only methyl-substituted histamine to significantly inhibit enzyme release was the type II agonist 4-methylhistamine, whereas the type I agonist 2-methylhistamine had no effect, suggesting that the histamine inhibition is via interaction with neutrophil type II receptors. In contrast, the histamine type II agonist dimaprit and its higher and lower analogs, which have little activity at type I or type II receptors, also inhibited βG release. Further, no correlation was found with histamine or its selective histamine receptor agonists and their specific activity at either type I or type II receptors. These data question whether both histamine and dimaprit have effects on lysosomal enzyme release that is distinct and separate from activation of type I and type II receptors.

Histamine also inhibits neutrophil βG release when the secretagogue is fMLP (21). In these experiments, the degree to which βG release was inhibited depended upon the histamine and fMLP concentrations, and was significantly potentiated if evaluated in the presence of the phosphodiesterase inhibitor IBMX (3-isobutyl-1-methylxanthine). Similarly, IBMX potentiated PGE_1 reduction of βG release. The observations with IBMX further imply that regulation of βG release is mediated by increased intracellular levels of cAMP. The fact that inhibition of βG release was dependent on both histamine and stimulator (fMLP) concentration further suggests that neutrophils may be modulated by an endogenous control system whose activity is dependent upon the intensity of the inflammatory stimuli. Such a conclusion agrees with reports by Tung and Lichtenstein (22) which evaluated modulation of basophil secretion by histamine; this will be discussed later.

Histamine's ability to inhibit βG release is decreased in leukocytes from patients with asthma (23) and atopic dermatitis (24). There is no evidence to suggest that the patients' cells had been partially degranulated, since total neutrophil βG content in asthma and atopic dermatitis patients is similar to that in normal subjects. The neutrophil cAMP response to histamine was similarly affected in these patients. Although histamine still inhibited βG release from leukocytes of asthma or atopic dermatitis patients, the effect is reduced 100-fold when compared to controls. Interestingly, this altered neutrophil response to histamine compares to the 100-fold increase in airway sensitivity to inhaled histamine seen in patients with asthma.

Other factors can modify the neutrophil response to histamine, and thereby regulate βG release. If neutrophils are incubated with live influenza viruses, the virus-treated cells have a diminished response to histamine (25). During influenza illnesses, airway epithelium is often injured by the direct cytotoxic action of the virus. The viral effects on histamine's regulation of lysosomal enzyme release may indicate another mechanism by which airway injury is increased during an influenza respiratory illness; that is, the loss of histamine modulation of βG release would promote greater neutrophil inflammatory capability.

2. Histaminase

Neutrophil granules also contain histaminase which catabolizes histamine (26). A nontoxic, dose-dependent release of neutrophil histaminase can be induced by C3b when bound to zymosan particles, erythrocytes, or Sephadex G-75 and by the calcium ionophore A23187; histaminase release occurs independent of βG secretion. Histaminase catabolizes histamine by generating an unstable intermediate imidazole-4-acetaldehyde which then spontaneously converts to imidazoleacetic acid (IAA). Histamine is a weak inhibitor of granulocyte release of histaminase. However, if neutrophils are incubated with IAA prior to activation by zymosan, there is a dose-dependent inhibition of histaminase release, but no effect on βG, myeloperoxidase, or lysozyme secretion. Therefore, although histamine does not significantly diminish neutrophil histaminase release (1000 times less effective than IAA), the IAA product of histaminase metabolism of histamine is a very potent inhibitor of this particular secretion process. Consequently, when histamine metabolizes histamine, the produce formed establishes a negative feedback inhibition of its own generation. Since eosinophils also contain histaminease (27), a similar mechanism may occur with this cell.

3. Collagenase

Neutrophil-derived collagenase may participate in collagen breakdown during inflammatory reactions. Collagenase is found in a latent or preactivated form within neutrophil cytoplasm; during inflammation collagenase is activated. The local concentration of collagenase is felt to reflect the intensity of the inflammatory reaction. Carrageenin-induced pleurisy or intraperitoneal injection of histamine or histamine-releasing compound 48/80 resulted in nearly total (90–98%) activation of cellular collagenase (28). In addition, both carrageenin-induced pleurisy and compound 48/80 increased the number of blood granulocytes, whereas histamine had no effect. While neither histamine type I nor type II antagonists (mepyramine and cimetidine, respectively) significantly inhibited leukocyte infiltration caused by compound 48/80 (presumably due to mast cell release of neutrophil chemotactic factor), they both prevented activation of collagenase. These observations suggest that although histamine release by compound 48/80 does not regulate leukocyte migration, it is a factor in activating granulocyte collagenase, which may thus potentiate the inflammatory response. This is another example of how histamine may act as an "indirect" messenger to further tissue injury.

4. Oxidative Metabolism

Superoxide anion (O_2^-) is the initial oxygen metabolite generated during the neutrophil respiratory burst, and is itself a potent proinflammatory agent. Further, O_2^- reacts to form other highly reactive oxygen metabolites which can be measured by chemiluminescence (CL) assays. When Lehmeyer and Johnston (29) studied the effects of anti-inflammatory drugs on the oxidative metabolism of phagocytes, they observed that histamine and other agents which elevate intracellular cAMP decreased aggregated IgG stimulation of O_2^- and CL. Histamine's suppressive effects were potentiated by theophylline, but were blocked when concentrations of cGMP were increased. The concentrations of histamine (1×10^{-5}–1×10^{-6} M) which suppressed O_2^- generation also inhibit neutrophil chemotaxis and lysosomal enzyme release.

Histamine also inhibits fMLP stimulation of neutrophil O_2^- generation and CL (30). Although the histamine type II antagonist cimetidine enhances neutrophil CL to fMPL and blocks the suppressive effects of histamine, 5–10 times higher concentrations of cimetidine than histamine are necessary to produce this effect. Since histamine also inhibits O_2^- generation in the cell-free xanthine-xanthine oxidase system, it is likely that a direct interaction occurs between histamine and O_2^-. These results suggest that histamine may interact both directly with neutrophils to alter O_2^- generation via histamine type II receptor-generated cAMP and nonspecifically as a noncellular scavenger of O_2^-. Therefore, histamine suppression of the neutrophil's respiratory burst is not entirely dependent upon histamine type II receptor-linked events.

Further attempts to clarify histamine regulation of neutrophil O_2^- generation found that the histamine effects were dependent on the particular cell activator. In studies making parallel analyses of neutrophil movement and metabolic activity, Seligman and associates (8) confirmed that histamine enhances chemokinesis and inhibits chemotaxis. Further, they found that histamine caused a stimulus-specific inhibition of membrane potential, O_2^- production, H_2O_2 formation, and release of βG. A similar effect was found with both histamine type I or type II agonists. In these studies, suppression of neutrophil functions by histamine or types I and II agonists occurred only when these agents were added prior to fMLP stimulation, and did not occur in cells activated by phorbol myristate acetate (PMA) or calcium ionophore. Finally, the histamine type II antagonist cimetidine was able to competitively antagonize these effects.

A precise interpretation of these results is difficult. However, the ability of both histamine types I and II agonists to mimic a histamine effect and of cimetidine to antagonize this effect, suggests the possibility of a single type of histamine receptor on neutrophils, at least in relationship to modulation of O_2^- generation (8). If such were the case, this particular receptor would have a lower affinity for histamine type II agonists and higher affinity for type I agonists than previously reported. In addition, only histamine type II antagonist binding to this postulated receptor would prevent the effect of histamine or its agonist analogs. It is a more likely possibility that the histamine type I agonist effects are not specific.

A more "expected" effect of histamine on neutrophil CL has been reported by Ozaki et al. (31). Here, both histamine and the type II agonist dimaprit inhibited fMLP-stimulated CL. Further, the histamine type II antagonists cimetidine and ranitidine, but not the type I antagonist mepyramine, blocked histamine's action. In contrast to findings of Seligman et al. (8), histamine type I agonists had no effect on CL, suggesting that regulation of this neutrophil function is mediated via histamine type II receptors. A similar type II histamine-receptor regulation of mononuclear cell CL to phytohemagglutinin has been reported (32,33). These findings corroborate the general principle that suggests histamine suppression of neutrophil inflammatory function is under type II receptor control.

Finally, histamine modulation of neutrophil activation and generation of oxygen metabolites provides an indirect mechanism of histamine regulation of leukocyte motility. When neutrophils generate oxygen metabolites and release lysosomal enzymes, a myeloperoxidase (MPO)/H_2O_2/halide complex is formed. This complex can regulate leukocyte chemotaxis and chemokinesis by inactivating certain leukoattractants through the oxidation of methionine (34). Stimuli affected by this product include complement-derived factors and synthetic peptides. This mechanism may also inactivate other mediators containing thioether groups. When histamine inhibits neutrophil activation and thus the formation of this complex, leukoattractants remain active and can thus potentiate granulocyte motility. Interestingly, the generation of a MPO/H_2O_2/halide system by neutrophils can also regulate the further secretion of histamine by mast cells (see below).

D. Alternative Histamine Receptors

In addition to histamine type I and type II receptors, two alternative histamine-binding sites have been proposed. Gespach and coworkers (35) recently described a subpopulation of histamine type II receptors which they define as

H_{2h} (histamine type II_h). These receptors mediate serotonin uptake by human platelets and are pharmacologically and biochemically distinct from histamine types I, II, and III (see below) receptors. The histamine type II_h receptor is characterized by a high affinity for type II receptor antagonists and an apparent link to the generation of intracellular cGMP.

A distinct non-histamine type I, non-histamine type II receptor has also been described by Arrang and associates (36) and defined as H_3. The histamine type III receptor is chemically stereoselective with structural requirements markedly different from types I and II receptors (37). Although initially identified on prejunctional nerve terminals in the rat brain, recent reports have located histamine type III receptors on other tissues, including guinea pig perivascular nerve terminals (38), human brain, guinea pig lung, and possibly skin and spleen (39). Since mast cells are abundantly present in bronchial mucosa, alveolar septal connective tissue, and pleura, it is possible that histamine type III receptors exist on these cells and modulate both synthesis and release of histamine. Although histamine type III receptors have yet to be identified on granulocytes, they may be responsible for histamine-neutrophil effects not identified under type I or II receptor control.

E. Neutrophil-Mast Cell Interaction

In 1985, Fantozzi and associates (40) suggested that a bidirectional control mechanism exists between neutrophils and mast cells. To demonstrate this relationship, it was initially noted that histamine inhibited neutrophil O_2^- generation by fMLP. To establish this possibility in an experimental setting, passively sensitized rat serosal mast cells were degranulated by acetylcholine in the presence of neutrophils; when fMLP was used to stimulate O_2^- production by neutrophils, which were isolated from this reaction mixture, the response was reduced. Moreover, this effect was blocked by cimetidine. In "reversing" the experimental design, fMLP activation of neutrophils caused a noncytotoxic histamine release from nonsensitized rat mast cells, an effect attributed to myeloperoxidase (MPO) release. These results suggest a neutrophil-mast cell bidirectional interaction that can inhibit one cell's function but activate the other.

Interestingly, the neutrophil-mast cell interaction appears to be stimulus dependent. For example, when Stendahl et al. (41) incubated neutrophils with serum-treated zymosan particles, the product generated by phagocytosis degranulated mast cells. From these results, they concluded that neutrophil MPO interacts with H_2O_2 and halide to then degranulate mast cells. In contrast, MPO was not required to release mast cell histamine when PMA was used to stimulate neutrophils (42). These studies suggest that a variety of neutrophil products can degranulate mast cells and that generation of these products is stimulus specific.

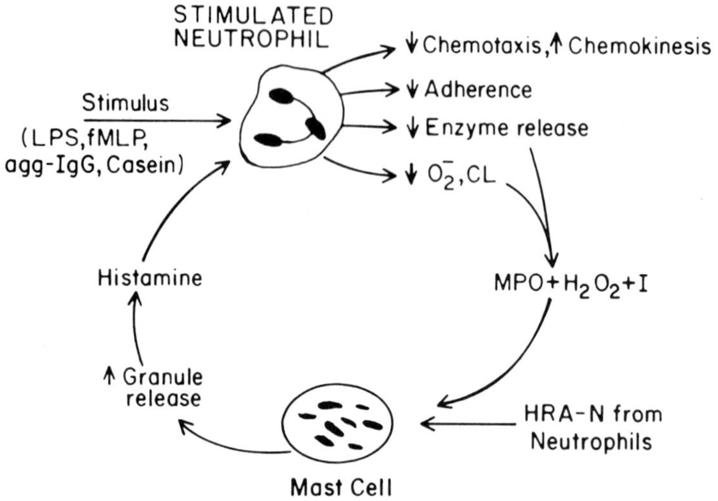

Figure 1 Histamine-neutrophil interaction. Histamine inhibits stimulated neutrophil function. In contrast, stimulated neutrophil products induce a noncytotoxic release of mast cell granules. This generates a bidirectional mechanism of down regulation of an inflammatory reaction.

Other interesting and potentially important neutrophil factors may influence mast cell histamine release. White and Kaliner (43) found that unstimulated neutrophils produce, or contain, histamine-releasing activity (HRA-N). The presence of HRA-N in neutrophils is not changed following zymosan stimulation or by the presence of atopic disease. Further, HRA-N is unique to neutrophils and not produced by mononuclear cells, platelets, or eosinophils. The investigators suggested that HRA-N may cause histamine release during late-phase reactions and in IgE-dependent allergic reactions, to thus perpetuate the late-phase allergic reaction which is associated with neutrophil infiltration. Precisely how neutrophils participate in the progression of late-phase reaction is not known. Nonetheless, the findings of White and Kaliner (43) suggest that recruited neutrophils can "deliver" HRA-N, which then causes more mediator release. Thus, the inflammatory process can become a self-perpetuating reaction. From what is presently known, histamine's role in late-phase allergic reactions is not established. Yet it is important to recall that in addition to its phlogistic properties, histamine can also suppress inflammation by activation of neutrophil and basophil histamine type II receptors. Eosinophils are also recruited during late-phase reactions. However, when neutrophils were coincubated with eosinophils from a patient with idiopathic hypereosinophilia syndrome, there was complete inhibition of HRA-N activity, suggesting an opposing eosinophil effect. These studies may show an additional mechanism by which inflammation is regulated and homeostasis achieved.

The interaction of mast cell–derived histamine and neutrophils is a complex, bidirectional process affecting a number of phases of inflammation (Fig. 1). By inhibiting neutrophil chemotaxis, enzyme release, and oxidative metabolism, mast cell or basophil-derived histamine can down regulate both the presence and participation of neutrophils in inflammation. Even though neutrophils can promote further release of histamine, and presumably other mast cell mediators via HRA-N, a negative feedback loop develops to curtail neutrophil participation in the inflammatory response. Maintenance of neutrophil hemostasis is a complicated, intricate process in which histamine is but one participant.

II. EOSINOPHILS

The eosinophil is now recognized as a major participant in tissue injury during immediate hypersensitivity reactions. Precisely how histamine influences eosinophil function has been difficult to ascertain because of difficulties in obtaining a sufficiently large number of purified eosinophils for study. Consequently, many studies have relied upon patients with hypereosinophilic syndromes as the source for purified eosinophils. Isolated cells from such patients may not represent normal eosinophil function. Nonetheless, it has been observed that histamine alters eosinophil motility, metabolic activity, cell surface receptors, and cellular cytotoxicity (Table 2). Although regulation of neutrophil function occurs principally via histamine type II receptors, the histamine receptor(s) modulating eosinophil activity is poorly defined.

A. Chemotaxis and Chemokinesis

1. In Vitro

Eosinophil involvement in immediate hypersensitivity begins with cell migration to a chemotactic factor; this response can be regulated at a number of areas: (1) generation of eosinophilic chemotactic activity, (2) selective chemotaxis of eosinophils, (3) the presence of inactivators and inhibitors of chemotactic stimuli, and (4) factors which alter eosinophil responsiveness to chemotactic stimuli through deactivation (44). Histamine appears to affect eosinophil motility in all four of these areas. Early studies on the ability of histamine, and its metabolite IAA, to regulate granulocyte motility reported specific chemotaxis of eosinophils (45–48), with a triphasic concentration-dependent modulation of this cell's migration (44). Low concentrations of histamine, 1-3 $\times 10^{-7}$ M, enhanced both eosinophil random and directed migration, whereas, high concentrations of

Table 2 Effect of Histamine on Eosinophil Function

Function	Stimulus	Effect	Receptor		
			H_1	H_2	non-H_1, non-H_2
cAMP	Histamine	↑		+	
Chemotaxis	Histamine (10^{-7} M)	↑			+
	EAS, C5a	↓		+	
Chemokinesis	Histamine ($< 10^{-7}$)	↑		+	
	($> 10^{-6}$)	↓		+	
	EAS, C5a	↑	+		
O_2^-	Histamine	↑	+		+?
	PMA, zymosan	↑	+		+?
Receptors					
C3b	Histamine	↑	+		
IgG	Histamine	0			
Cytotoxicity (C′ = dependent	Histamine	↑	+		

histamine, 4 × 10^{-6} M or greater, inhibited cell movement. Intermediate ranges of histamine, 3 × 10^{-7}-1.25 × 10^{-6} M, induced chemotactic migration. The eosinophil response to histamine was concluded to be a change in true chemotaxis and not simply increased chemokinesis. Finally, preincubation of eosinophils with histamine deactivates the cell's chemotactic response to subsequent histamine gradients (49).

Studies by Clark et al. (48) and also Turnball and Kay (3) observed marked variations in eosinophil chemotactic activity to histamine. Variations in eosinophil responsiveness appeared dependent not only on the source of cells, but differed among eosinophils from the same subject. To clarify these findings, the following observations were made. Gallin et al. (5) found that the degree of histamine-induced chemotaxis was dependent on the percentage of eosinophils in the leukocyte preparation being evaluated—the more eosinophils present, the greater the relative chemotactic response. Further, high concentrations of histamine (1 × 10^{-6}-1.0 × 10^{-5} M) altered eosinophil morphology by stimulating eosinophil orientation, and pseudopod and cell spreading. These effects, however, were not homogeneous, as the eosinophil reaction to histamine varied with time and the extent of the response (47).

In part, this variability in activity may be accounted for by the source of eosinophils for study. Often eosinophils were used in low purity (10-60%) and from a variety of patient sources, including individuals with idiopathic hypereosinophilia. When Wadee and coworkers (50) evaluated highly purified suspensions of eosinophils (90–95%) from eosinophilic patients, no change in either chemotaxis or chemokinesis was found to histamine. These findings suggest that observed differences in eosinophil chemotaxis to histamine may be due to (1) the type of motility assay system utilized, (2) a lack of eosinophil purity, (3) the patient source of eosinophils, or (4) the existence of eosinophil subpopulations.

The existence of eosinophil subpopulations, or heterogeneity, was initially proposed by Clark and coworkers (3,46,48). Their supposition was based upon observations that eosinophils do not migrate en masse to chemotactic factors as expected, and, moreover, that the response to histamine varied with different individuals (see discussion of eosinophil heterogeneity below).

The variability in eosinophil responsiveness is also seen when the effects of histamine type I and type II antagonists are evaluated on histamine chemotaxis (3,44,49). For example, Clark et al. (3) found that eosinophil chemotaxis to histamine was not altered by either type I or type II receptor antagonists. Further, deactivation to histamine-induced chemotaxis was not blocked by either type I or type II antagonists, thus suggesting this effect arose via a non-type I, non-type II receptor. To explain these observations, the following possibilities were considered: Human eosinophils have a third type of histamine receptor (non-type I, non-type II) and/or eosinophils are a heterogeneous cell population varying in response to histamine.

In contrast to difficulties encountered in characterizing eosinophil chemotaxis to histamine, the ability of histamine to modulate this cell's attraction to other stimuli is more clearly defined; in general, histamine suppresses stimulated eosinophil chemotaxis and this effect is blocked by type II receptor antagonists. Using highly purified populations of eosinophils, Clark et al. (48) and Wadee et al. (50) measured in vitro eosinophil chemotaxis to endotoxin-activated serum and C5a in the presence of histamine. Histamine inhibited chemotaxis to these attractants even though a concurrent increase in chemokinesis occurred. In addition, histamine inhibited eosinophil chemotaxis to eosinophil chemotactic tetrapeptides (ECF-A), eosinophilic chemotactic factor of anaphylaxis, both in vitro and in vivo in humans and marmosets (51). Histamine inhibition of eosinophil chemotaxis appeared to be mediated by type II receptors and an increase in cAMP; preexposure of eosinophils to the type II antagonist metiamide, but not the type I antagonists diphenylhydramine, blocked histamine inhibition (50). However, eosinophil's chemotactic sensitivity to histamine type I and type II antagonists was found to vary, again suggesting a heterogeneity of this granulocyte population (48). In contrast, enhancement of chemokinesis by histamine appears to be mediated by histamine type I receptors (3).

Indirect modulation of eosinophil-directed movement can be achieved through histamine's interaction with other leukocytes (52). When mononuclear cells were incubated with histamine at concentrations which did not affect eosinophil chemotaxis, a factor was generated which inhibited eosinophil chemotaxis to activated complement components, casein, or ECF-A. Both diphenhydramine and metiamide blocked the ability of histamine to stimulate release of this immobilizing factor from mononuclear cells, but did not modify eosinophil migration when added to cell-free histamine-stimulated mononuclear cell supernates. Therefore, the antagonists appeared to block the initial interaction between histamine and mononuclear cells. Histamine-stimulated secretion of this mononuclear cell factor, which modulates eosinophil motility, may be an important factor in the conflicting reports on histamine effects on eosinophil motility, particularly when in vitro experiments are conducted with mixed leukocyte suspensions.

2. In Vivo

Evaluation of the in vivo responses of eosinophils to histamine have proved difficult (45,47,51,53-57). Whereas some studies report that histamine induced a localized influx of eosinophils, others detected only a systemic, but not localized, eosinophilia to histamine (5). Initially, Litt (58) suggested that the low pH found with large concentrations of histamine was responsible for peripheral blood and lymph node eosinophilia. However, when Bryant and Kay (59) and Gallin et al. (5) used skin windows to evaluate eosinophil recruitment to large doses of histamine (1×10^{-5}-1×10^{-3} M), they found the eosinophil response to histamine was greater in atopic than in nonatopic subjects. This work supports the conclusion that skin-window eosinophilia is not related to the acidic pH found with large concentrations of histamine. Further, it was observed that the skin-window response to histamine was independent of circulating levels of eosinophils and less than that observed with antigen.

In guinea pigs, Pincus (60) found polymyxin B induced peritoneal eosinophilia. Although polymyxin B causes mast cell degranulation, this antibiotic is not by itself chemotactic for eosinophils. When guinea pigs were treated with diphenhydramine, but not metiamide, the peritoneal eosinophilia to polymoxin B was blocked. Further, histamine alone did not induce peritoneal eosinophilia. Pincus' results suggest that mast cell degranulation and not just the presence of histamine is necessary for peritoneal eosinophil infiltration. However, histamine enhances this process through a histamine type I receptor response which may relate to increased vascular permeability.

To further determine the participation of histamine in cutaneous anaphylaxis, Woodward et al. (61) studied eosinophil accumulation in ovalbumin-sensitized guinea pigs. When antigen initiated the immediate hypersensitivity reaction, neither the histamine type I nor type II antagonists pyrilamine or cimetidine, respectively, inhibited eosinophil accumulation. However, when the antagonists were used in combination, eosinophilia was significantly reduced.

Expanding on these studies and evaluating the effect of histamine on eosinophil participation in immediate hypersensitivity reactions, the following experiments were performed (62). Conjunctival application of histamine caused a dose-dependent eosinophil infiltration in sensitized guinea pigs. In this system, cimetidine blocked eosinophil infiltration induced by low-to-intermediate doses of histamine ($< 0.5\%$ solution). In contrast, pyrilamine decreased the number of eosinophils in both epithelial and subepithelial regions responding to all histamine concentrations. The combination of the two drugs was indistinguishable from pyrialmine alone. The authors concluded that histamine in the absence of other mast cell derived factors will attract eosinophils to the conjuctiva, and this response is mediated by type I receptors which increase vascular permeability. With antigen activation of mast cell release, both histamine type I and type II antagonists are necessary to block the effect, indicating a more complex mechanism of cellular attraction than simply an effect on vascular permeability.

When uveitis was used as a model, Mindel and associates (63) did not observe histamine-enhanced eosinophil infiltration. In this model, the type II histamine agonist dimaprit had a dual effect. First, dimaprit and nordimaprit induced eosinophilic infiltration unrelated to types I and II histamine receptor activity. Second, this effect was inhibited by dimaprit's histamine type II agonist activity, such that the presence of a type II antagonist blocked dimaprit's type II agonist activity and enhanced its type II receptor-independent effect. Whether these results reflect a difference in the organ being evaluated or that these two histamine derivatives act through a nonhistamine mechanism can not be determined from the reported studies.

B. Oxidative Metabolism

Histamine, 1×10^{-7}-1×10^{-6} M, but not its metabolite IAA, stimulated normal human eosinophils and guinea pig peritoneal exudate eosinophils to generate O_2^-; however, there was considerable variability in this cellular response to histamine (64). Chlorpheniramine strongly inhibited guinea pig eosinophil production of O_2^- by zymosan, PMA, or histamine stimulation. In contrast, the histamine type II receptor blocker cimetidine had little effect on either resting or stimulated O_2^- generation. The observation that histamine type I antagonists inhibit eosinophil O_2^- generation to zymosan and PMA suggests that maximum O_2^- production may occur only when histamine interacts with eosinophils. If this is correct, it creates an intriguing condition whereby histamine potentiates the effects of eosinophil-derived inflammation by O_2^-. In contrast, neutrophils were not activated by any concentration of histamine.

C. Complement Receptors

From in vitro experiments, it is also apparent that histamine enhances eosinophil expression of C3b but not IgG receptors (65). Histamine does not have a similar effect on monocytes or neutrophils. The histamine-dependent increase in eosinophil C4b receptors was dose and time dependent, and was also found with IAA (66). The increased appearance of C3b receptors to histamine may represent: (1) generation of new receptors, (2) presentation of "hidden" receptors, (3) association of C3b receptor subunits, or (4) an increase in the binding affinity of existing receptors (67). Histamine enhancement of eosinophil C3b receptors was found to be histamine type I dependent and was blocked by chlorpheniramine and mepyramine, but not by the type II antagonists buriamide and metiamide (68). This suggests another example of how histamine "arms" the eosinophil for its enhanced participation in the immune response.

D. Eosinophil Cytotoxicity

Possibly as a consequence of increased C3b receptors, histamine induces an increase in complement (C′)-dependent eosinophil cytotoxicity to schistosomula of *Schistosoma mansoni* in the human (69). When eosinophils were exposed to histamine followed by incubation with (1) antibody alone, (2) antibody plus C′, or (3) C′ alone, schistosomula death was greatest in the reaction mixtures which contained C′. Histamine alone did not influence antibody-dependent killing. Interestingly, while C′ was required for histamine-enhanced cytotoxicity, limiting the C′ concentration increased the histamine effect on schistosomula killing. In contrast, histamine enhanced C-independent, antibody-dependent eosinophil cytotoxicity in the rat (70).

Histamine has an intriguing effect on the eosinophil's potential for participation in inflammation. Histamine acts on the eosinophil to (1) mobilize, (2) stimulate and increase oxidative metabolism, (3) enhance the number of C3b membrane receptors, and (4) accelerate C′-dependent parasite death. These histamine-dependent activities appear to be mediated via histamine type I or combined type I/type II receptor responses. The neutrophil, in contrast, is not similarly affected by histamine. Because eosinophilia is frequently associated with mast cell–dependent reactions, histamine may play a unique role in potentiating this cell's participation in these responses.

E. Eosinophil-Induced Histamine Release

Eosinophils can elicit histamine release from mast cells. Activated eosinophils release peroxidase (EPO) and H_2O_2, which then combine to interact with mast cells (71). Mast cell histamine release occurs with low concentrations of EPO (25-30 mU) complexed with H_2O_2 and iodine, and is greater than secretion induced by neutrophil MPO. In addition, EPO complexes with mast cell granules, and in the presence of H_2O_2 and iodine, can further induce mast cell degranulation. This interaction can set off a positive feedback loop. Therefore, eosinophils

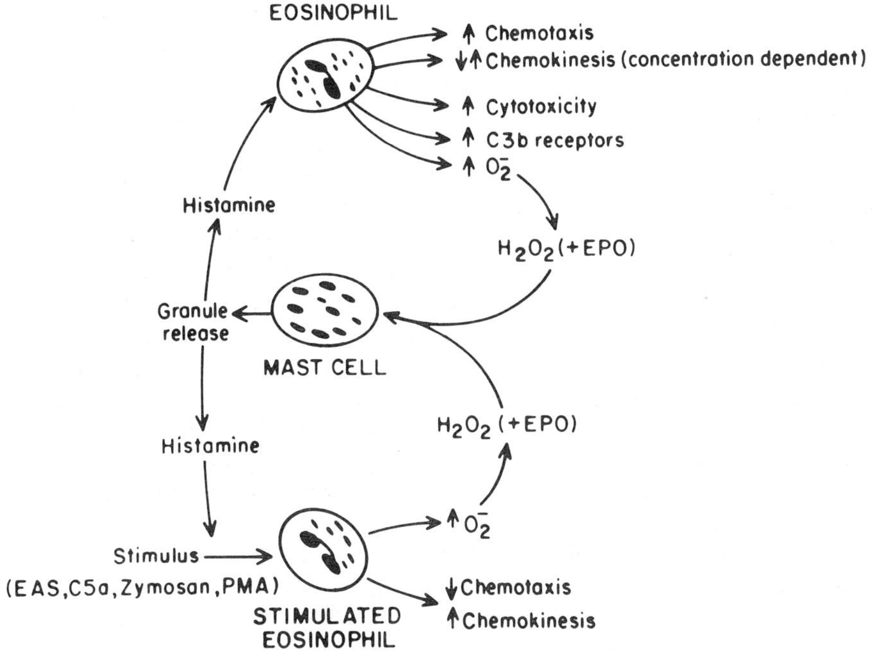

Figure 2 Histamine-eosinophil interactions. Histamine stimulates proinflammatory eosinophil functions which in turn can enhance further mast cell release of histamine. Only stimulated eosinophil chemotaxis appears to be inhibited by cell interaction with histamine.

attracted to the inflammatory site, possibly by histamine, release EPO and H_2O_2 (following stimulation by histamine or other activators), which can form an EPO/H_2O_2/halide system to stimulate further histamine release (Fig. 2). This process has the potential to become a self-perpetuating reaction. Thus, eosinophil-histamine interactions may initiate a cyclical, proinflammatory process, which would be beneficial if the stimulus were a parasite infection, but detrimental in hypersensitivity reactions such as anaphylaxis, allergic rhinitis, and asthma.

F. Eosinophil Heterogeneity

Conflicting results and wide variations in eosinophil-histamine responses of individual subjects have been reported by many (3,44,46,48,49,67). To explain these results, it was suggested that peripheral blood eosinophils may act as a heterogeneous population of cells when exposed to histamine (3,5,44,48). Bryant and coworkers (72) also found considerable variability in the eosinophil's chemotactic response to histamine, which depended on the patient's clinical diagnosis. In some patients, the chemotactic response of eosinophils to histamine formed a bell-shaped curve with maximal chemotaxis at 1×10^{-5} M and a decreased response at higher and lower doses. Cells from other patients, however, showed a linear, dose-dependent decrease of histamine chemotaxis. The majority of blood eosinophil isolates from patients in whom eosinophilia arose in association with asthma, parasite infection, or pulmonary eosinophilia (diseases with exogenous antigens and/or elevated IgE levels), had a linear response to histamine. In contrast, cells from patients whose disease was not associated with these conditions (e.g., neoplasia) had a bell-shaped response curve to histamine.

It is now well recognized that eosinophils are a heterogeneous population of cells, as noted by variations in cell density, which also reflects, or influences, functional activities (73-75). Therefore, it will be essential to reevaluate histamine's effects on eosinophils in relationship to cell density. An increased percentage of peripheral blood eosinophils are hypodense in patients with asthma, allergic rhinitis, parasitic infections, and certain types of hypereosinophilia (76-79). Further, hypodense eosinophils are functionally more active (80-83), and may therefore have very different responses to histamine than normodense eosinophils from normal subjects. Only when the eosinophil response to histamine is evaluated in relationship to cell density will we have a more complete knowledge or understanding of this relationship.

III. BASOPHILS

Although basophils secrete histamine which may initiate immediate hypersensitivity reactions, histamine may also regulate basophil function through a feedback loop (Fig. 3). The precise mechanism by which histamine accomplishes this is difficult to ascertain, as experiments of basophil function are most often conducted with mixed leukocyte suspensions.

A. Histamine Regulation of Chemotaxis

Although histamine is not chemotactic for basophils (4), it inhibits basophil chemotaxis to C5a, but not to fMLP or chemotactic factor from mitogen-stimulated human leukocytes derived chemotactic factor (LDCF) (Table 3). Histamine suppression of basophil chemotaxis is antagonized by the high doses of the type II antagonist metiamide. Although basophils respond to agonists such as dimaprit, PGE_1, IBMX, and dibutyryl cAMP with an increase in intracellular cAMP (22,84), it is difficult to know if increased cAMP affects basophil function in the same manner as observed in other granulocytes. If histamine inhibits basophil chemotaxis to C5a by increasing cAMP, it would also be expected to reduce cell movement to fMLP and LDCF. This variability in response to histamine suggests

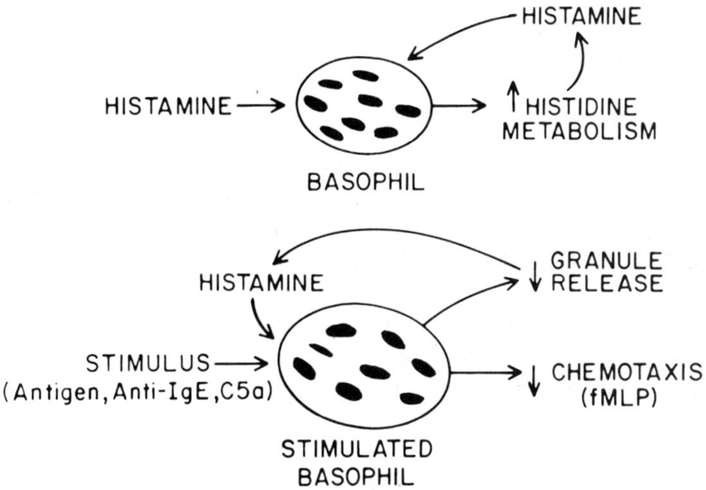

Figure 3 Histamine-basophil interaction. Although extracellular histamine enhances further histamine generation via increased histidine metabolism, it also inhibits stimulated basophil chemotaxis and granule release resulting in an anti-inflammatory effect.

Table 3 Effect of Histamine on Basophil Function

Function	Stimulus	Effect	Receptor		
			H_1	H_2	non-H_1, non-H_2
cAMP	Histamine	↑		+	
Chemotaxis	Histamine	0			
	C5a	↓		+?	
	fMLP, LDCF	0			
Histamine release	Antigen, anti-IgE	↓		+	
Histidine uptake	Histamine	↑	+		

that basophils, like eosinophils, may be a heterogeneous population of cells with some subpopulation(s) of cells responsive and others unresponsive to histamine.

B. Histamine-Regulation of Basophil Secretion

Antigen-dependent basophil histamine release involves glycolysis, requires calcium, and may be accompanied by an initial increase in intracellular cAMP (22). Interestingly, preincubation of leukocytes with histamine inhibited basophil histamine release to antigen and anti-IgE (85-87). This histamine effect operates during basophil activation rather than during the release phase (88) and is mediated through type II receptors (89,90). Cimetidine did not block histamine inhibition of basophil degranulation unless present prior to initiation of basophil histamine release by antigen or other secretogogue. Histamine type II antagonists (cimetidine, buriamide, metiamide, and ciotidine) consistently enhanced antigen-induced histamine release from basophils, whereas type I antagonists had no effect on this process (84). Further support that the negative feedback loop is mediated by a histamine type I receptor comes from studies showing that the type II agonist dimaprit also reduces basophil histamine release (89). Therefore, it is proposed that the effect of histamine type II antagonists on histamine inhibition of basophil degranulation is due to a blocking of the capacity of released histamine to act on other basophil type II receptors and in all likelihood does not have a self-feedback mechanism. Agents which block histamine metabolism but not type II receptors (aminoguanidine and amodiaquine) do not enhance histamine release (84).

Histamine type II receptor regulation of basophil histamine release depends on several factors. Tung and Lichtenstein (22) found the ability by which cAMP stimulating agonists (including type II receptor agonists) inhibit histamine release was inversely proportional to the concentration of antigen used to initiate the response. Moreover, Bergstrand and associates (91) found that regulation of histamine release was dependent on the concentration of the inhibitor (type II agonists). When stimulated histamine release from basophils was very low dimaprit suppression was great. In contrast, when the same concentration of dimaprit was evaluated in conditions of high basophil histamine release suppression was small. Furthermore, the capacity of various concentrations of histamine agonists to inhibit histamine release varied between individuals regardless of the degree of stimulated histamine release obtained. Finally, Hofman and coworkers (90) reported that effect of type I and type II receptor antagonists on histamine release was dependent on the antagonist concentration, the presence of exogenous histamine in the medium, the degranulation stimulus, and the type of target cells. Therefore, to evaluate the effectiveness of histamine release, many factors must be considered.

Confirmation that negative histamine feedback regulates the immediate hypersensitivity reaction in vivo is not established and the importance of the basophil response to histamine is not known. Peters et al. (92) found no differences in the basophil response to dimaprit between asthmatic and normal subjects when correlations were examined between dimaprit inhibition of histamine release in relationship to airway reactivity, allergic status, or baseline pulmonary function. Although the role of basophils in airway disease has not been fully established, it was suggested that basophils participate in the late-phase reactions of the nose (93). Failure, or an impairment, of histamine to modulate this basophil activity in the late-phase response would potentiate the release process and hence late allergic reactions in the nose. Peters et al. (94) have suggested that mast cells and mast cell mediators are primarily responsible for immediate-phase allergic reactions and initiation of the events which lead to the late phase in the lung; in contrast to basophils, histamine and type II agonists have no effect on human lung mast cell function. Study of the histamine-mast cell interaction in a highly purified cell suspension has been limited and compromised by cell heterogeneity. Nonetheless, most data suggest that the mast cell, unlike the basophil, is not responsive to histamine.

C. Histamine Metabolism

Although histamine appears to inhibit basophil chemotaxis and secretion through type II receptor activation, Stewart and Kay (95) have found that histamine acting through the type I receptor may enhance basophil uptake of histidine. High concentrations (1×10^{-3} M) of histamine were required to see this effect and type I antagonists (1×10^{-5} M) partially blocked the response. Histamine analogs did not increase histidine uptake. By this intriguing interaction, it would appear that high concentrations of histamine promote increased metabolism of histidine for further synthesis of histamine, thus resulting in a positive feedback mechanism for continued proinflammatory effects.

IV. CONCLUSIONS

Histamine interacts with neutrophils, eosinophils, and basophils; the net result of this interaction is complex. If there is a consistent pattern which emerges from our present information, it is that anti-inflammatory effects of histamine on granulocyte function follow type II receptor activation. Here histamine interacts with type II receptors and inhibits a variety of granulocyte functions, including chemotaxis, lysosomal enzyme release, and histamine release. In contrast, activation of histamine type I receptors can stimulate eosinophil chemotaxis, chemokinesis (at high histamine concentrations or by another stimulus), and oxidative metabolism, and can increase C3b receptors and cell cytotoxicity to promote this granulocyte's participation in inflammation.

However, a "completed" portrait of the histamine-granulocyte interactions and how this response influences inflammation is not fully ascertained. Although histamine can initiate inflammation by its actions on vascular permeability, smooth muscle contraction, and vasodilation, it also has the ability to down regulate the inflammatory response. What finally determines the net result of histamine on the overall inflammatory resonse has yet to be fully determined. Is it the number of various receptors activated, specificity to the stimulus, quantity of histamine, or predominance of cell type involved in the reaction that determines the complex interaction of histamine with granulocytes? These questions need further investigation. Yet current efforts to unravel the role of histamine in the inflammatory process have provided yet another example of how nature's intricate balance serves to maintain and establish homeostasis and host protection.

ACKNOWLEDGMENT

Supported in part by grants from the NIA AI 10404, 15685, and 23181.

REFERENCES

1. Weinstein, Y., K.L. Melmon, H. Bourne, and M. Sela, Specific leukocyte receptors for small endogenous hormones. J. Clin. Invest. 52:1349–1361 (1973).
2. Anderson, R., A. Glover, and A. R. Rabson, The *in vitro* effects of histamine and metiamide on neutrophil motility and their relationship to intracellular cyclic nucleotide levels, J. Immunol. 118:1690–1696 (1977).
3. Clark, R. A. F., J. A. Sandler, J. I. Gallin, and A. F. Kaplan, Histamine modulation of eosinophil migration, J. Immunol. 118:137–145 (1977).
4. Lett-Brown, and E. J. Leonard, Histamine-induced inhibition of normal human basophil chemotaxis to C5a, J. Immunol. 118:815–818 (1977).
5. Gallin, J. I., A. M. Weinstein, E. B. Cramer, and A. P. Kaplan, Histamine modulation of human eosinophil locomotion *in vitro* and *in vivo*. In The Eosinophil in Health and Disease, Mahmoud, A. A. F., Austen, K. F., and Simon, A. S., Eds. Grune & Stratton, New York (1980), pp. 185–203.
6. Hill, H. R., R. D. Estensen, P. G. Quie, N. A. Hogan, and A. D. Goldberg, Modulation of human neutrophil chemotactic responses by cyclic 3′, 5′-guanosine monophosphate and cyclic 3′,5′-adenosine monophosphate, Metabolism 24:447–456 (1975).
7. Zigmond, S. H., and J. G. Hirsch, Leukocyte locomotion and chemotaxis. New methods for evaluation and demonstration of a cell-derived chemotactic factor, J. Exp. Med. 137:387–393 (1973).

8. Seligman, B. E., M. P. Fletcher, and J. I. Gallin, Histamine modulation of human neutrophil oxidative metabolism, locomotion, degranulation, and membrane potential changes, J. Immunol. 130:1902–1909 (1983).
9. Hill, H. R., and P. G. Quie, Raised serum-IgE levels and defective neutrophil chemotaxis in three children with eczema and recurrent bacterial infections. Lancet 1:183–187 (1974).
10. Patrone, F., F. Dallegri, G. Lanzi, and C. Sacchetti, Reversal by cimetidine of histamine-induced inhibition of true chemotaxis in neutrophil polymorphonuclears, Res. Exp. Med. 176:201–205 (1980).
11. Radermecker, M., and M.-P. Maldague, Depression of neutrophil chemotaxis in atopic individuals: An H_2 histamine receptor response. Int. Arch. Allergy Appl. Immunol. 65:144–152 (1981).
12. Hirasawa, N., K. Ohuchi, M. Watanabe, and S. Tsurufuji, Role of endogenous histamine in post-anaphylactic phase of allergic inflammation in rats, J. Pharmacol. Exp. Ther. 241:967–973 (1987).
13. Rigal, D., J. C. Monier, and G. Souweine, The effects of histamine on leukocyte migration test in man, Cell. Immunol. 46:360–372 (1979).
14. Thulin, H., J. M. Hanifin, and R. Bryant, Leukocyte adherence in atopic dermatitis diminished responses to histamine and isoproternol, Acta Dermatol. (Stockh.) 60:235–238 (1980).
15. Petty, H. R., and J. W. Francis, Polymorphonuclear leukocyte histamine receptors: Occurrence in cell surface clusters and their redistribution during locomotion, Proc. Natl. Acad. Sci. U.S.A. 83:4332–4335 (1986).
16. Zurier, R. B., N. G. Weissmann, S. Hoffstein, S. Kammerman, and H. H. Tai, Mechanism of lysosomal enzyme release from human leukocytes: II. Effects of cAMP and cGMP, autonomic agonists, and agents which effect microtubule function, J. Clin. Invest. 53:297–309 (1974).
17. Busse, W. W., and J. Sosman, Histamine inhibition of neutrophil lysosomal enzyme release: An H_2 histamine receptor response, Science 194:737–738 (1976).
18. Busse, W. W., W. Cooper, and C. Anderson, Dimaprit inhibition of zymosan-stimulated beta-glucuronidase release from human granulocytes, Agents Actions 10:15–18 (1980).
19. Marone, G., L. L. Thomas, and L. M. Lichtenstein, The role of agonists that activate adenylate cyclase in the control of cAMP metabolism and enzyme release by human polymorphonuclear leukocytes, J. Immunol. 125:2277–2283 (1980).
20. Vickers, M. R., K. Milliner, D. Martin, and C. R. Ganellin, Histamine-induced inhibition of lymphocyte proliferation and lysosomal enzyme release from polymorphs may not be mediated via H_1- or H_2-receptors, Agents Actions, 12:630–634 (1982).
21. Fantozzi, R., S. Bruenlleschi, S. Cambi, P. Blandina, E. Masini, and P. F. Mannaioni, Autocoid and B-adrenergic agonist modulation of N-formyl methionyl-leucyl-phenylalanine evoked lysosomal enzyme release from human neutrophils, Agents Actions, 14:441–450 (1984).

22. Tung, R. S., and L. M. Lichtenstein, Cyclic AMP agonist inhibition increases at low levels of histamine release from human basophils, J. Pharmacol. Exp. Ther. 218:642–646 (1981).
23. Busse, W. W., and J. Sosman, Decreased H_2 histamine response of granulocytes of asthmatic patients, J. Clin. Invest. 59:1080–1084 (1977).
24. Busse, W. W., and S. D. H. Lantis, Impaired H_2 histamine granulocyte response in active atopic eczema, J. Invest. Dermatol. 73:184–187 (1979).
25. Busse, W. W., W. Cooper, D. M. Warshauer, E. C. Dick, H. L. Wallow, and R. Albrecht, Impairment of isoproterenol, H_2 histamine, and prostaglandin E_1 response of human granulocytes after inoculation *in vitro* with live influenza vaccines, Am. Rev. Respir. Dis. 119:561–569 (1979).
26. Herman, J. J., J. K. Brenner, and H. R. Colten, Inhibition of histamine release from human granulocytes by products of histaminase activity, Science 206:77–78 (1979).
27. Zeiger, R. S., Yurdin, D. L., and H. R. Colten, Histamine metabolism. II. Cellular and subcellular localization of the catabolic enzymes, histaminase and histamine methyl transferase, in human leukocytes, J. Allergy Clin. Immunol. 58:172–179 (1975).
28. Wojtecka-Lukasik, E., and S. Maslinski, Histamine 5-hydroxytryptamine and compound 48/80 activate PMN-leucocyte collagenase of the rat, Agents Actions 14:451–453 (1984).
29. Lehmeyer, J. E., and R. B. J. Johnston, Jr., Effect of anti-inflammatory drugs and agents that elevate intracellular cyclic AMP on the release of toxi oxygen metabolites by phagocytes: Studies in a model of tissue-bound IgG, Clin. Immunol. Immunopathol. 9:482–490 (1978).
30. Tarnok, I., and Z. Tarnok, Interaction of cimetidine and histamine with superoxide generated in a cell-free system and in neutrophils, Agents Actions 20:324–326 (1987).
31. Ozaki, Y., S. Kume, and T. Ohashi, Effects of histamine agonists and antagonists on luminol-dependent chemiluminescence of granulocytes, Agents Actions 15:182–188 (1984).
32. Meretey, K., M. I. K. Fekete, U. Bohm, and A. Falus, Effect of H_1 and H_2 agonists on the chemiluminescence of human blood mononuclear cells induced by phytohaemagglutinin, Immunopharmacology 9:175–180 (1985).
33. Meretey, K., U. Bohm, and A. Falus, Action of histamine on PHA chemiluminescence response of blood mononuclear cells in autoimmune patients, Agents Actions 18:254–257 (1986).
34. Clark, R. A., S. Szot, K. Venkatasubramanian, nd E. Schiffman, Chemotactic factor inactivation by myeloperoxidase-mediated oxidation of methionine, J. Immunol. 124:2020–2026 (1980).
35. Gespach, C., J. M. Launay, S. Emani, D. Bondoux, and C. Dreux, Biochemical and pharmacological characterization of histamine-mediated up-regulation of human platelet serotonin uptake. Evidence for a subclass of histamine H_2 receptors ($H_2\lambda$) highly sensitive to H_2 receptor antagonists, Agents Actions 18:115–119 (1986).

36. Arrang, J. M., M. Garbarg, and J.-C. Schwartz, Autoinhibition of brain histamine release mediated by a novel class (H_3) of histamine receptor, Nature 302:832–837 (1983).
37. Arrang, J. M., J. C. Schwartz, and W. Schumack, Stereoselectivity of the histamine H_3-presynaptic autoreceptor, Eur. J. Pharmacol. 117:109–114 (1985).
38. Ishikawa, S., and N. Sperelakis, A novel class (H_3) of histamine receptors on perivascular nerve terminals, Nature 327:158–160 (1987).
39. Arrang, J. M., M. Garbarg, J. C. Lancelot, J. M. Leconte, H. Pollard, M. Robba, W. Schumack, and J. C. Schwartz, Highly potent and selective ligands for histamine H_3-receptors, Nature 327:117–123 (1987).
40. Fantozzi, R., S. Bruenlleschi, L. Giuliattini, P. Blondina, P. Masini, G. Lavallo, and P. F. Mannaioni, Mast cell and neutrophil interactions: A role for superoxide anion and histamine, Agents Actions 16:260–264 (1985).
41. Stendahl, O., L. Molin, and M. Lindroth, Granulocyte-mediated release of histamine from mast cells. Effect of myeloperoxidase and its inhibition by anti-inflammatory sulfone compounds, Int. Arch. Allergy Appl. Immunol. 70:277–284 (1983).
42. Coble, B. L., M. Lindroth, L. Molin, and O. Stendahl, Histamine release from mast cells during phagocytosis and interaction with activated neutrophils, Int. Arch. Allergy Appl. Immunol. 75:32–34 (1984).
43. White, M. V., and M. A. Kaliner, Neutrophils and mast cells. I. Human neutrophil-derived histamine-releasing activity, J. Immunol. 139:1624–1630 (1987).
44. Goetzl, E. J., Modulation of human eosinophil polymorphonuclear leukocyte migration and function, Am. J. Pathol. 85:419–436 (1976).
45. Parish, W. E., Substances that attract eosinophils *in vitro* and *in vivo* and that elicit blood eosinophils, Antibodies Chemother. 19:233–270 (1974).
46. Clark, R. A. F., J. I. Gallin, A. P. Kaplan, The selective eosinophil chemotactic activity of histamine, J. Exp. Med. 142:1462–1476 (1975).
47. Turnbull, L. W., and A. B. Kay, Eosinophils and mediators of anaphylaxis: Histamine and imidazole acetic acid as chemotactic agents for human eosinophil leucocytes, Immunology 31:797–802 (1976).
48. Clark, R. A. F., J. I. Gallin, and A. F. Kaplan, The nature of histamine control of eosinophil localization. in Leucocyte Chemotaxis (Gallin, J. I., and Quie, P. G., Eds.), Raven Press, New York (1978), pp. 195–210.
49. Jones, D. G., and A. B. Kay, Chemotactic activity of guinea pig eosinophils for the ECF-A acidic tetrapeptides, histamine, histamine metabolites, and the effect of H_1- and H_2-receptor antagonists, Int. Arch. Allergy Appl. Immunol. 55:277–282 (1977).
50. Wadee, A. A., R. Anderson, and R. Shea, In vitro effects of histamine on eosinophil migration, Int. Arch. Allergy Appl. Immunol. 63:322–329 (1980).
51. Turnball, L. W., D. P. Evans, and A. B. Kay, Human eosinophils, acidic tetrapeptides (ECF-A) and histamine, Immunology 32:57–63 (1977).

52. Kownatzki, E., G. Till, M. Gogelmann, G. Terwort, and D. Gemsa, Histamine induces release of an eonsinophil immobilizing factor from mononuclear cells, Nature 270:67–69 (1977).
53. Vaughn, J., The function of the eosinophil leukocyte, Blood 8:1–15 (1953).
54. Speirs, R. S., Physiological approaches to an understanding of the function of eosinophils and basophils, Ann. N.Y. Acad. Sci. 59:706–731 (1955).
55. Archer, R. K., The eosinophil response in the horst to intramedullary and intradermal injections of histamine, ACTH and cortisone, J. Pathol. 72:87–94 (1956).
56. Eidinger, D., S. R. Wilkinson, and D. A. Rose, A study of cellular responses in immune reactions utilizing the skin window technique, J. Allergy Clin. Immunol. 35:77–85 (1964).
57. Vegad, J. L., and M. C. Lancaster, Eosinophil leukocyte-attracting effect of histamine in the sheep skin, Indian J. Exp. Biol. 10:147–148 (1972).
58. Litt, M., Studies in experimental eosinophilia: XI. Dependence of eosinophils, apparently induced by histamine, on acidity, Int. Arch. Allergy Appl. Immunol. 50:473–487 (1976).
59. Bryant, D. H., and A. B. Kay, Cutaneous eosinophil accumulation in atopic and non-atopic individuals: The effect of an ECF-A tetrapeptide and histamine, Clin. Allergy 7:211–217 (1977).
60. Pincus, S. H., Production of eosinophil-rich guinea pig peritoneal exudates, Blood 52:127–134 (1978).
61. Woodward, D. F., C. S. Speda, S. B. Hawley, and A. L. Nieves, Histamine H_1- and H_2-receptor involvement in eosinophil infiltration and the microvascular changes associated with cutaneous anaphylaxis, Agents Actions 17:121–125 (1985).
62. Woodward, D. F., C. S. Speda, S. B. Hawley, and A. L. Nieves, Conjunctival eosinophil infiltration evoked by histamine and immediate hypersensitivity, Invest. Opthal. Visual Sci. 27:1495–1503 (1986).
63. Mindel, J. S., A. H. Friedman, T. Haimov, A. B. Kharlamb, and J. M. Freilich, Eosinophil chemotaxis and anterior uveitis from topical dimaprit and nordimaprit, Invest. Opthal. Visual Sci. 27:1504–1511 (1986).
64. Pincus, S. H., A.-M. DiNapoli, and W. R. Schooley, Superoxide production by eosinophils: Activation by histamine, J. Invest. Dermatol. 79:53–57 (1982).
65. Anwar, A. R. E., and A. B. Kay, The ECF-A tetrapeptides and histamine selectively enhance human eosinophil complement receptors, Nature 269: 522–524 (1977).
66. Anwar, A. R. E., and A. B. Kay, Enhancement of human eosinophil complement receptors by pharmacologic mediators, J. Immunol. 121:1245–1250 (1978).
67. Kay, A. B., The role of the eosinophil, J. Allergy Clin. Immunol. 64:90–104 (1979).
68. Anwar, A. R. E., and A. B. Kay, H_1-receptor dependence of histamine-induced enhancement of human eosinophil C3b rosettes, Clin. Exp. Immunol. 42:196–199 (1980).

69. Anwar, A. R. E., J. R. McKean, S. R. Smithers, and A. B. Kay, Human eosinophil- and neutrophil-mediated killing of schistosomula of *Schisto-soma mensoni in vitro*: I. Enhancement of complement-dependent damage by mast cell-derived mediators and formyl methionyl peptides, J. Immunol. 124:1122–1129 (1980).
70. Capron, M., J. Rousseaux, C. Mazingue, H. Bezin, and A. Capron, Rat mast cell-eosinophil interaction in antibody-dependent eosinophil cytotoxicity to *Schistomsa Mansoni* schistosomula, J. Immunol. 121:2518–2525 (1978).
71. Henderson, W. R., E. Y. Chi, and S. J. Klebanoff, Eosinophil peroxidase-induced mast cell secretion, J. Exp. Med. 152:265–279 (1980).
72. Bryant, D. H., L. W. Turnbull, and A. B. Kay, Eosinophil chemotaxis to an ECF-A tetrapeptide and histamine: The response in various disease states, Clin. Allergy 7:219–226 (1977).
73. Pincus, S. H., W. R. Schooley, A. M. DiNapoli, and S. Border, Metabolic heterogeneity of eosinophils from normal and hypereosinophilic patients, Blood 58:1175–1181 (1981).
74. Winquist, I., T. Olofsson, I. Olsson, A. Persson, and T. Hallberg, Altered density, metabolism and surface receptors of eosinophils in eosinophilia, Immunology 47:531–539 (1982).
75. Prin, L., J. Charon, M. Capron, P. Gosset, H. Taelman, A. B. Tonnel, and A. Capron, Heterogeneity of human eosinophils. II. Variability of respiratory burst activity related to cell density, Clin. Exp. Immunol. 57:735–742 (1984).
76. Fukuda, T., S. L. Dunnette, C. E. Reed, S. J. Ackerman, M. S. Peters, and G. J. Gleich, Increased numbers of hypodense eosinophils in the blood of patients with bronchial asthma, Am. Rev. Respir. Dis. 132:981–985 (1985).
77. Kauffman, H. E., B. van der Belt, J. G. R. deMonchy, H. Bollens, G. H. Köeter, and K. deVries, Leukotriene C_4 production by normal density and low-density eosinophils of atropic individuals and other patients with eosinophilia, J. Allergy Clin. Immunol. 79:611–619 (1987).
78. Shult, P. A., M. Lega, S. Jadidi, R. Vrtis, T. Warner, F. M. Graziano, and W. W. Busse, The presence of hypodense eosinophils and diminished chemi-luminescence respond in asthma, J. Allergy Clin. Immunol. 81:429–437 (1988).
79. Frick, W., J. B. Sedgwick, and W. W. Busse, Hypodense eosinophils in aller-gic rhinitis, J. Allergy Clin. Immunol. 82:119–125, 1988.
80. Beswick, P. H., and A. B. Kay, The effects of an ECF-A and formyl methi-onyl chemotactis peptides on oxidative metabolism of human eosinophils and neutrophils, Clin. Exp. Immunol. 43:399–407 (1981).
81. Learn, D. B., and E. P. Brestel, A comparison of superoxide production by human eosinophils and neutrophils, Agents Actions, 12:485–488 (1982).
82. Prin, L., M. Capron, A. B. Tonnel, O. Bletry, and A. Capron, Heterogeneity of humans peripheral blood eosinophils: Variability in cell density and cyto-toxic ability in relation to the level and the origin of hypereosinophilia, Int. Arch. Allergy Appl. Immunol. 72:336-346 (1983).

83. Khalife, J., M. Capron, J.-Y. Cesbron, P.-C. Tai, H. Taelman, L. Prin, and A. Capron, Role of specific IgE antibodies in peroxidase (EPO) release from human eosinophils, J. Immunol. 137:1659–1664 (1986).
84. Tung, R., A. Kagey-Sobotka, M. Plaut, and L. M. Lichtenstein, H_2 antihistamine augment antigen-induced histamine release from human basophils *in vitro*, J. Immunol. 129:2113–2115 (1982).
85. Lichtenstein, L. M., and E. Gillespie, The effects of the H_1 and H_2 antihistamines on "allergic" histamine release and its inhibition by histamine, J. Pharm. Exp. Ther. 192:441–450 (1975).
86. Lichtenstein, L. M., G. Marone, L. L. Thomas, and F. J. Malveaux, The role of basophils in inflammatory reaction, J. Pharm. Exp. Ther. 195:65–69 (1978).
87. Norn, S., H. Parmin, and P. S. Skov, H_2 antihistamine (cimetidine) and allergic-inflammatory reactions, Allergy 35:357–361 (1980).
88. Bourne, H. R., K. L. Melmon, and L. M. Lichtenstein, Histamine augments leukocyte adenosine 3′5′-monophosphate and blocks antigenic histamine release, Science, 173:743–745 (1971).
89. Rising, T. J., and S. Lewis, A species comparison of the histamine H_2-receptor on mast cells and basophils, Agents Actions, 12:263–267 (1982).
90. Hofman, J., Z. Siergiejko, B. Kucyewska, and S. Chyrek-Borowska, The effect of H_1 and H_2 receptor blockers on immunological and nonspecific histamine release from isolated target cells, Arch. Immunol. Ther. Exp. 32:599–604 (1984).
91. Bergstrand, H., A. Björnsson, J. M. Frick, B. Lundquist, and B. A. Peterson, Anti-IgE-induced histamine release from human basophilic leukocytes: Depends on nature and concentration of inhibitor and secretagogue, Allergy, 37:503–512 (1982).
92. Peters, S. P., R. S. Tung, M. Chatham, E. R. Bleecher, and L. M. Lichtenstein, Inhibitability and enhanceability of basophil histamine release in asthmatic and normal subjects, Int. Arch. Allergy Appl. Immunol. 76:344–349 (1985).
93. Naclerio, R. M., D. Proud, A. G. Togias, N. F. Adkinson, Jr., D. A. Meyers, A. Kagey-Sobotka, M. Plaut, P. S. Norman, and L. M. Lichtenstein, Inflammatory mediators in late antigen-induced rhinitis, N. Engl. J. Med. 313: 65–70 (1985).
94. Peters, S. P., R. M. Naclerio, R. P. Schleimer, D. W. MacGlashan, U. Pipkorn, and L. M. Lichtenstein, The pharmacologic control of mediator release from human basophils and mast cells, Respiration 50(Suppl. 2):116–122 (1986).
95. Stewart, J., and A. B. Kay, Histamine increases histidine uptake by basophils, Clin. Exp. Immunol. 40:423–426 (1980).

Part II
Diseases with Abnormal Histamine-Induced Lymphocyte Function

7

Abnormal Leukocyte Responses to Histamine in Atopic Subjects: Clues to the Pathogenesis of the Atopic Diathesis

DENNIS J. BEER *Boston University School of Medicine, Boston, Massachusetts*

ROSS E. ROCKLIN *Boehringer Ingelheim Pharmaceuticals, Inc., Ridgefield, Connecticut, and New England Medical Center Hospital, Boston, Massachusetts*

I. INTRODUCTION

The occurrence of allergic rhinitis and/or asthma in many individuals with a familial background of such disorders, and the presence in the serum of these subjects of passive transfer activity to the relevant allergen led Coca and associates (1,2) to promote the term atopy for the propensity to develop an altered state of reactivity after natural exposure to specific allergens. As presently used, atopy connotes a familial tendency to manifest singly, or in combination, such conditions as rhinitis, asthma, urticaria, and eczematous (infantile or atopic) dermatitis. The passive transfer serum factor in these individuals has been identified as immunoglobulin E (IgE). The importance of specific IgE in the pathogenesis of the atopic diathesis is that this immunoglobulin isotype is homocytotropic for tissue mast cells and basophils, and thereby makes these cells the target for specific antigen. The binding of antigen to the Fab portions of IgE on these metachromatic cells results in the release of numerous potent inflammatory mediators (including histamine), which are the effector molecules causing the symptoms of allergic disease.

The atopic state is characterized by hyperactivity of IgE-synthesizing B cells, and by a decreased sensitivity to negative signals that are able to down regulate an inflammatory response. In this chapter, we will review recent investigations that have demonstrated abnormal leukocyte responses to histamine in atopic subjects and relate these abnormalities to the pathogenesis of the atopic state.

II. CORRELATIONS BETWEEN FUNCTIONAL AND PHENOTYPIC EXPRESSION OF HISTAMINE TYPE II RECEPTORS ON T LYMPHOCYTES

As reviewed in a previous chapter, a functionally distinct subset of CD8+ human T cells with suppressor capabilities has been defined by the presence of functional histamine type II (H_2) receptors. Martinez et al. (3) and Beer et al. (4) demonstrated decreased suppressor-cell activity in response to histamine in an atopic population. In the latter study (4), blood mononuclear cells were activated by histamine (10^{-5}-10^{-3} M) or 20 μg/ml of concanavalin A (Con A) for 24 hr, and after mitomycin C treatment, were cocultured with autologous mitogen-stimulated mononuclear cells. Suppressor-activity was measured as the percentage of suppression of mitogen-induced tritiated thymidine incorporated into cellular deoxyribonucleic acid (DNA). As shown in Figure 1, cells isolated from the atopic group were less able to generate histamine-induced suppressor activity than those isolated from the normal control group; however, there was some overlap between individual subjects in both groups. At each of the three concentrations of histamine employed, mononuclear cells from the atopic subjects generated significantly less mean suppressor activity than did mononuclear cells from normal controls. A histamine concentration of 10^{-3} M was required to induce the same degree of suppressor activity in the atopic group as that produced by 10^{-5} M histamine in the normal control group. The factors of age, sex, presence of asthma, and severity of symptoms did not differentiate the atopic subjects with regard to their ability to generate histamine-induced suppressor activity. This defect in suppressor cell response appeared to be specific for histamine, since Con A-induced suppressor activity in these subjects was not statistically different from such activity in the normal controls. This latter finding was in agreement with the work of Martinez et al. (3).

Several other groups of investigators have analyzed the suppressive effect of histamine on in vitro lymphocyte mitogenesis in atopic subjects (5-7). Wang and Zweiman (5) noted equivalent histamine-induced suppression in atopic and normal subjects. Strannegard and Strannegard (6) and Ogden et al. (7) found that lymphocytes from atopic individuals had increased sensitivity to histamine-induced suppression. The disparity in the results between the latter studies and

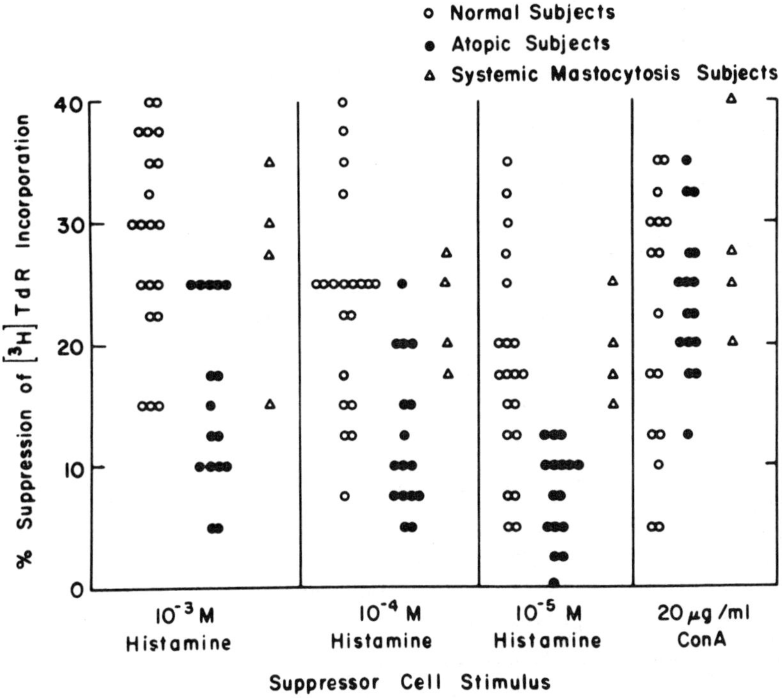

Figure 1 Suppressor activity of histamine and concanavalin A (Con A) in atopic subjects and controls. Activity was expressed as the percentage of suppression of tritiated thymidine [^{3}H]TdR incorporated into cellular DNA. Concanavalin A–induced suppressor activity was similar in all three groups. Despite the overlap of the percentages of histamine-induced suppression in individual subjects in the atopic population with percentages in the normal group, the atopic population as a whole had reduced histamine-induced activity ($p < 0.005$). Suppressor activity in the control group of patients (nonatopic patients with systemic mastocytosis) was similar to that in the normal control group.

those of Martinez et al. (3) and Beer et al. (4) may be accounted for by differences in the ages and clinical aspects of the patient populations studied, the concomitant use of pharmacotherapy and/or immunotherapy, or differences in experimental design.

In order to investigate whether the diminution in histamine-activated suppressor-cell function in atopic individuals was associated with alterations in phenotypic expression of histamine receptors, Beer et al. (4) used flow-cytometric analysis to enumerate specific histamine type I (H_1) and type II histamine receptors on T lymphocytes (8). As shown in Figure 2, T cells possess-

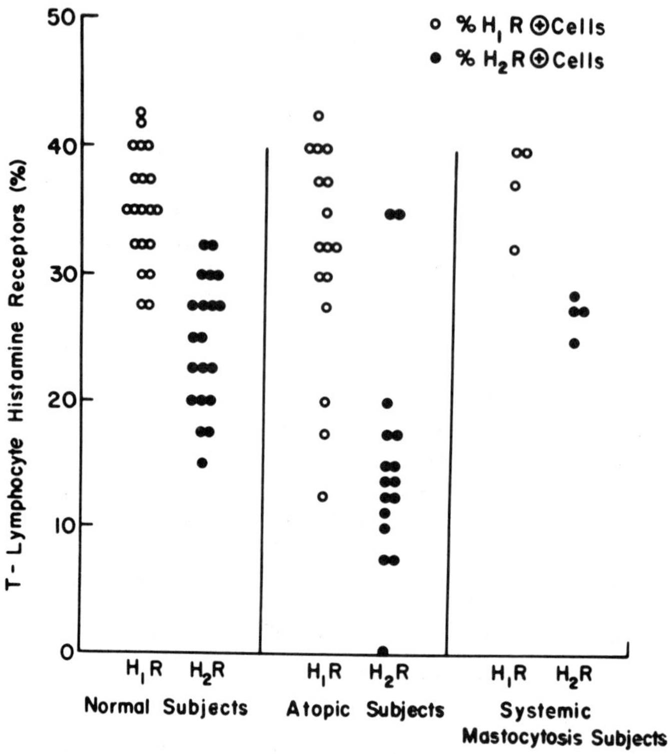

Figure 2 Percentage of T lymphocytes bearing histamine type I and type II receptors. The percentage of T cells bearing histamine type I receptors was similar in all three populations. Despite the overlap of the percentages of T lymphocytes bearing type II receptors in individual subjects in the atopic population with those in the normal group, the atopic population as a whole had a reduced percentage of these T cells ($p < 0.001$). Expression of the histamine type II receptor in the mastocytosis patients was similar to that in the normal controls.

ing type II histamine receptors were reduced significantly in atopic subjects, as compared with T cells from normal controls. The mean percentage of cells bearing type I receptors for histamine was identical in both groups. In the atopic population, regression analysis showed a significant correlation between the degree of histamine (10^{-4} M)-induced suppressor cell activity and the phenotypic expression of type II receptors (Fig. 3). The abnormality in histamine type II receptor expression in the atopic subjects may have reflected either a reduction in the number of T lymphocytes bearing the receptor or an abnormality in the binding affinity for histamine of the receptors themselves. The flow-cytometric technique was not sensitive enough to distinguish between these possibilities.

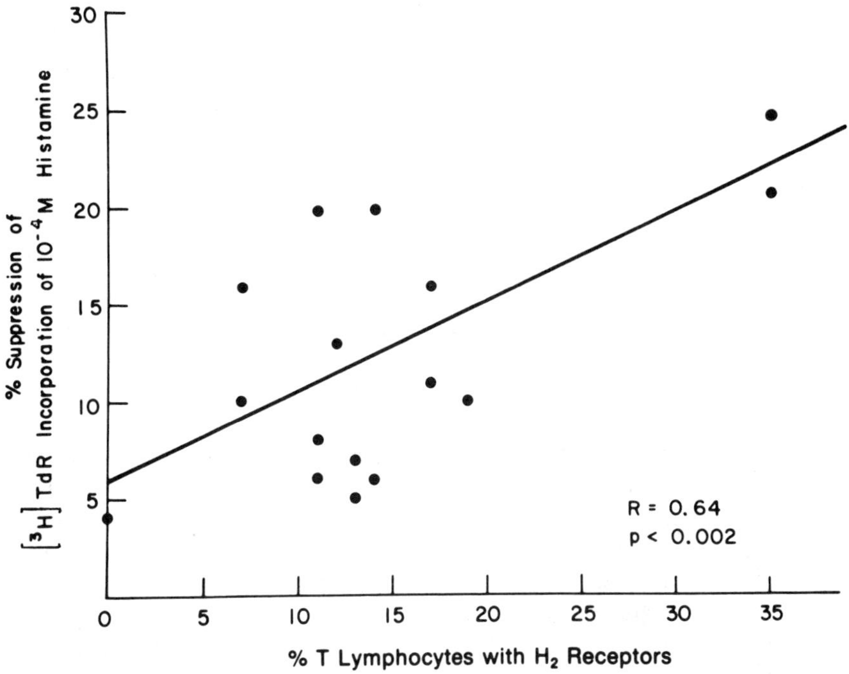

Figure 3 Regression analysis of histamine-induced suppression and percentage of T lymphocytes possessing histamine type II receptors in the atopic subjects. The line of best fit had a y intercept of 3.8 and a slope of 0.47. The correlation coefficient ($r = 0.64$) was statistically significant ($p < 0.002$).

One possible explanation for both the diminished histamine-induced suppressor activity and the type II receptor expression on T lymphocytes in the atopic population was that these findings represented secondary changes resulting from chronic in vivo stimulation of T cells by circulating histamine. Further experiments performed in parallel with the above studies (4) argued against this possibility. Mononuclear cells from nonatopic patients with systemic mastocytosis (a disease characterized by chronically elevated circulating histamine) exhibited histamine-induced suppressor activity (see Fig. 1) and expressed levels of histamine type II receptors on their T cells (see Fig. 2) that were indistinguishable from those of the normal control group. These latter findings mitigated against the observed abnormalities in atopic subjects as being secondary to in vivo desensitization or receptor down regulation. Rather, the data derived from the mastocytosis control group suggested that the suppressor-cell abnormalities observed in allergic subjects were related to a primary defect inherent to the atopic diathesis.

Table 1 Binding Characteristics of [^{3}H]Pyrilamine to Human T-cell Subsets from Normal and Atopic Subjects

	K_D (nM)[a]	Number of receptors/cell
Normal		
CD4	1.4 ± 1.1	6,838
CD8	1.3 ± 1.8	35,697
Atopic		
CD4	1.6 ± 2.1	8,005
CD8	1.8 ± 2.2	7,199

[a]Mean data ± SEM for 10 separate experimental subjects.

Having demonstrated a defect in histamine-induced suppressor activity in association with decreased histamine type II receptor expression on T lymphocytes from atopic individuals, Beer et al. (9) determined if there was a corresponding deficit in histamine type I phenotype and function in T cells of atopics. Paired aliquots of T cells from normal and atopic donors were studied in parallel for histamine type I receptor binding as measured by a radiolabeled type I receptor antagonist (tritiated pyrilamine) binding assay (10) and for histamine-induction of the CD4 cell-derived lymphokines, lymphocyte migration inhibitory factors (these lymphokines are discussed in detail elsewhere in this book) (11,12).

Table 1 depicts the "Ligand" computer program (13)-generated characteristics of tritiated pyrilamine binding to human T-cell subsets. The dissociation constants (K_D) for histamine type I receptor binding on CD4 lymphocytes from normal and atopic subjects were 1.4 ± 1 nM and 1.6 ± 2.1 nM, respectively. The K_D for histamine type I receptor binding on CD8 cells were similar. For the CD4 subpopulation, the mean number of histamine type I receptors per cell was 6838 and 8005 for normal and atopic individuals, respectively. For the CD8 subpopulation, the mean number of histamine type I receptors per cell was 35,697 and 7199 for normals and atopics, respectively.

The measurement of histamine type I receptor-bearing cell-derived histamine-induced lymphocyte migration inhibitory activity was quantitated in a modified Boyden chamber assay (11). Mononuclear cells from normals and atopics were incubated with histamine (10^{-4} M) and cimetidine (10^{-4} M). The conditioned cell-free supernatants were harvested, applied to a Sephadex G-100 column, and the column fractions were assayed for T-cell migration inhibitory activity. In each chromatogram, there were two areas of migration inhibitory activity which corresponded to molecular weights of 75 kDa ($LyMIF_{75K}$) and 35 kDa ($LyMIF_{35K}$). The generation of $LyMIF_{75K}$ and $LyMIF_{35K}$ activities were equivalent in normals and atopics.

Collectively, the present data and that described previously concerning histamine-induced suppressor activity (4) demonstrated that the phenotypic and functional differences in histamine type II receptor-bearing CD8 cells between normals and atopics does not extend to the type I receptor-bearing CD4 lymphocyte subset. As yet, the observed deficit in the number of histamine type I receptor sites present on CD8 cells of atopics has not been shown to have a functional correlate.

III. LYMPHOCYTE-MONOCYTE DYSFUNCTION AND MONONUCLEAR CELL SENSITIVITY TO PROSTAGLANDINS

As discussed in an earlier section of this book, proper functioning of the histamine-induced suppressor cell system involves obligatory interactions between lymphocytes and monocytes (14,15). A monokine, interleukin-1 (IL-1), has been shown to be obligatory for the activation of suppressor lymphocytes in response to histamine (14). In addition, type II receptor-bearing T lymphocytes when activated with histamine in the presence of IL-1 elaborate the lymphokine histamine-induced suppressor factor (HSF), which has been shown

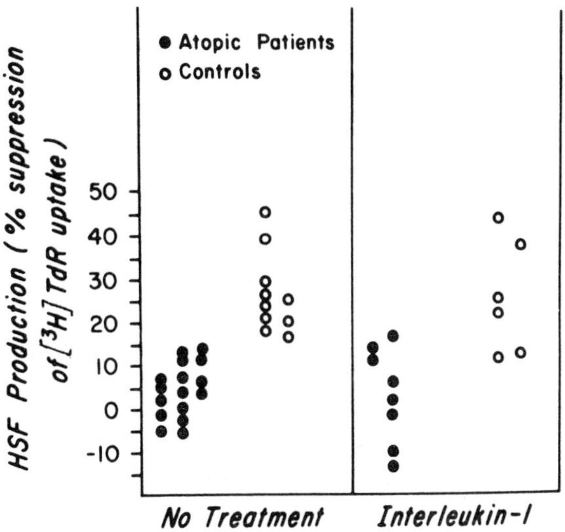

Figure 4 Histamine-induced suppressor factor (HSF) production by mononuclear cells from atopic and control subjects. The mean amount of HSF activity was lower in atopics than controls ($p < 0.01$). Interleukin-1 added to cultures did not improve the atopic response.

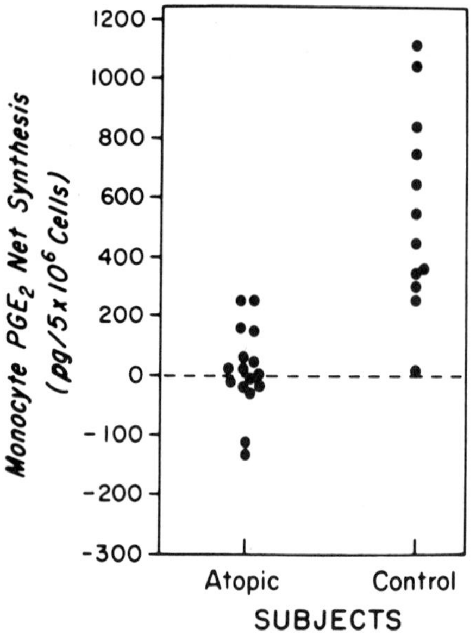

Figure 5 Prostaglandin E_2 (PGE_2) production by histamine-induced suppressor factor (HSF)–stimulated monocytes obtained from atopic patients and normal subjects. The mean net synthesis of PGE_2 by atopic monocytes was significantly reduced ($p < 0.01$) compared to that of control monocytes.

to augment the production of prostaglandins by monocytes (15,16). These latter compounds are thought to be intimately involved in the effector stage of this reaction and may directly suppress lymphocyte proliferation or lymphokine production, or further activate suppressor T cells (16,17).

Matloff et al. (18), investigating lymphocyte-monocyte dysfunction in atopic subjects, provided further evidence for an underlying defect in the immunoregulatory system of mononuclear cells of atopic subjects. Blood mononuclear cells were isolated from asymptomatic (out-of-season) atopic subjects and from normal controls and were incubated in the absence or presence of histamine (10^{-4} M) for 24 hr. Cell-free supernatants were harvested and assayed for the presence of histamine-induced suppressor factor. As shown in Figure 4, mononuclear cells from the atopic subjects generated significantly less HSF activity than cells from the nonatopic controls. This latter response was not corrected by the addition of exogenous IL-1 during the generation phase of the coculture assay. This suggested that deficient IL-1 production by monocytes from atopic individuals was not the cause of reduced HSF production. Although it was possible that lymphocytes from atopics failed to respond to IL-1 in an

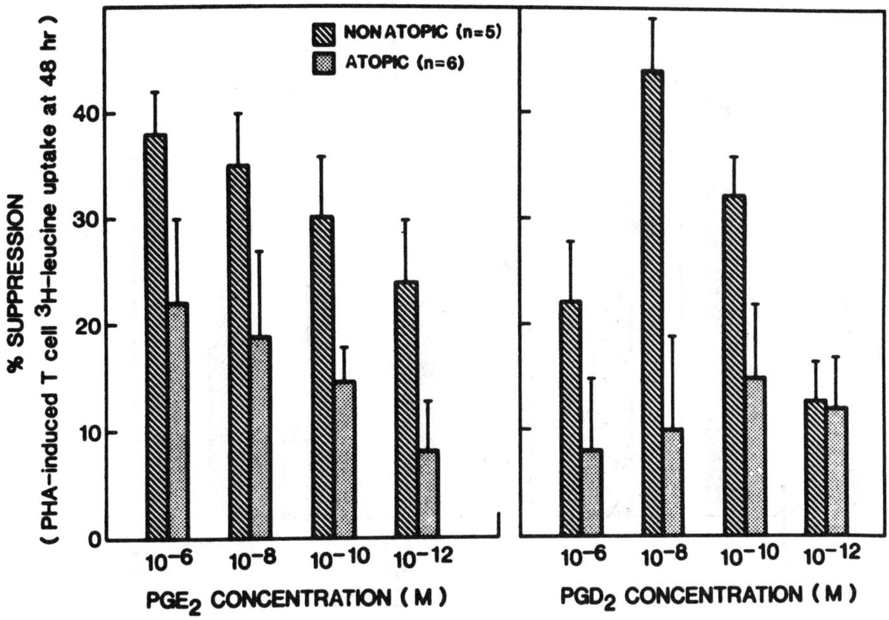

Figure 6 Dose-dependent suppression by PGE_2 and PGD_2 of PHA-induced [^{3}H]leucine uptake by nonatopic and atopic T cells. T-enriched cell populations were cultured for 48 hr with PHA and 10^{-6} and 10^{-12} M PGE_2 or PGD_2. Suppression of [^{3}H]leucine uptake by atopic cells by PGE_2 and PGD_2 was significantly less than that for nonatopic cells. Bars represent the mean ± SE percent suppression.

appropriate fashion, the finding of normal Con A-induced suppressor responses (an IL-1-dependent event (14)) in these individuals made this unlikely.

Matloff et al. (18) next investigated the adequacy of the second stage of histamine-induced suppression. Monocytes were isolated from atopics and normal control subjects, suspended in control or HSF-containing supernatants derived from one common pool, and cultured for 24 hr. The cell-free culture supernatants were harvested and assayed for their content of prostaglandin E_2 (PGE_2) by radioimmunoassay. As shown in Figure 5, monocytes form atopics produced significantly less PGE_2 in response to HSF than did control monocytes. The explanation for the decreased PGE_2 production by monocytes from atopics was not determined, but could have been related to reduced amounts of available substrate or altered arachidonic acid metabolic pathways.

Expanding upon disordered regulation of the immune and inflammatory responses of atopic subjects, Rocklin et al. (19) evaluated the effect of PGE_2

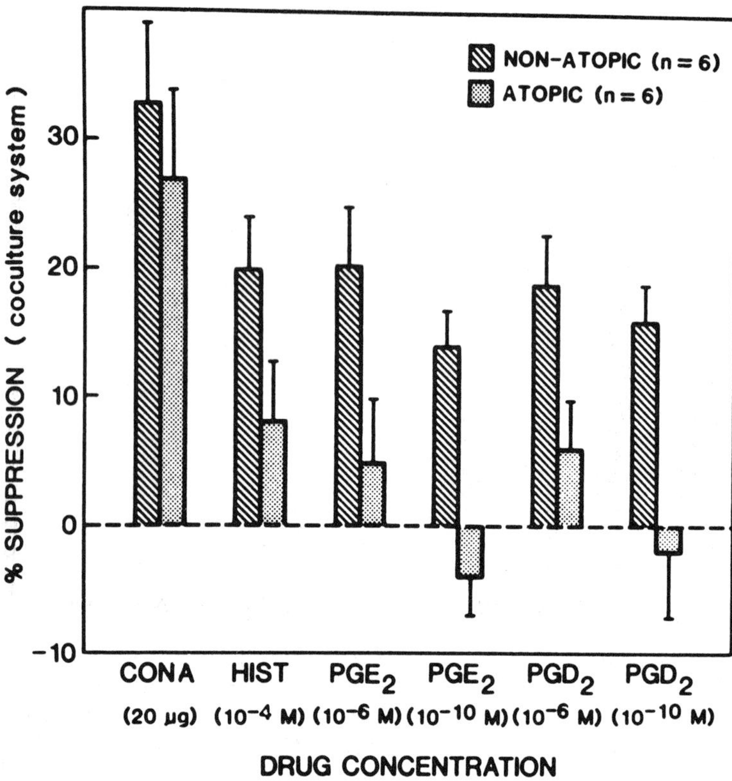

Figure 7 Coculture suppressor response by nonatopic and atopic mononuclear cells (MNCs). MNCs were preactivated by Con A (20 μg/ml), histamine (10^{-6} M), PGE_2 (10^{-4} M), and PGD_2 (10^{-6} or 10^{-10} M) for 48 hr, and then were cocultured with Con A–stimulated autologous indicator cells and suppression of lymphocyte proliferation was measured. Both PGE_2 and PGD_2 were capable of generating suppressor-cell activity in nonatopic MNCs. In contrast, atopic MNCs did not generate significant suppressor cell activity in response to PGE_2 (as well as histamine), but did develop normal suppressor-cell response to Con A. Bars represent the mean ± SE percent suppression.

and PGD_2 on several lymphocyte responses. Both PGE_2 and PGD_2 inhibited, in a dose-dependent manner (10^{-12}-10^{-6} M), mitogen-stimulated protein synthesis (as measured by tritiated leucine uptake) by T cells from normal individuals. Prostaglandin E_2- and PGD_2-induced suppression of tritiated leucine uptake by T cells from atopic subjects was significantly less than that for normal control cells (Fig. 6). Moreover, when mononuclear cells were preactivated with PGE_2 and PGD_2 in the first stage of a suppressor coculture assay and then combined in coculture with lectin-stimulated autologous indicator cells only the mononuclear cells from normal donors demonstrated significant suppressor-cell activity. Mononuclear cells from atopic donors did not generate significant suppressor activity in response to PGE_2 or PGD_2 (Fig. 7). These data, combined with those above showing decreased HSF generation and decreased PGE_2 production by monocytes suggested that mononuclear leukocytes from atopic individuals were less able to generate negative signals and less sensitive to the down regulating effects of these signals. In vivo, this disordered regulation could amplify the inflammatory components of the atopic diathesis.

IV. GRANULOCYTE RESPONSES TO HISTAMINE

Whether antigen is administered intranasally, intrabronchially, or intradermally, it causes pathophysiologic responses in atopic persons. The reaction occurring within minutes has been termed the early- or immediate-phase response. A subsequent reaction without additional exposure to antigen occurring within hours of the early reaction has been termed the late-phase response. This late-phase response has been observed in the skin (20,21), the lung (22,23), and the nose (24,25). This late-phase atopic response reflects tissue inflammation occuring after antigen exposure and recruitment of granulocytes ia a major component of this late-phase inflammatory response. Histamine, found to be present in both the early- and late-phase reactions, has a dual role in the late-phase inflammatory response. Although histamine can amplify an inflammatory reaction by its actions on vascular tone and permeability, it also has the ability to down regulate the inflammatory reaction. As reviewed in Chapter 6 by Sedgwick and Busse, histamine via interaction with type II receptors inhibits a variety of granulocyte functions including chemotaxis and lysosomal enzyme release. Defects in these down regulatory properties of histamine which have been reported in atopic subjects (26-28) account in part for the exaggerated inflammatory responses that these individuals display.

Adherence is one of the innate properties of leukocytes and is a requisite step in the process of chemotaxis. Thulin et al. (26) showed that histamine via interaction with a type II receptor inhibited leukocyte adherence. This group found that leukocytes from atopics were significantly less sensitive than those from normals to histamine-mediated inhibition of adherence. This diminished histamine type II receptor function of leukocytes from atopic subjects was paralleled by a lack of response to the beta agonist, isoproterenol. These findings suggested abnormal regulation in atopics of the adenylate cyclase/cyclic adenosine monophosphate (cAMP) system which may be part of the pathogenesis of the atopic diathesis (29).

Histamine has been shown to inhibit lysosomal enzyme (β-glucuronidase) release from neutrophils (30,31). Similar to the effects of catecholamines and prostaglandins of the E series, this inhibition of zymosan- or n-formyl-methionyl-leucyl-phenylalanine (fMLP)–induced lysosomal enzyme release has been associated with increases in intracellular concentrations of cyclic AMP (30,31). Busse and associates (27,28) have demonstrated an inability of histamine to increase intracellular cyclic AMP and down regulate β-glucuronidase release in leukocytes from patients with asthma and atopic dermatitis. Although not proven, it is possible that this decreased responsiveness to histamine may be contributing to the inflammatory component of these disorders.

V. CONTROL OF IMMUNOGLOBULIN E PRODUCTION

Antibody responses of the IgE isotype, like other immunoglobulin classes, are regulated by a finely tuned network of complex cellular and molecular interactions. The relevant cells in this immunologic network consists of B-lymphocyte precursors of IgE antibody–secreting cells, macrophages, and T lymphocytes. In this scheme, the T lymphocyte plays the most sophisticated regulatory role. There are helper and suppressor T cells capable of mutually interacting with one another as well as with IgE antibody–secreting cells.

The atopic state is characterized by hyperactivity of IgE-synthesizing B cells (32–34). Several observations in humans have suggested that suppressor T cell dysfunction may contribute to the increased production of IgE in the atopic diathesis. First, there is a frequent association of increased serum IgE levels with primary immunodeficiency disorders, each usually characterized by partial T-cell deficiency (35,36). In certain patients with ataxia-telangiectasia, Wiskott-Aldrich, and DiGeorge syndromes there is significant elevation of the serum IgE levels, presumably because there are sufficient numbers of helper/inducer T lymphocytes to initiate immunoglobulin synthesis, but insufficient numbers of suppressor T cells to inhibit it. Second, in disorders such as the hyper-IgE syndrome and severe atopic dermatitis with elevated serum IgE, there is a reduction in the number of cytotoxic/suppressor T cells of the CD8 phenotype (37). And third, there are elevated serum IgE levels in recipients of allogeneic bone marrow transplants during acute graft-versus-host disease. This is temporarily correlated with a deficiency in circulating suppressor T cells (38).

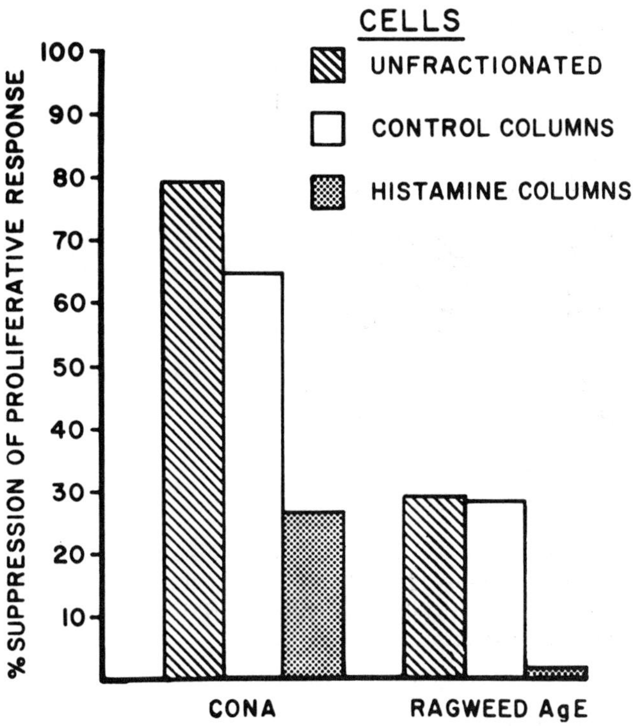

Figure 8 Generation of suppressor cells after chromatography over insolubilized conjugates of histamine or control columns. Mononuclear cells from patients treated with immunotherapy were chromatographed, and the nonretained cells were used to generate suppressor cells induced by ragweed or concanavalin A. Histamine columns, but not control columns, greatly depleted cells capable of exerting suppressor activity in response to antigen and, to a much lesser degree, in response to a nonspecific stimulus (concanavalin A).

The relation between histamine-induced suppressor-cell dysfunction in association with decreased histamine type II receptor expression and the regulation of in vivo biosynthesis of IgE is not clear. However, in view of the T-cell dependence of IgE antibody production, hyperproduction of specific IgE observed in the atopic diathesis might be a consequence of this altered regulatory function. In humans, it has been demonstrated that atopic individuals have reduced proportions of T cells with surface membrane receptors for the Fc portion of IgG, and that after successful immunotherapy, the proportion of these T cells

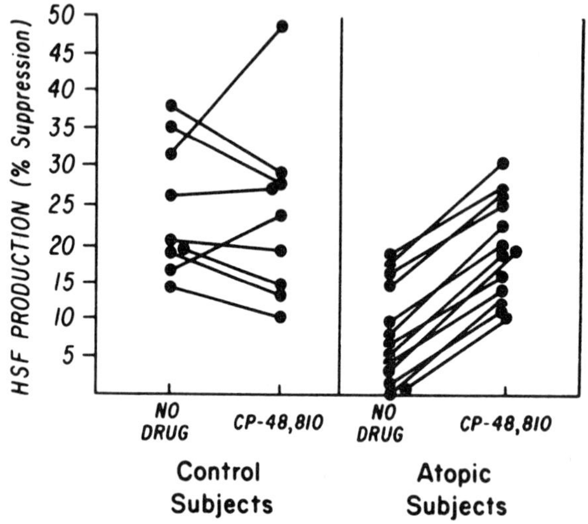

Figure 9 Effect of Fanetizole mesylate (2.5×10^{-4} M) on histamine-induced suppressor factor (HSF) production by mononuclear cells from control and atopic subjects. Fanetizole mesylate significantly enhanced HSF production by mononuclear cells from atopic subjects.

reached normal values (39). Cells within the latter subpopulation have been demonstrated to regulate immunoglobulin synthesis by suppressing T-dependent B-cell differentiation (40). In the context of the above studies (4,18), it has been shown that T lymphocytes bearing histamine type II receptors and expressing suppressor activity following stimulation with histamine also possess receptors for IgG (41). It is possible then that the observed abnormalities in atopic subjects reflect a global in vivo deficiency in antigen-nonspecific and/or antigen-specific suppressor-cell activity, either or both of which may be necessary for the dampening of IgE antibody production.

Indirect evidence for this hypothesis is provided by a study by Rocklin et al. (42), in which it was demonstrated that ragweed antigen-specific suppressor T lymphocytes could be detected in ragweed-allergic individuals after 6 and 12 months of immunotherapy, but not prior to therapy. When lymphocytes were taken from treated patients and passed over columns containing insolubilized histamine, antigen-specific suppressor T cells that could be activated by ragweed antigen were deleted (Fig. 8). These results indicated that antigen-specific suppressor T cells belonging to the subpopulation of lymphocytes bearing histamine receptors were generated during immunotherapy, and failure to detect these cells in untreated patients may be a reflection of a basic defect leading to the atopic diathesis.

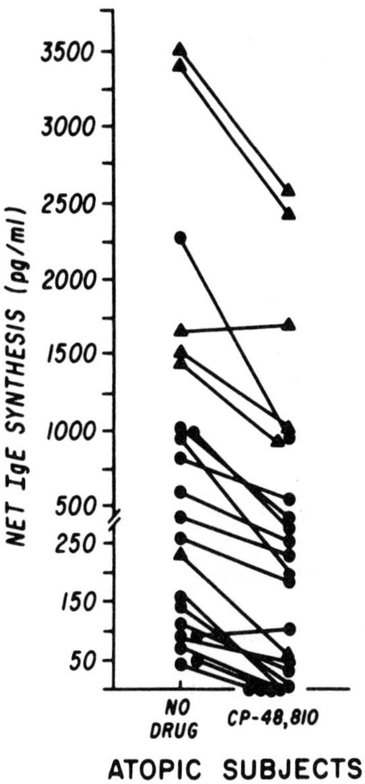

Figure 10 Effect of Fanetizole mesylate (2.5×10^{-4} M) on de novo IgE synthesis by atopic patients without eczema (●—●) and patients with eczema (▲—▲). Fanetizole mesylate significantly reduced spontaneous in vitro IgE production in atopic subjects.

Rocklin et al. (43) analyzed the effect of Fanetizole mesylate, a new immunostimulating drug similar in activity to levamisole, on histamine-induced suppressor activity and IgE synthesis in vitro. When this compound was added with histamine to mononuclear cells from atopic subjects during the generation stage of the coculture assay, their ability to suppress the subsequent mitogen-induced lymphocyte proliferation response was equivalent to that of suppressor cells from normal donors. As shown in Figure 9, the restorative effect of Fanetizole mesylate was a consequence of enhanced production of HSF. It was not related to enhancement of prostaglandin production. In addition, in vitro IgE synthesis by mononuclear cells from atopics was reduced significantly in the presence of Fanetizole mesylate (Fig. 10). This compound was found not to be

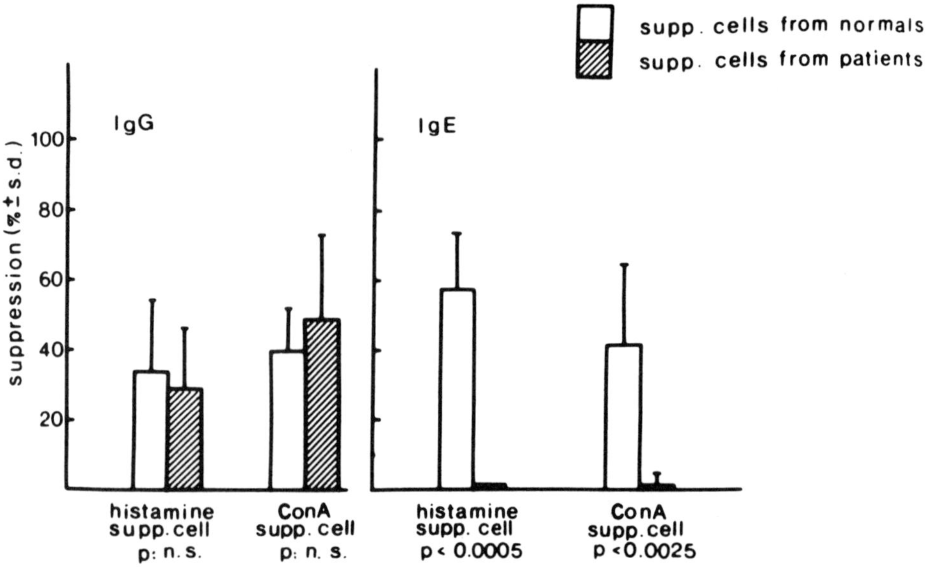

Figure 11 Percentage of suppression of IgG (left panel) and IgE (right panel) in vitro synthesis of normal cells by suppressor cells (histamine or Con A–induced) from nonatopic individuals (open bar) or atopic patients (hatched bar).

cytotoxic for B cells, and in fact the drug did not significantly alter pokeweed mitogen-induced IgG synthesis by atopic or normal mononuclear cells. These results suggested that Fanetizole mesylate could partially correct an in vitro immunoregulatory defect in atopic individuals and could reduce IgE production. Whether this represented cause and effect has not been determined and clinical trials of this drug in the treatment of allergic subjects have not been published.

More direct evidence for a relationship between the decreased histamine-induced suppressor-cell activity and the increased production of IgE in atopics has been provided in a study by Hebert et al. (44). These investigators harvested blood lymphocytes from untreated grass-sensitive, asymptomatic (out-of-season) atopic subjects and from nonatopic donors, and treated these cells with media alone (control), with histamine (10^{-3} M), or with 10 μg/ml Con A. After irradiation, these suppressor cells were added to cultures of blood lymphocytes from nonatopics stimulated with pokeweed mitogen. The effect of these suppressor cells on the in vitro IgG and IgE synthesis was then determined by a reverse hemolytic plaque assay. Histamine-induced suppressor-cell activity from normal donors caused a significant suppression of pokeweed mitogen-driven IgG and IgE synthesis by normal cells. Although histamine-activated suppressor cells from atopic subjects significantly suppressed pokeweed mitogen-induced IgG production of normal cells, they did not suppress IgE production (Fig. 11). In addition, Con A-induced suppressor cells from nonatopic donors behaved like those induced by histamine in significantly suppressing the pokeweed mitogen-driven IgG and IgE synthesis. When generated from atopic patients, Con A-activated suppressor cells decreased the IgG, but not the IgE production (Fig. 11). This study (44) suggested a defective Con A-induced suppressor activity toward IgE production in atopics which had not been reported to be the case when the nonspecific response to phytohemagglutin had been examined (3,4).

VI. CONCLUSIONS

Traditionally, histamine has been considered primarily as an effector molecule in immediate-type hypersensitivity responses. Over the past 2 decades, it has become apparent that histamine and other small molecular weight mediators such as prostaglandins and beta-mimetic catecholamines are part of the physiologic process that regulates both immune and inflammatory events. In particular, histamine, by interaction with type II receptors, generally induces either directly or indirectly (elaboration of a suppressor factor) an inhibitory signal to mononuclear cells and granulocytes which participate in inflammatory reactions.

The atopic state is characterized by disordered regulation of IgE synthesis and a decreased sensitivity to inhibitory signals that are able to down regulate an inflammatory response. In this context, the abnormal mononuclear cells and granulocyte responses to histamine in atopic subjects that were detailed in this chapter can be viewed as contributing to the pathogenesis of atopy. Further understanding of this and other immunoregulatory defects in the atopic diathesis may lead to new therapeutic approaches. At one level, as exemplified by the in vitro studies with Fanetizole mesylate (43), such knowledge might enable the prevention or suppression of IgE synthesis. At another level, approaches may be devised to augment the effects of inhibitory signals on the inflmmatory component of the allergic diathesis.

ACKNOWLEDGMENTS

This work was supported by U.S. Public Health Service Grants HL-32802 and AI-16362 and by a Trudeau Scholar Award from the American Lung Association.

We thank Sharon Davignon for her expert assistance in the preparation of this manuscript.

REFERENCES

1. Coca, A. F., and R. A. Cooke, On the classification of the phenomena of hypersensitiveness, J. Immunol. 8:163–182 (1923).
2. Coca, A. F., and E. F. Grove, Studies in hypersensitiveness. XIII. A study of the atopic reagins, J. Immunol. 10:445–464 (1925).
3. Martinez, J. D., J. Santos, D. J. Stechschulte, and N. I. Abdou, Nonspecific suppressor cell function in atopic subjects, J. Allergy Clin. Immunol. 64: 485–490 (1979).
4. Beer, D. J., M. E. Osband, R. P. McCaffrey, N. A. Soter, and R. E. Rocklin, Abnormal histamine-induced suppressor-cell function in atopic subjects. N. Engl. J. Med. 306:454–458 (1982).
5. Wang, S. R., and B. Zweiman, Histamine suppression of human lymphocyte responses to mitogens, Cell. Immunol. 36:28–36 (1978).
6. Strannegard, I. L., and O. Strannegard, Increased sensitivity of lymphocytes from atopic individuals to histamine-induced suppression, Scand. J. Immunol. 6:1225–1231 (1977).
7. Ogden, B. E., G. G. Krueger, and H. R. Hill, Lymphocyte suppressor activity in atopic eczema, Clin. Exp. Immunol. 35:269–275 (1979).
8. Osband, M. E., E. B. Cohen, R. P. McCaffrey, and H. M. Shapiro, A technique for the flow cytometric analysis of lymphocytes bearing histamine receptors, Blood 56:923–925 (1980).
9. Beer, D. J., K. Armour, K. Doyle, W. Cameron, and R. E. Rocklin, Normal phenotypic and functional expression of histamine type I (H_1) receptors on $T4^+$ lymphocytes from atopic individuals, Clin. Res. 34:276A (1986).
10. Cameron, W., K. Doyle, and R. E. Rocklin, Histamine type I (H_1) receptor radioligand binding studies on normal T cell subsets, B cells, and monocytes, J. Immunol. 136:2116–2120 (1986).
11. Berman, J. S., R. G. McFadden, W. W. Cruikshank, D. M. Center, and D. J. Beer, Functional characteristics of histamine receptor-bearing mononuclear cells. II. Identification and characterization of two histamine-induced human lymphokines that inhibit lymphocyte migration, J. Immunol. 133: 1495–1504 (1984).
12. Berman, J. S., W. W. Cruikshank, D. M. Center, A. C. Theodore, and D. J. Beer, Chemoattractant lymphokines specific for the helper/inducer T-lymphocyte subset, Cell. Immunol. 95:105–112 (1985).
13. Munson, P. J., and D. Rodbard, "Ligand": A versatile computerized approach for characterization of ligand-binding systems, Anal. Biochem. 107: 220–239 (1980).
14. Beer, D. J., C. A. Dinarello, L. J. Rosenwasser, and R. E. Rocklin, Human monocyte-derived soluble product(s) has an accessory function in the generation of histamine and concanavalin A-induced suppressor T cells, J. Clin. Invest. 70:393–400 (1982).
15. Beer, D. J., L. J. Rosenwasser, C. A. Dinarello, and R. E. Rocklin, Cellular interactions in the generation and expression of histamine-induced suppressor activity, Cell. Immunol. 69:101–112 (1982).

16. Rocklin, R. E., I. Kiselis, D. J. Beer, P. Rossi, F. Maggi, and J. Bellanti, Augmentation of prostaglandin and thromboxane production *in vitro* by monocytes exposed to histamine-induced suppressor factor (HSF), Cell. Immunol. 77:92–98 (1983).
17. Staszak, C., and J. S. Goodwin, Is prostaglandin a mediator for the inhibitory action of histamine, hydrocortisone, and isoproterenol, Cell. Immunol. 54:351–461 (1980).
18. Matloff, S. M., I. K. Kiselis, and R. E. Rocklin, Reduced production of histamine-induced suppressor factor (HSF) by atopic mononuclear cells and decreased prostaglandin E_2 output by HSF-stimulated atopic monocytes, J. Allergy Clin. Immunol. 72:359–364 (1983).
19. Rocklin, R. E., L. Thistle, and C. Audera, Decreased sensitivity of atopic mononuclear cells to prostaglandin E_2 (PGE_2) and prostaglandin D_2 (PGD_2). J. Immunol. 135:2033–2039 (1985).
20. Dolovich, J., F. E. Hargreave, R. Chalmers, K. J. Shier, J. Gauldie, and J. Bienenstock, Late cutaneous allergic responses in isolated IgE-dependent reactions, J. Allergy Clin. Immunol. 52:38–46 (1973).
21. Solley, G. O., G. L. Gleich, R. E. Jordon, and A. L. Schroeter, The late phase of the immediate wheal and flare skin reaction: its dependence upon IgE antibodies, J. Clin. Invest. 58:408–420 (1976).
22. Pepys, J., and B. J. Hutchcroft, Bronchial provocation tests in etiologic diagnosis and analysis of asthma, Am. Rev. Resp. Dis. 112:829–859 (1975).
23. Robertson, D. G., A. T. Kerigan, F. E. Hargreave, R. Chalmers, and J. Dolovich, Late asthmatic responses induced by ragweek pollen allergen, J. Allergy Clin. Immunol. 54:244–254 (1974).
24. Dvoracek, J. E., J. W. Yunginger, E. B. Kerr, R. E. Hyatt, and G. J. Gleich, Induction of normal late-phase reactions by insufflation of ragweed-pollen extract, J. Allergy Clin. Immunol. 73:363–368 (1984).
25. Naclerio, R. M., D. Proud, A. G. Togias, N. F. Adkinson, Jr., D. A. Meyers, A. Kagey-Sabotka, M. Plaut, P. S. Norman, and L. M. Lichtenstein, Inflammatory mediators in late antigen-induced rhinitis, N. Engl. J. Med. 313:65–70 (1985).
26. Thulin, H., J. M. Hanifin, and R. Bryant, Leukocyte adherence in atopic dermatitis: Diminished response to histamine and isoproterenol, Acta Derm. Venereol. (Stockh.) 60:235–238 (1980).
27. Busse, W. W., and J. Sosman, Decreased H_2 histamine response of granulocytes of asthmatic patients, J. Clin. Invest. 59:1080–1087 (1977).
28. Busse, W. W., and S. D. H. Lantis, Impaired H_2 histamine granulocyte response in active atopic eczema, J. Invest. Dermatol. 73:184–187 (1979).
29. Szentivanyi, A., The beta-adrenergic theory of the atopic abnormality in asthma, J. Allergy 42:203–232 (1968).
30. Zurier, R. B., N. G. Weissmann, S. Hoffstein, S. Kammerman, and H. H. Tai, Mechanism of lysosomal enzyme release from human leukocytes: II. Effects of cAMP and cGMP, autonomic agonists, and agents which effect microtubule function, J. Clin. Invest. 53:297–309 (1974).

31. Fantozzi, R., S. Brunelleschi, S. Cambi, P. Blandina, E. Masini, and P. F. Mannaioni, Autacoid and β-adrenergic agonist modulation of N-formyl-methionyl-leucyl-phenylalanine evoked lysosomal enzyme release from human neutrophils, Agents Actions 14:441–450 (1984).
32. Tada, T., Regulation of reagenic antibody formation in animals, Prog. Allergy 19:122–194 (1975).
33. Ishizaka, K., and T. Ishizaka, Mechanisms of reagenic hypersensitivity and IgE antibody response, Immunol. Rev. 41:109–148 (1978).
34. Katz, D. H., Control of the IgE antibody production by suppressor substances, J. Allergy Clin. Immunol. 62:44–55 (1978).
35. Waldmann, T. A., S. H. Polmar, S. T. Balestra, M. C. Jost, K. M. Bruce, and W. D. Terry, Immunoglobulin E in immunologic deficiency diseases. II. Serum IgE concentration of patients with acquired hypogammaglobulinema, thymoma and hypogammaglobulinemia, myotonic dystrophy, intestinal lymphagiectasia, and Wiskott-Aldrich syndrome, J. Immunol. 109:304–310 (1972).
36. Leung, D. Y. M., and R. S. Geha, Regulation of the human IgE antibody response. Int. Rev. Immunol. 2:75–125 (1987).
37. Strannegard, O., and I.-L. Strannegard, T lymphocyte numbers and function in human IgE-mediated allergy, Immunol. Rev. 41:149–170 (1978).
38. Geha, R. S., J. M. Rappaport, F. J. Twarog, R. Parkman, F. S. Rosen, Increased serum immunoglobulin E levels following allogeneic bone marrow transplantation, J. Allergy Clin. Immunol. 66:78–81 (1980).
39. Canonica, G. W., M. C. Mingari, G. Melioli, M. Colombatti, and L. Moretta, Imbalances of T cell subpopulations in patients with atopic diseases and effect of specific immunotherapy, J. Immunol. 123:2669–2672 (1979).
40. Moretta, L., S. R. Webb, C. E. Grossi, P. M. Lydyard, and M. D. Cooper, Functional analysis of two human T-cell subpopulations: Help and suppression of B-cell responses by T cells bearing receptor for IgM or IgG, J. Exp. Med. 146:184–200 (1977).
41. Rocklin, R. E., J. Breard, S. Gupta, R. A. Good, and K. L. Melmon, Characterization of the human blood lymphocytes that produce a histamine-induced suppressor factor, Cell. Immunol. 51:226–237 (1980).
42. Rocklin, R. E., A. L. Sheffer, D. K. Greineder, and K. L. Melmon, Generation of antigen-specific suppressor cells during allergy desensitization, N. Engl. J. Med. 302:1213–1219 (1980).
43. Rocklin, R. E., Z. Hemady, S. Matloff, I. Kiselis, and M. Lima, Correction of an *in vitro* immunoregulatory defect in atopic subjects by the immunostimulating drug Fanetizole mesylate (CP-48, 810), Int. J. Immunopharmacol. 6:1–8 (1984).
44. Hebert, J., R. Beaudoin, M. Girard, A. Beaulieu, L. Perelmutter, and C. Tremblay, The regulatory effect of histamine on the immune response. III. Defect on *in vitro* IgE production in atopics, Ann. Allergy 53:138–142 (1984).

8

Autoimmune Thyroid Disease

ROBERT VOLPÉ *University of Toronto and the Wellesley Hospital, Toronto, Ontario, Canada*

I. INTRODUCTION

Over the past 2 decades, our laboratory has been devoted to the pursuit of the immunoregulatory disturbance(s) which may form the basis of human autoimmune thyroid disease (AITD). Clearly, AITD encompasses clinically disparate disorders. On the one hand, Graves' (Basedow's, Parry's) disease (GD) is primarily associated with hyperthyroidism whereas on the other hand Hashimoto's thryoiditis (HT) and its variants are most commonly manifested by either a euthyroid goiter or a hypothyroid state. Not only may the clinical expression of these conditions be markedly different, but there are also some genetic, pathogenetic, pathologic, and immunologic elements that differ between them (1,2). In my view, therefore, the autoimmune thyroid diseases cannot be considered merely a spectrum of the same condition (1,2). The genetic differences result in different pathways leading to what should be considered separate entities however closely they are related to one another. However, there are certain features which are similar, if not identical, in the various disorders, and thus certain principles may be applied to them all.

Graves' disease is currently defined as a form of hyperthyroidism with a diffuse goiter, due to the stimulation of the thyrotrophin (TSH) receptor by a TSH-receptor antibody termed thyroid-stimulating antibody (TSAb). An appropriate new designation would be autoimmune thyrotoxicosis (1). The second major autoimmune thyroid disorder, namely, autoimmune thyroiditis, was first described by Hashimoto in 1912 (3). He reported patients with goiter in whom the thyroid histology was characterized by diffuse lymphocytic infiltration, atrophy of the parenchymal cells, fibrosis, and eosinophilic change in parenchymal cells. In the chronic fibrous thyroiditis variant, fibrosis predominates and lymphocytic infiltration is less marked. In the lymphocytic thyroiditis of childhood and adolescence, Askanazy cells and germinal centers are less obvious than in the adult form. The titers of thyroid antibodies are generally lower in this group when compared to adults, and indeed are often negative (4). Postpartum thyroiditis is another variant of autoimmune thyroiditis occurring as a transient clinical disorder, commencing 2-6 months following a pregnancy, although it sometimes does culminate in a chronic form (5). In idiopathic myxedema, now clearly due to autoimmune thyroiditis, the gland is characterized by atrophy rather than by hypertrophy. The atrophic, asymptomatic form is clinically occult and is often discovered only at autopsy. Although there are subtle genetic and pathogenetic differences between these variants, the generic term autoimmune thyroiditis is appropriate for the entire group. Evidence will be cited below describing the participation of an autoimmune process in these conditions, primarily related to a defect in immunoregulation. The overlap between GD and HT has long been recognized. Indeed, both diseases frequently aggregate in the same family. There are several reports of identical twins, one with GD and the other with HT. In fact, both GD and HT can coexist in the same thyroid gland and the clinical expression will depend upon which condition predominates (1).

Increasing evidence from our laboratory (6-13) and from others (14-20) favors the view that the underlying disorder in human AITD is a genetically induced antigen-specific defect in suppressor T-lymphocyte function. The major elements of this hypothesis are depicted schematically in Fig. 1. As will be noted below, this hypothesis is not universally accepted and other hypotheses will be discussed briefly. However, this author feels that the current evidence favoring the above hypothesis is increasingly compelling and no other seems to accord as well with clinical observations, available research data, and reasoned interpretation.

While there is now positive evidence bearing on each point depicted in Figure 1, an argument was advanced as early as 1970-1972 (21,22) (before such evidence was available) suggesting that there must be a specific defect in "immune surveillance" to account for AITD. The theoretical possibilities which might account for the development of an organ-specific autoimmune disease

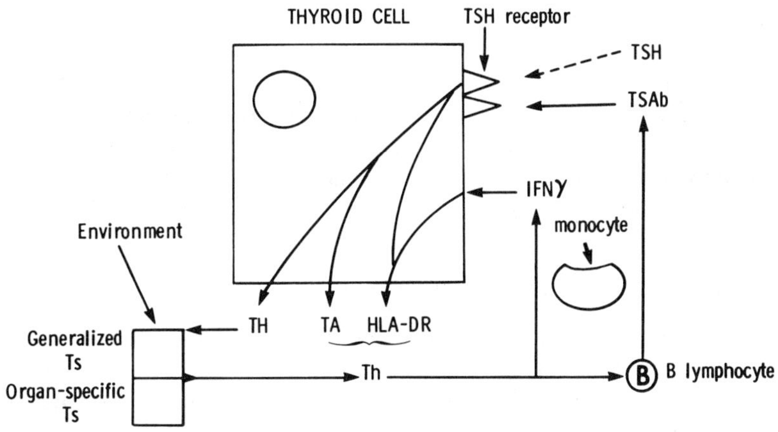

Figure 1 Hypothesis for the pathogenesis of Graves' disease (GD). The basic factor necessary for the development of GD is considered to be an HLA-related genetically induced organ-specific defect in suppressor T lymphocyte (T_S) function. Precipitating factors from the environment (e.g., stress, infection, drugs, aging, trauma) may cause a reduction in generalized T_S. The resultant is to reduce suppression of a thyroid-directed helper T-lymphocyte (Th) population. In the presence of monocytes and the specific antigen, the specific Th will then produce interferon-γ (IFN-γ), and will also stimulate specific B lymphocytes to produce thyroid-stimulating antibody (TSAb). TSAb, like TSH, stimulates the TSH receptor and will result in increased thyroid hormone (TH) production and increased thyroid antigen (TA); e.g., microvillar antigen, expression. IFN-γ causes HLA-DR expression on the thyroid cell surface and this effect is enhanced by TSAb (TSH). Thus, antigen presentation by the thyroid cell occurs directly (requiring the presence of the antigen and HLA-DR expression); this activates and stimulates the specific Th further, and the cycle is repeated. Moreover, excess thyroid hormone acts on generalized T_S, reducing their number and function, further stimulating Th and adding to the cycle, thus perpetuating the disease. Without the specific T_S abnormality, however, continued cycling does not occur, and the process would soon culminate. Similar, slightly different mechanisms are postulated for Hashimoto's thyroiditis. (From Ref. 57, used with permission.)

would be: (1) an antigenic stimulus (however initiated) which would precipitate and/or even maintain the disorder; (2) a precipitating antigenic stimulus, but coupled with an underlying immune abnormality; (3) mutation of appropriate T and/or B lymphocytes to form an abnormal clone or clones of lymphocytes committed to, and interactive with, a particular target organ—these would be autonomous and not subject to normal immunoregulation; and (4) a specific inherent defect in immunoregulation. In the latter hypothesis, all that would be additionally required to precipitate the disease would be (a) the presence of the antigen, without any need for it to be abnormal in any way, (b) the appearance and/or availability of appropriate thyroid-directed clones of helper T lymphocytes and B lymphocytes, and (c) perturbation of the general immune system by such factors, e.g., as stress, trauma, infection, drugs, and aging, which would be then superimposed on the organ-specific abnormality. In this hypothesis, there would be no need for any antigenic abnormality, as will be discussed below.

II. IS THERE ANY ANTIGENIC ABNORMALITY?

In a recent review of his concept of a multigenic basis for the pathogenesis of spontaneous autoimmune thyroiditis, Wick (23) has reviewed the intrinsic functional changes within the thyroid cells of the obese strain (OS) chicken, which develops a spontaneous hereditary autoimmune thyroiditis. This genetic abnormality in the thyroid cells is manifested by thyroid hyperfunction and autonomy, and cannot be suppressed by high doses of thyroxine. Moreover, Wick (23) has reviewed the evidence that thyroiditis can be induced by passive transfer of antithyroglobulin into susceptible chickens, but not into histocompatible chickens. This suggests that the thyroid gland in these animals is particularly susceptible to an autoimmune attack. (It should be added that Wick went on to review the evidence that the immune system was also functionally deranged, and that the thyroid cell abnormality was not necessarily responsible for the thyroiditis, or at least was not the sole abnormality.) Incidentally, it appeared from the data described by Wick that the appearance of spontaneous autoimmune thyroiditis in the OS chicken depends upon an aberration of the immune system encoded by genes located both inside and outside of the major histocompatibility complex (MHC). As noted above, the final genetic factor proposed by Wick was a thyroid cell factor, as demonstrated by the alterations noted earlier in this paragraph; i.e., some disturbance in the target cell antigen.

Is this true in humans as well? It certainly has been postulated that viral infections of the thyroid gland may alter the antigenic structure of the thyroid antigens, thus changing "self" to "nonself," and thus precipitating autoimmune attacks. Wick (23) has mentioned this possibility in his review. Indeed, viruses have been described in the thyroid cells in Hashimoto's thyroiditis (24,25), but similar viruses have also been observed in normal thyroid glands (25). Bottazzo et al. (26) have also made this suggestion, proposing that viruses may stimulate intrathyroidal T lymphocytes to produce intereferon-γ, which in turn would induce the thyroid cells to exhibit HLA-DR on their cell membranes, thus allowing them to present antigen. This was considered by Bottazzo to be the primary inductive step in inducing autoimmune thyroid disease (27). Indeed, Belfiore et al. (28) and Neufeld et al. (29) have demonstrated that viral transfection of thyroid cells in culture can induce weak thyrocyte HLA-DR expression. In addition, it has also been shown that thyroid cells can present an influenzal peptide to influenza-specific T lymphocytes sharing the same HLA-DR antigen (30). Moreover, it is certainly true that diseased thyroid glands contain T lymphocytes that can recognize autologous thyroid cells expressing HLA-DR (31).

However, Mowat (32) has pointed out that viral infections stimulate predominantly interferon-α and -β production, whereas interferon-γ can be produced only by mitogenic or antigenic stimulation of primed lymphocytes. Moreover, he expressed reservations about the possible pathologic role of target cell HLA-DR expression. In addition, Iwatani et al. (31) in our laboratory have shown that the expression of HLA-DR antigen on thyroid cells in culture depends on the presence not only of helper T lymphocytes, but also of monocytes. If the latter two types of cells are removed from the preparations, HLA-DR expression on the thyroid cells is prevented.

Furthermore, there is nothing peculiar about the GD thyroid cells that do express HLA-DR in vivo, but lose this expression in about 3 days of tissue culture. (This would be unlikely to happen if viruses were transfecting the thyroid cells.) Thereafter their response to mitogens, mediated only through the response of passenger lymphocytes in the cultures, is no different from that of normal thyroid cells (31). Indeed, the supernatants from lymphocytes from patients with either active, untreated GD on the one hand, or hypothyroid HT on the other, produced less interferon-γ and thyrocyte HLA-DR expression following *nonspecific* mitogenic stimulation than did normal lymphocytes. In contrast, lymphocytes from patients with GD or HT are capable in coculture of stimulating directly autologous thyroid cells (which have been previously allowed to lose their HLA-DR expression) to again express aberrant HLA-DR expression; this occurs much more sharply and quickly than with normal lymphocytes. This is due to the fact that the GD and HT T lymphocytes are already sensitized to the thyroid antigen.

Grubeck-Loebenstein et al. (33) have shown that thyrocytes from nontoxic goiter (NTG) and GD in allogeneic mixtures stimulated the mixed lymphocyte reaction (MLR) similarly, whereas in autologous MLR the stimulatory activity of thyrocytes was significantly higher in GD than in NTG. Intrathyroidal T-cell lines proliferated specifically in response to autologous thyrocytes in GD but did not do so in NTG. Thus, thyroid lymphocytic infiltrates appear to be thyroid specific only in GD but not in NTG. It may well be that in NTG, local antigenic stimulation by thyrocytes may induce secondary immunization processes locally, whereas the intrathyroidal T lymphocytes recognize autoantigen in GD but not in NTG. Thus, it would appear that NTG cannot be considered a primary autoimmune disorder. It is also clear from these data that class II antigen expression is not specific for autoimmune thyroid disease and is not sufficient by itself to maintain the on-going process. Similar studies should be carried out in papillary carcinoma of the thyroid, in which lymphocytic infiltration is likely to prove secondary to local antigenic perturbation.

Moreover, Davies et al. (34) have shown that thyroid cells from normal persons have the capacity for stimulating T lymphocytes after lectin-induced thyrocyte HLA-DR expression. From all the data above, it seems evident that thyrocyte HLA-DR expression is a secondary phenomenon; i.e., secondary to the initial immune assault itself. It is, however, possible that it might help to potentiate the T-lymphocyte response once the immune process is initiated, but it is equally clear that it will not continue once the underlying process itself abates. Leclère et al. (35) have shown that in subacute thyroiditis, the thyroid follicular cells express HLA-DR, yet chronic autoimmune thyroiditis does not develop. Moreover, xenotransplantation of GD thyroid tissue into nude, athymic mice results in a loss of thyrocyte HLA-DR expression, and a return to normal of the thyroid cells. This is neither consistent with a viral nor with any other alteration of thyroid-cell antigenicity (36–38). Thus, HLA-DR expression on thyroid cells is not itself a potentiating factor, at least when acting alone. However, Figure 1 suggests means by which it may act as a potentiating factor for as long as the basic immunoregulatory perturbation persists, but no longer.

It has been suggested further that other infective organisms may play a role in initiating autoimmune thyroid disease. The most commonly suggested organism for this is *Yersinia enterocolitica*, although other organisms have also been mentioned (39–43). The reason for this is the presence of cross reactivity between antigens from these microorganisms and thyroid cell membrane antigens, including the TSH receptor (42,43). These examples of cross reactivity undoubtedly represent "molecular mimicry"; however, it does not necessarily follow that this molecular mimicry plays any significant role in the induction of organ-specific autoimmune disease. One example will suffice to put this matter into perspective. In Northern Europe, where *Yersinia* infections are relatively common, the incidence of anti-*Yersinia* antibodies in patients with Graves' disease is 60%; however, in North America, where *Yersinia* infections are very rare, the incidence of anti-*Yersinia* antibodies in patients with Graves' disease is the same as it is in Northern Europe. Moreover, in overt *Yersinia* infections, the incidence of clinical thyroid disease is not increased (41). This suggests strongly that the appearance of these antibodies against *Yersinia* in such patients has no pathologic significance, since one would otherwise expect that there would be a much higher incidence of antibodies to this microorganism in patients with autoimmune thyroid disease in those countries where the infection is much more rampant. A recent suggestion that patients with GD have or have had active *Yersinia* infection (43) does not take into account the above logical consideration that molecular mimicry can act in either or both directions (the autoantigen versus the microorganism antigen). The above considerations favor the view that the autoantigen has been the primary antigen involved in AITD, and the appearance of antibodies to *Yersinia* is an artefact related to the homology between the two antigens. Nevertheless, Adams (44) has raised the possibility that infecting viruses with HLA-DR3 like antigenicity may be involved in the emergence of "forbidden" clones of B lymphocytes directed against the target (thyroid) tissue, but his views are highly speculative and will be discussed further below.

All of the above data taken together suggest strongly that there is no antigenic abnormality in primary autoimmune thyroid disease. There does not appear to be any unique feature of the thyroid cells in AITD which makes them more susceptible to interferon-γ stimulation or more vulnerable to the onslaught of autoimmune thyroid disease by the immune system (31). Moreover, direct comparisons of the antigens involved in AITD have shown no differences from those in normal thyroid glands (45–47).

III. AUTOIMMUNE THYROID DISEASE DUE TO THE MUTATION OF T AND/OR B LYMPHOCYTES TO AN ABNORMAL "AUTONOMOUS" CLONE(S)

Adams (48) has claimed that antibodies to thyroglobulin and to thyroid microsomes (thyroperoxidase) are natural antibodies, whereas thyroid-stimulating antibody (TSAb) of GD is an abnormal antibody produced by a mutant forbidden B-lymphocyte clone; this abnormal clone would then not be subject to normal immunoregulation. However, there are no data to support such a claim, and it is not safe to assume that there is any fundamental difference between the production of one thyroid autoantibody versus another.

It has already been demonstrated that peripheral blood lymphocytes from many normal persons are capable of producing antithyroglobulin and antimicrosomal antibodies in vitro when appropriately stimulated (49,50); similarly, normal T lymphocytes are capable of producing thyroid-specific helper factor in vitro under appropriate circumstances (51). Thus, the appropriate clones are clearly available normally, but apparently held in check by normal immunoregulation. While the production of TSAb from peripheral blood lymphocytes of normal persons has not been similarly demonstrated, that may well be due to the lack of an extremely sensitive technique capable of demonstrating very small concentrations of TSAb rather than due to any fundamental difference between the various antibodies.

It has been claimed that B lymphocytes producing antithyroglobulin and antimicrosomal antibodies are autonomous (52,53). If this were true, it would be a point in favor of the Adams hypothesis for the pathogenesis of AITD. However, it is evident that the production of these autoantibodies by the AITD B lymphocytes remains regulated by T lymphocytes; the B lymphocytes require helper T lymphocytes so as to produce the thyroid autoantibodies (11), and are appropriately suppressed by suppressor T lymphocytes (11-13,16-19). Thus, the AITD B lymphocytes respond to the appropriate signals in a normal fashion, and are clearly not autonomous.

While similar in vitro studies have not been performed using TSAb as the endpoint, as mentioned above, this appears to be a result of the difficulty in measuring TSAb in lymphocyte supernatants. In vivo, however, it would appear that the production of TSAb is under similar control. For example, it is well recognized that TSAb declines after patients with Graves' disease are treated with antithyroid drugs (54). There is now evidence that antithyroid drugs exert their immunomodulatory effects via direct effects on the thyroid cells (55-58), and not on the immunocytes. The reduction in thyroid cell activity (see below) then reduces thyrocyte-T lymphocyte signaling, with a consequent reduction in activated helper T lymphocytes (59), and an increase in total (60) and activated (61) suppressor T lymphocytes. This then results in a reduction in the B-lymphocyte production of TSAb. Once again, these B lymphocytes are responding normally to appropriate signaling. Indeed, this may lead to disappearance of TSAb from the blood and prolonged immunologic remission may take place—surely evidence for lack of autonomy of TSAb-producing B lymphocytes. (The nature of remissions will be discussed more fully below.)

Thus, the available evidence does not favor the view that mutations of lymphocytes to form abnormal clones constitutes the route by which AITD develops. In our view, random mutations of lymphocytes to form clones capable of producing autoantibodies are normal and frequent events, and random with respect to time, although apparently with some genetic restriction (thus not all normal persons will have the capacity to produce certain autoantibodies). What appears to be necessary to induce AITD is a disturbance in the regulation or control of autoantibody production.

IV. IMMUNOREGULATION IN AUTOIMMUNE THYROID DISEASE

As has been mentioned above, there is now evidence that helper T lymphocytes can produce organ-specific helper factor even when the lymphocytes are derived from normal peripheral blood (51). It is also evident that helper T lymphocytes are necessary to stimulate B lymphocytes to produce immunoglobulin G (IgG) thyroid autoantibodies (11,13). Moreover, it has been demonstrated that helper T lymphocytes derived from the thyroid glands of patients with autoimmune thyroid disease are in part committed to the thyroid; i.e., are organ-specific helper T lymphocytes (62,63). It is also evident that there are nonspecific helper T lymphocytes in addition to the specific or committed T lymphocytes (63).

This also appears to be true for suppressor T lymphocytes which may comprise both specific and nonspecific cells. While the specific suppressor T lymphocytes would be capable of inhibiting specific populations of helper T lymphocytes and B lymphocytes, nonspecific suppressor T lymphocytes are also capable of influencing these events. Effector T lymphocytes, responsible for direct cytotoxicity, are also controlled by suppressor T lymphocytes.

Several mechanisms have been proposed to explain the disorder of immunoregulation seen in AITD, including loss of suppressor T-lymphocyte function (6–20), intrinsic T-cell hyperactivity (64,65) (already discussed), inappropriate contrasuppressor cell function (66,67), decreased suppressor-inducer function (68), defective clonal inactivation of immature self-reactive B lymphocytes, or emergence of a mutant clone (44,48) (already discussed). Evidence to be presented below favors the first of these hypotheses.

A. Defect in Organ-Specific Suppressor T-Lymphocyte Function

Studies of suppressor T lymphocyte numbers and functions in autoimmune thyroid disease have been two pronged; i.e., those of generalized (nonspecific) suppressor T-lymphocyte function, and conversely, studies of antigen-specific suppressor T-lymphocyte numbers and functions. In human autoimmune thyroid disease, much of the evidence with respect to an antigen-specific suppressor T-lymphocyte defect has come from studies of a modified migration inhibitory factor (MIF) test using preparations of T lymphocytes (6–10,14,15). The procedure has been criticized on the grounds that it is difficult to standardize, and that it does not directly relate to autoantibody production. However, the MIF test indicates the production of a T-lymphocyte lymphokine in response to antigen, and thus can be considered as an index of (helper) T-lymphocyte sensitization. Since such antigen-specific T-helper sensitization may be an important first step in specific autoantibody production, studies of this stage may be helpful in understanding the immunoregulatory abnormality in organ-specific autoimmune disease. In this context, Okita et al. (6) have shown that preparations of peripheral blood T lymphocytes from patients with GD or HT will produce MIF in response to thyroid antigen. If normal T lymphocytes are added to the sensitized T lymphocytes in ratios from 1:1 to 1:9 (normal:sensitized), then MIF production is abolished. If, however, one adds populations of T lymphocytes from one patient with GD or HT to the T lymphocytes of another similar patient, MIF production in response to thyroid antigens continues. Treatment of the normal T lymphocytes with irradiation (1000 rad) (8), mitomycin C, or cimetidine (a histamine type II) (H_2) receptor blocker) (7), procedures designed to abolish suppressor T lymphocyte function, were also capable of preventing the normal T lymphocytes from abolishing MIF production under the circumstances noted above. (The role of histamine type II receptors on suppressor T lymphocytes will be discussed below.) Thus, these experiments suggested that it was the addition of the normal suppressor T lymphocytes that led to the abolition of MIF production by the T-lymphocyte population from patients with AITD in response to thyroid antigen. On the other hand, T lymphocytes from patients with GD or HT were unable to ameliorate MIF production by lymphocytes from other similar patients, thus suggesting that there was a defect in suppressor T-lymphocyte function in these disorders. Moreover, these effects were seen equally in both GD and HT, without any relationship to thyroid function. Indeed, this apparent defect in specific suppressor T-lymphocyte activity lasted in the majority of patients with Graves' disease many years after ^{131}I therapy (10). More recently, Topliss et al. (9) have presented evidence indicating that this suppressor T-lymphocyte defect is disease specific. While Ludgate et al. (69) were unable to reproduce these results using a direct MIF procedure, Vento et al., using an indirect MIF procedure, amply confirmed the above findings (14,15). While they initially compared autoimmune hepatitis with autoimmune thyroiditis, they repeated all of the experiments reported by Okita et al. (6,7) and Topliss et al. (8,9), with parallel results. Recently, Corazza et al. (70) applied this same technique to the study of celiac disease, and concluded that it too was due to a specific defect in suppressor T-lymphocyte function.

Further evidence has accumulated supporting an organ-specific defect in suppressor T-lymphocyte function in AITD. Noma et al. (16,17) have thus provided evidence that there is an antigen-specific disorder in suppressor T-lymphocyte function in HT, using a plaque-forming assay for the production of anti-thyroglogulin. These results have been confirmed by Mori et al. (19), who have shown that antigen-specific histamine type II receptor–bearing suppressor T lymphocytes are relatively deficient in HT (similar to the findings of Okita et al. (7)). (See further detail below.) Tao et al. (18) have also used a plaque-forming assay to demonstrate similarly an antigen-specific deficiency in suppressor T-lymphocyte function in HT. Balasz et al. (20), using a separate procedure, were also able to show an antigen-specific suppressor T-lymphocyte disturbance in a patient with GD whose identical twin was discordant for this disorder. Benveniste et al. (11) have likewise shown evidence that there is a partial or a relative qualitative or quantitative defect in an antigen-specific suppressor T-lymphocyte population in HT by studying autoantibody production (by an ELISA technique) by thyroid-derived lymphocytes. Ueki et al. (71) have recently shown that the suppressor function of intrathyroidal T8-positive cells was remarkably reduced in the glands of patients with GD.

In our own laboratory, Iitaka et al. (13) have studied this question once again by culturing subsets of lymphocytes from patients with AITD. CD8 (suppressor/cytotoxic) and CD4 (helper/inducer) cells were separated from T lymphocytes by the panning method. Patient's B cells and autologous CD4 cells were cultured for 7 days with or without autologous or allogeneic CD8 cells in the presence of either pokeweed mitogen (PWM) or *Staphylococcus aureus* strain Cowan I (SAC) plus human thyroid microsomal antigen. Immunoglobulin-secreting cells producing antithyroid microsomal antibody (AMA) and total IgG were detected by the ELISA spot assay. With PWM stimulation, the suppressor effect of autologous or allogeneic CD8 cells from patients with positive serum AMA on the induction of AMA (of IgG type)–secreting cells was significantly less effective than that of CD8 cells from normal subjects. CD8 cells from patients *with negative serum AMA* suppressed the induction of AMA-secreting cells as well as normal CD8 cells. CD8 cells from both patients and normal subjects suppressed the induction of IgG-secreting cells equally well.

On the other hand, with the combination of SAC and thyroid microsomal antigen stimulation, CD8 cells from both normal subjects and patients scarcely suppressed the induction of IgG-secreting cells. However, CD8 cells from both normal subjects and patients with *negative* serum AMA did suppress the induction of AMA-secreting cells, suggesting the induction of thyroid microsomal antibody–specific suppressor cells. CD8 cells from patients with *positive* serum AMA did not suppress AMA-secreting cells as much as did CD8 cells from either normal subjects or from AITD patients negative for serum AMA. Iitaka et al. (13) were also able to demonstrate that this disorder in AITD suppressor T-lymphocyte function was not due to any disturbance in suppressor-inducer CD4 cells, since the same CD4 cells were able to induce potent suppressor effector activity in CD8 cells from normal subjects. Moreover, the fact that CD8 cells from both patients and normal subjects suppressed the induction of IgG-secreting cells efficiently and equally indicates that generalized suppressor function even in CD8 cells from patients with positive serum AMA is not impaired despite the defect in AMA-specific suppressor function. Since allogeneic and autologous suppressor T lymphocytes produced equal results under these circumstances, it seemed appropriate to compare results when either allogeneic or autologous CD8 cells were added to the AITD CD4 and B cells.

The finding that generalized suppressor T-lymphocyte function was normal in the CD8 cells from patients with positive serum AMA is contrary to the previous report by Davies and Platzer (72), who have shown that patients with AITD have a defect in suppressor T-cell function, not only for antithyroglobulin antibody, but also for IgG production, as determined by ELISA of culture supernatants. On the other hand, our results are in accord with other reports (16,18,19).

The evidence described above that the antigen-specific defect in suppressor T-lymphocyte function in AITD is partial (11,13,19) may well account for the various previous reports of autologous systems in which suppressor T-lymphocyte function has been shown to be present in AITD; in these papers, the authors have generally inferred from such data that there is no abnormality of suppressor T-cell function in AITD (73). However, while there is indeed demonstrable antigen-specific suppressor T-cell function in AITD, it is significantly less than in lymphocytes from normal persons when these are compared (13,19).

1. The Role of the Histamine Type II Receptor-Bearing Suppressor T Lymphocytes

Rocklin (74) has shown that histamine suppresses guinea pig skin test reactivity and macrophage inhibitory factor production, and these inhibitory effects can be blocked by histamine type II receptor antagonists, but not by type I histamine receptor antagonists. Further studies by the same group suggested that suppressor cells bearing histamine type II receptors may play a role in modulating the production or release of migration inhibitory factor by effector cells (75).

To elucidate the association of histamine type II receptor-bearing cells with allosuppressor function in normal T lymphocytes, our own group has studied the immunoregulatory effect of both histamine type I and type II receptor antagonists on normal T lymphocytes before mixing them with T lymphocytes from patients with AITD; their effect on the production of MIF by sensitized T lymphocytes of patients with GD in response to thyroid antigen was then observed (7).

Cimetidine was used as the histamine type II receptor antagonist, whereas chlorpheniramine was used as the type I receptor antagonist. Solutions of these drugs were freshly prepared in each experiment at a concentration (10^{-3} M) used in previous in vitro studies.

There was a significant difference between the migration index (derived by dividing the area of migration in the presence of thyroid antigen by the area of migration in the absence of thyroid antigen) between the results of T lymphocytes from normal persons versus those from patients with Graves' disease; those from patients with GD manifested a highly significant inhibition of migration in response to thyroid antigen. This response was antigen specific. However, when untreated normal T lymphocytes were mixed with patient T lymphocytes in various ratios, the migration indices of this mixture was found to be in the normal range; i.e., the normal T lymphocytes abolished the ability of the Graves' lymphocytes to respond to the thyroid antigen, and thus produce MIF. In contrast, when cimetidine-treated normal T lymphocytes and patient T lymphocytes were mixed in the same ratios, the migration indices of these mixtures once again were abnormal, and were similar to those of patient's T lymphocytes alone. In other words, cimetidine-treated normal T lymphocytes had no suppressor effect on the Graves'-sensitized T lymphocytes (Fig. 2).

However, when chlorpheniramine-treated normal T lymphocytes were mixed with GD patient's T lymphocytes in various ratios, the migration inhibition of patient's T lymphocytes in the presence of thyroid antigen was abolished; this was similar to the abolition of the migration inhibition of sensitized T lymphocytes when untreated normal T lymphocytes were added in the same

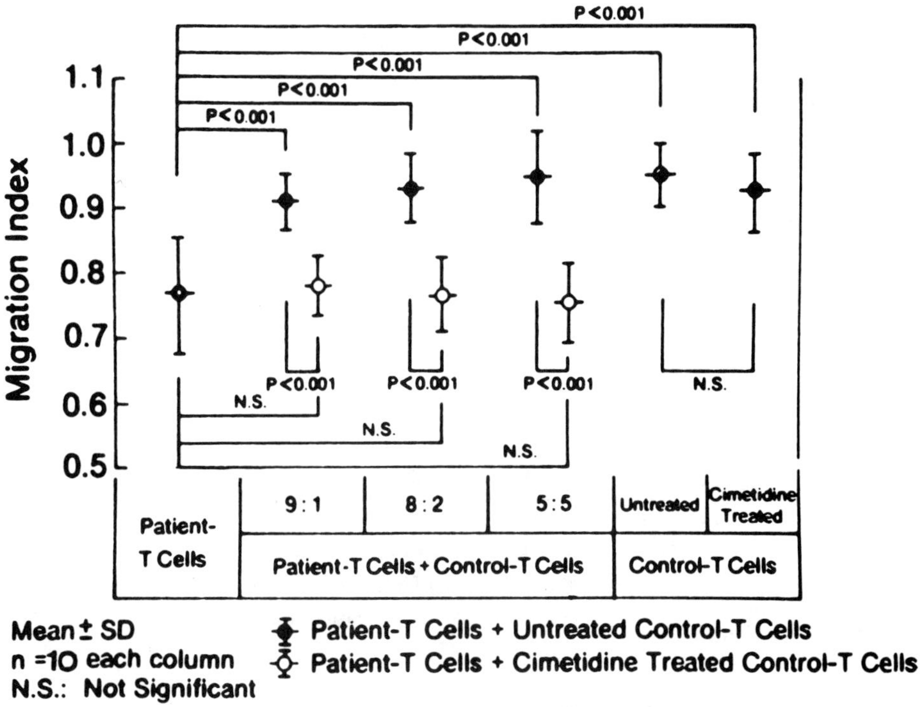

Figure 2 Normal T lymphocytes when mixed in various ratios with patient T lymphocytes abolished migration inhibitory factor (MIF) production. Pretreatment of the normal T lymphocytes with cimetidine (a histamine type II receptor antagonist) led to a loss in their ability to suppress MIF production by the sensitized T lymphocytes of GD patients. (From Ref. 7, used with permission.)

ratios. In other words, chlorpheniramine had no influence on the suppressive effect of normal T lymphocytes on the production of MIF by sensitized T lymphocytes in response to the specific antigen (7) (Fig. 3).

These findings suggested that an abnormal histamine type II receptor response of suppressor T lymphocytes in GD may contribute to the immunoregulatory defect underlying the pathogenesis of this disorder. This is further supported by studies demonstrating an alteration in the function of normal T lymphocytes pretreated with mitomycin C or low-dose irradiation (procedures which affect allosuppressor cells, but not allohelper cells). Thus, mitomycin C-treated or irradiated normal T lymphocytes lose their ability to suppress the production of MIF by sensitized T lymphocytes (6–8). These findings also strongly suggest that the loss of the suppressor function of normal T lympho-

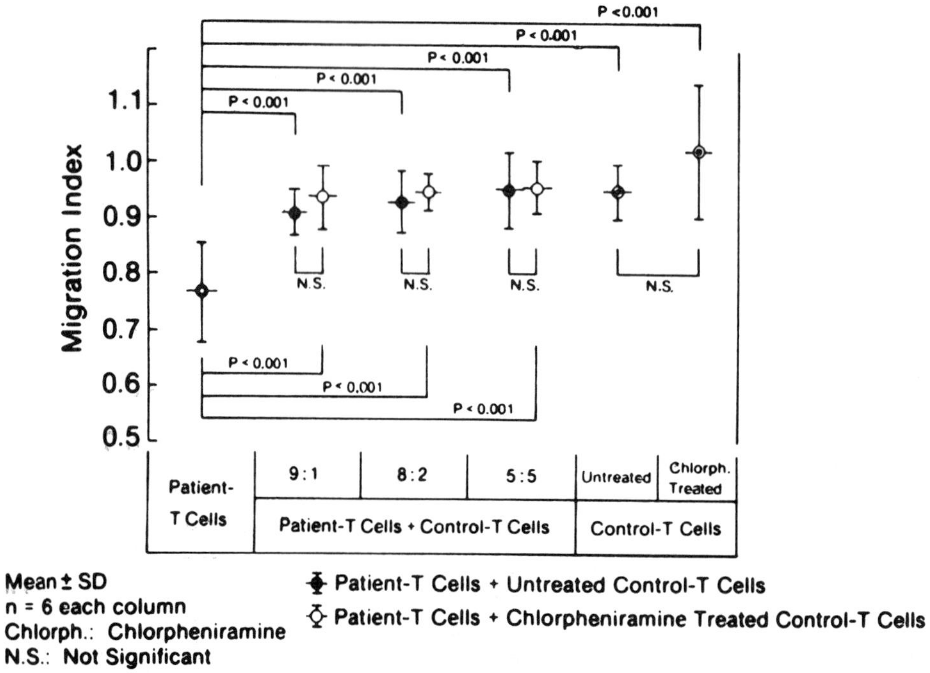

Figure 3 In contrast to cimetidine, pretreatment of normal T lymphocytes with chlorpheniramine (a histamine type II receptor antagonist) did not alter their ability to suppress MIF production by GD T lymphocytes. (From Ref. 7, used with permission.)

cytes is directly related to the blockade of type II histamine receptors by cimetidine (7). It should also be noted that cimetidine did not influence the individual migration indices of normal T lymphocytes when employed alone in the test, indicating that specific antigen sensitization is a prerequisite for the elaboration and release of MIF by helper T lymphocytes (7) (Fig. 4).

Mori et al. (19) have likewise studied suppressor T-lymphocyte function in autoimmune thyroid disease. They used the generation of thyroglobulin plaque-forming cells and protein A plaque-forming cells to investigate the function of lymphocytes from patients with autoimmune thyroid disease. T and B lymphocytes were mixed in cultures without mitogenic or antigenic stimulation so as to identify baseline effects of T lymphocytes in the system. Thyroglogulin plaque-forming cells were found in 44% of the patients who had high titers of antithyroglobulin in their sera. Thyrglobulin-specific and nonspecific immuno-

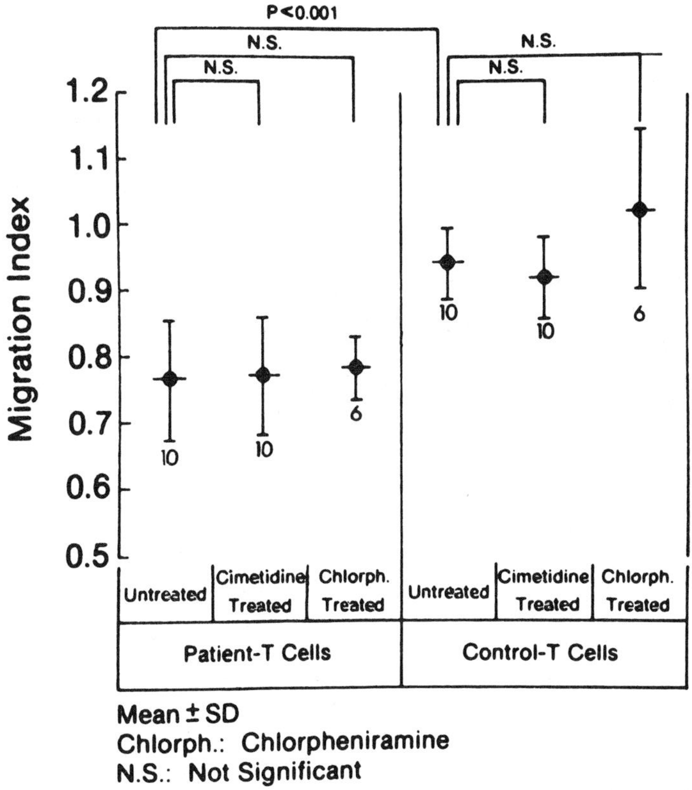

Figure 4 The mean migration index (MI) of GD patients was significantly different from that of normal controls ($p < 0.001$). Pretreatment with cimetidine or chlorpheniramine did not influence the MIs of normal or patient T lymphocytes when used individually. (From Ref. 7, used with permission.)

regulation by T lymphocytes from patients with autoimmune thyroid disease as well as from normal subjects was studied using B lymphocytes from the patients in the mixed lymphocyte subset system. Normal T lymphocytes inhibited thyroglobulin plaque-forming cell induction, but patient's T cells did not, whereas the same extent of helper effects was found on protein A plaque-forming cell induction by the addition of either patient or normal T lymphocytes. In this study, histamine type II receptor-positive T lymphocytes were separated from histamine type II receptor-negative T lymphocytes by using cimetidine/carrier protein conjugate attached to polystyrene plates. The T lymphocytes were then suspended in phosphate-buffered saline poured on the plates, and at the end of

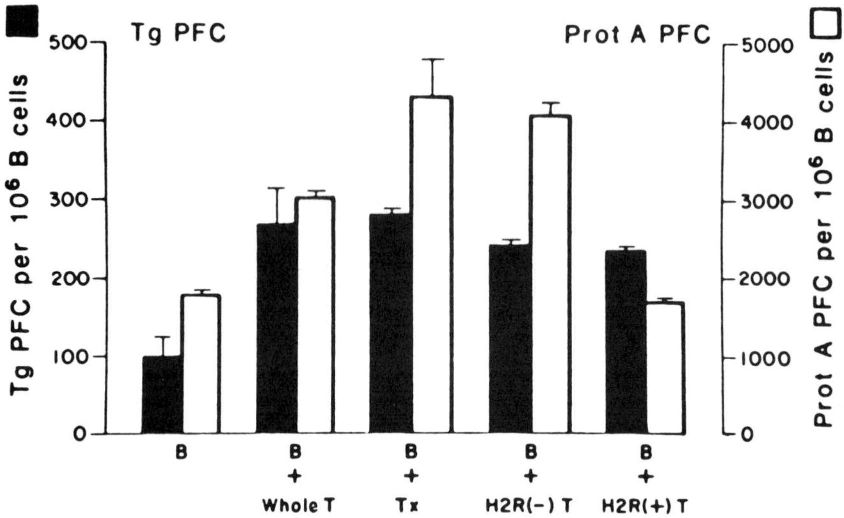

Figure 5 Defect of thyroglobulin (Tg)–specific suppressor T cells in autoimmune thyroid disease. Patient B cells (0.5×10^6) were incubated for 6 days with different kinds of autologous T cells (2×10^6); whole T cells, T cells removed (Tx), $H_2R(-)$ T cells, and $H_2R(+)$ T cells. Triplicate tube cultures were set up, and results are expressed as the mean ± SD from duplicate plaque assays. (From Ref. 19, used with permission.) H_2R = histamine type II.

an incubation period, the histamine type II receptor–negative cells were removed by gently swirling the plate and collecting the supernatant by decanting it. After washing with further phosphate-buffered saline, the histamine type II receptor–positive T-cell fraction was removed by pipetting vigorously and washing the plates with phosphate-buffered saline. The percentage of histamine type II receptor–positive cells was 95% in the type II receptor–positive group and 5% in the type II–receptor negative group. It was found that autologous histamine type II receptor–bearing T lymphocytes from patients with AITD inhibited protein A plaque-forming cell induction, as would be expected of normal suppressor T lymphocytes. However, they did not specifically inhibit thyroglogulin plaque-forming cell induction (any more than T lymphocytes negative for histamine type II receptors) when added to an autologous T plus B lymphocyte (from autoimmune thyroid disease patients) system. T lymphocytes negative for histamine type II receptors induced both thyroglobulin and protein A plaques (Fig. 5).

These data indicate that in vitro thyroglobulin-specific T-cell regulation could be studied in the T plus B lymphocyte system by using B cells from patients with autoimmune thyroid disease with high thyroglobulin antibody titers in their serum. Thyroglobulin-specific suppressor T lymphocytes appear to be present in all individuals and to be involved in the regulation of thyroglobulin antibody production. However, normal (allogeneic) T lymphocytes were able to suppress both protein A and thyroglobulin-specific plaques, whereas either allogeneic or autologous T lymphocytes from patients with AITD suppressed thyroglobulin-specific plaques considerably less than the normal T lymphocytes, but suppressed the protein A plaques equally well as normal T lymphocytes.

These data are consistent with the view that a deficiency of a histamine type II receptor–positive T-cell subset allows increased thyroglobulin plaque-forming cells to be produced in thyroid autoimmunity. This is not to say that the molecular abnormality in the antigen-specific suppressor T lymphocytes in autoimmune thyroid disease is a defect in the histamine type II receptor on these cells. However, that remains a distinct possibility. What is clear, however, is that histamine type II receptor integrity is certainly necessary for normal suppressor T-lymphocyte functioning.

B. Generalized Suppressor T-lymphocyte Function and Numbers

While there is thus now a considerable body of evidence supporting the view that there is an organ-specific defect in suppressor T-lymphocyte function in autoimmune thyroid disease, the magnitude of such an organ-specific defect must be minimal; it would therefore not be expected that there would be any generalized suppressor T-lymphocyte disorder in patients with AITD. Such a generalized disturbance would be expected to result in multiple clinical disorders of immunoregulation. Moreover, such a generalized disturbance in suppressor T-lymphocyte function would not be in accord with genetic observations in which AITD appears much more commonly in patients where the propositi also have AITD rather than other organ-specific autoimmune disorders (76). Nevertheless, a review of the literature shows that, in general, there does appear to be a reduction in the numbers and function of generalized suppressor T lymphocytes in the hyperthyroid phase of Graves' disease; however, these tend to normalize as thyroid function itself improves (77,78). With some exceptions, results have usually been reported to be normal in euthyroid HT. Indeed, however, one report indicated that there is a reduction in suppressor T-lymphocyte numbers in euthyroid nonendemic goiter (79). However, unpublished work from our laboratory has failed to show any such abnormality in either HT or nontoxic goiter.

Since suppressor T-lymphocyte numbers and function tended to return to normal following treatment of GD, the most likely interpretation is that hyperthyroidism itself has adverse effects on generalized suppressor T-lymphocyte (T_S) numbers and function. This view has been disputed by Weetman and McGregor (80), but evidence from our own laboratory makes it clear that severe hyperthyroidism does indeed cause a reduction in T_S numbers. Gerstein et al. (78) in our laboratory have demonstrated that in active, untreated GD, there is a reduction in the Leu 2a+15+ subset, a subset considered to be relatively pure suppressor T lymphocytes. Moreover, this reduction is much more significant when the total serum triiodothyronine values are greater than 7 nmol/L. One year following radioactive iodine therapy delivered as primary treatment for hyperthyroidism, these lymphocyte subset values had returned to normal. Since radioactive iodine can scarcely be considered an immunosuppressive drug, the only variable appeared to be that of the hyperthyroid state itself. Moreover, several of the patients still had very high titers of TSAb and other thyroid autoantibodies at the end of the year following radioactive iodine therapy; i.e., their organ-specific abnormality was still manifest, and yet their lymphocyte subsets had then returned to normal. Thus, it seemed evident that hyperthyroidism per se (or some factor relating closely thereto) did have a deleterious effect on suppressor T-lymphocyte numbers, and that this might have been additive or superimposed on the antigen-specific suppressor T-lymphocyte defect; it thus may be an important factor in causing self-perpetuation of the disease.

It is also clear that there is an increased number of Ia-bearing (HLA-DR bearing) T lymphocytes in patients with organ-specific autoimmune disease, and this is most particularly evident in active, untreated Graves' disease (59). However, there is a sharp reduction in activated (Ia-bearing) helper T lymphocytes following either radioactive iodine therapy (59) or antithyroid drug therapy (61); by the same token, Karlsson et al. (61) have shown a sharp increase in activated suppressor T lymphocytes in the early phases following the institution of antithyroid drug therapy. Since evidence from our own laboratory indicates that antithyroid drug therapy does not have any direct effect on antigen presentation by the thyroid cells (58), it may be assumed that the above effect results from an amelioration of the hyperthyroid state itself. There is also a sharp reduction in natural killer (NK) cell activity with states of excess thyroid hormone (81).

Not only does hyperthyroidism have an effect on suppressor T-lymphocyte function and on the immune system in general, but there are many other factors in the environment which have similar effects. Thus, such environmental factors as stress, infection, drugs, trauma, and aging will perturb the generalized suppressor T-lymphocyte/helper T-lymphocyte ratio, and could readily act as initiating factors in precipitating AITD. While it has been shown that there is no increase in the incidence and magnitude of stresses suffered by patients before the onset of GD compared to a normal control population (82), those authors failed to take into account the patient's genetic susceptibility by virtue of their organ-specific disturbance in immunoregulation to deal with further alterations in their immune system. This is dealt with in part in a recent editorial in the journal the *Lancet* on the relation of emotion and immunity (83).

We would therefore postulate that in patients with AITD, there is a genetically induced partial defect in antigen-specific suppressor T-lymphocyte function. This may be multigenic in origin, and there may be some genetic restriction in terms of the availability of all of the components. Precipitating factors from the environment, such as stress, e.g., infection, drugs, and trauma, may cause a reduction in generalized suppressor T-lymphocyte function and numbers which becomes additive and superimposed on the organ-specific suppressor T-lymphocyte defect. The results would be to reduce suppression of a thyroid-directed helper T-lymphocyte population. The specific helper T-lymphocyte population will then (in the presence of monocytes and, of course, the specific antigen) produce interferon-γ, and will also stimulate specific B lymphocytes to produce thyroid autoantibodies. In the case of HT particularly, cytotoxic T lymphocytes would also be amplified. In the case of GD, thyroid-stimulating antibody, like TSH, would stimulate the TSH receptor, and would result in increased thyroid hormone production as well as increased antigenic expression. Interferon-γ will cause thyrocyte HLA-DR expression, and this effect is enhanced by TSAb and TSH, although the latter agents will not induce HLA-DR expression initially. Thus, antigen presentation by the thyroid cells occurs directly (requiring the presence of the antigen and HLA-DR expression); this presentation activates and stimulates the specific helper T-lymphocyte population further and the cycle is repeated. Moreover, in the case of GD, excess thyroid hormone acts on generalized suppressor T lymphocytes, reducing their numbers and function (78), further stimulating specific helper T lymphocytes and adding to the cycle, and thus perpetuating the disease. In the case of hypothyroid HT, increased TSH would continue to stimulate antigen production, and also be a self-perpetuating factor (56). Without the specific suppressor T lymphocyte abnormality, however, continued cycling would not occur and the process would soon be terminated.

C. Anti-idiotypes in Immunoregulation

It has been suggested that anti-idiotypic antibodies might play a role in immunoregulation. That is, antibodies against TSAb might neutralize TSAb, and thus prevent the clinical manifestations of Graves' disease. Pashke et al. (84) have recently made a case for this notion, and Raines et al. (85) have made a similar proposal, but could only demonstrate such antibodies in a very small minority of patients with GD (although, when present, they seemed to correlate inversely with the presence of TSH receptor antibodies).

This proposal, however, meets with a number of objections. First, anti-idiotypic antibodies are usually a magnitude weaker than the primary antibody, and it would be unlikely that this would form an effective line of immunoregulation. Second, the presence of this type of regulatory pathway would not likely be associated with a reduction of immunologic activity; yet, nevertheless, intrathyroidal lymphocytes decline or even disappear when patients go into remission. Third, the experiments conducted by Paschke et al., which have been interpreted by those authors as suggesting the presence of anti-idiotypic antibodies capable of blocking TSAb activity, can be interpreted in other ways. These authors mixed serum samples with low thyrotrophin receptor antibody (TRAb) and high TRAb values, and this resulted in a lower biologic activity than would be expected by calculating the mean value of biologic parameters. They interpreted this as indicating the presence of anti-idiotypic antibodies, and proposed that these could then modulate disease activity. However, their experiments could also be interpreted as suggesting that TRAb activity may vary with different dilutions. This has been previously suggested by Zakarija and McKenzie (86) in a case of neonatal GD disease which was delayed for a considerable length of time, presumably by blocking antibodies. When the passively transferred serum gradually became diluted over the passage of time, the biologic activity was markedly altered.

When all of the currently available evidence is taken together, it would appear that the role of anti-idiotypic antibodies (while certainly not dismissed) is not a major one in terms of immunoregulation, and is not likely to be the major pathway of remission in Graves' disease.

V. VARIATIONS IN THE CLINICAL COURSE AND REMISSION OF AITD

It is certainly evident that there are profound variations in the serologic expression and clinical course of AITD. While it is beyond the scope of this chapter to discuss these variations in detail, it may be speculated that variations of the immune status of a patient results from alterations in the generalized immune system secondary to environmental factors; this would be superimposed on the organ-specific abnormality of suppressor T-lymphocyte function, and would be sufficient to account for these variations. Mention has been made above of the potentiating elements which will come into play once AITD has been initiated, and this would add a further factor in maintaining or varying the disease expression.

Remissions have been known to occur in both HT and GD. Presumably they occur in the same manner as described above; namely, in patient with a relatively minor or moderate partial defect in antigen-specific suppressor T-lymphocyte function in whom the generalized immune status has been ameliorated to the point where there is an insufficient organ-specific abnormality in the immune system to maintain the disease. Hence, remission occurs. Weetman

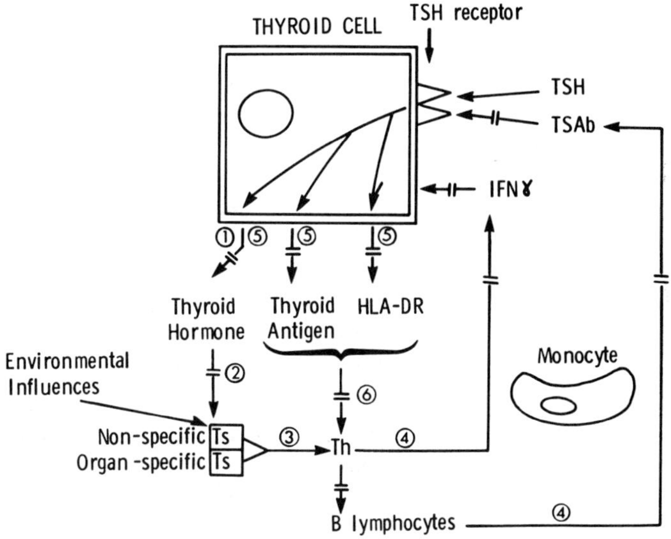

Figure 6 Induction of remission in GD with ATDs. The sequence depicted in Figure 1 is interrupted by ATDs acting on the thyroid cells directly. The primary action is to reduce thyroid hormone production (1). This normalization of function releases the inhibition of nonspecific Ts and that function returns to normal (2). The additive effect on the basic organ-specific Ts defect is thus lost. Suppression of the specific Th population is brought about (3) in the subset of patients who do not have a severe organ-specific T_S defect. This results in a reduction of IFN-γ production and reduced Th stimulation of B lymphocytes to produce TSAb (4). The combined reduction of TSAb and IFN-γ will reduce thyroid antigen and HLA-DR expression, i.e., antigen presentation by the thyroid cell; there will also be reduced thyroid hormone production (5). The reduced hormone production will further reduce T_S inhibition, reducing Th activity; reduced antigen presentation will have the same effect (6). This beneficial cycle will then repeat itself, but will not occur in those patients with a severe organ-specific T_S defect. An additional mechanism of ATD action on the thyroid cell might be to reduce antigen presentation directly. (From Ref. 57, used with permission.)

and McGregor, however (80), have proposed that antithyroid drugs (ATDs) work directly on the immune system to induce remissions in GD. However, this proposal is somewhat difficult to accept, since if this is a pharmacologic effect of these drugs, then one would expect that all patients having a similar pharmacologic effect in terms of normalization of thyroid function would also have a concomitant ameliorating effect on their immune system, with reduction of

TSAb production. However, this is clearly not the case. This and other discrepancies have stimulated the suggestion that ATDs act through modulation of thyroid cell activity to induce such remissions (55-57), and there is now evidence favoring this view. Totterman et al. (55) have demonstrated that antithyroid therapy for GD has resulted in a marked decline in the number of activated T helper/inducer cells and a transient increase in activated T suppressor/cytotoxic cells. These and other markers of T-cell activation were also reduced by methimazole in the thyroid-infiltrating lymphocytes, whereas methimazole did not alter HLA-DR expression of T lymphocytes in vitro. Indeed, Aguayo et al. have shown that ATD do not reduce interferon-γ production by peripheral blood mononuclear cells (87). They have also shown (58,87) that ATDs do not reduce thyrocyte expression of HLA-DR, microsomal antigen, or thyroglobulin, whether the thyroid cells are from normal thyroid glands or from GD. Thus, it would appear that ATDs act by reducing thyroid cell activity, ameliorating hyperthyroidism, and thus reduce the impact of hyperthyroidism on the immune system. This in turn would improve generalized suppressor T-lymphocyte function (in those persons having a less severe antigen-specific suppressor T-lymphocyte disturbance), and thus reduce thyroid-directed helper T-lymphocyte function. This in turn would reduce TSAb production and also might reduce interferon-γ production. There would be a decline in TSAb which would reduce the stimulation of the thyroid cell and bring about further normalization of thyroid function; the reduced production of interferon-γ occurring as a result would also have the effect of reducing antigen presentation to the thyroid cell, thus further reducing T-lymphocyte stimulation and activation. The continuing cycle could well be seen to go on to remission (Fig. 6). While the question of the pathogenesis of exophthalmos is obviously a closely related matter to that of AITD, space precludes a detailed discussion of this topic and the reader is referred elsewhere for my own views about this matter (1).

VI. CONCLUSIONS

There is now considerable evidence for a genetically induced antigen-specific defect in suppressor T lymphocytes as the basis for AITD, derived from several laboratories and via different types of experimental techniques. The defect may involve histamine type II receptors on these cells, although more evidence is necessary to determine whether this is the primary disturbance. In addition, there is now evidence for additive effects on reducing generalized suppressor T-lymphocyte numbers and/or function by environmental factors as well as hyperthyroidism itself, and these effects would be superimposed upon the organ-specific defect. Such effects on generalized suppressor T-lymphocyte numbers may act as precipitating and self-perpetuating factors, in Graves' disease at least. Presentation of the antigen on the thyroid cell via HLA-DR expression on its cell membrane does occur as a result of interferon-γ production by T lymphocytes. This in turn appears to be secondary to the initial specific immune assault and is not a primary inductive step. However, it may be important as an amplifying intermediate factor, but cannot perpetuate the process in the absence of the underlying immune disorder. There is, however, no evidence for an underlying antigenic abnormality or stimulus in human autoimmune thyroid disease, and the initiating event would appear to be due to perturbation of the generalized immune system superimposed on the organ-specific abnormality. Variations in the serologic and clinical expression of AITD would appear to depend on the severity of the original organ-specific disturbance in suppressor T-lymphocyte function, plus the added factor of environmental influences playing upon generalized suppressor T-lymphocyte function and numbers. Remission in GD brought about by antithyroid drugs may well be via their effect on modulating the thyroid cell activity; this will then reduce thyrocyte-immunocyte signaling, allowing remission to occur in those patients with a partial organ-specific defect in suppressor T lymphocytes.

ACKNOWLEDGMENTS

Work cited from the author's laboratory has been supported by the Medical Research Council of Canada (MT859) and the Angus Foundation, Wellesley Hospital, Toronto, Ontario, Canada.

REFERENCES

1. Volpé, R., Autoimmune thyroid disease. In Autoimmunity in Endocrine Disease, (Volpé, R., Ed.), Marcel Dekker, New York (1985), pp. 109–285.
2. Volpé, R., Autoimmune thyroid disease–A perspective, Mol. Biol. Med. 3:25–51 (1986).
3. Hashimoto, H., Zur Kenntnis der Lymphomastosen Veranderung der Schildruse (Strume Lymphomatosa), Arch. Klin. Chir. 97:219–248 (1912).
4. Loeb, P. D., A. L. Drash, and F. M. Kenny, Prevalence of low titer and "negative" antithyroglobulin antibodies in biopsy-proven juvenile Hashimoto's thyroiditis, J. Pediatr. 82:17–21 (1973).
5. Amino, H., and K. Miyai, Postpartum autoimmune endocrine syndrome. In Autoimmune Endocrine Disease (Davies, T. F., Ed.), Wiley-Interscience, New York (1983), pp. 247–272.
6. Okita, N., V. V. Row, and R. Volpé, Suppressor T lymphocyte deficiency in Graves' disease and Hashimoto's thyroiditis, J. Clin. Endocrinol. Metab. 52:528–533 (1981).
7. Okita, N., J. How, D. Topliss, M. Lewis, V. V. Row, and R. Volpé, Suppressor T lymphocyte dysfunction in Graves' disease: Role of H-2 histamine receptor-bearing suppressor T lymphocytes, J. Clin. Endocrinol. Metab. 53: 1002–1007 (1981).

8. Topliss, D. J., N. Okita, M. Lewis, V. V. Row, and R. Volpé, Allosuppressor T lymphocytes abolish migration inhibition factor production in autoimmune thyroid disease: Evidence from radiosensitivity experiments, Clin. Endocrinol. 15:335–341 (1981).
9. Topliss, D. J., J. How, M. Lewis, V. V. Row, and R. Volpé, Evidence for cell-mediated immunity and specific suppressor T lymphocyte dysfunction in Graves' disease and diabetes mellitus, J. Clin. Endocrinol. Metab. 57:700–705 (1983).
10. How, J., D. J. Topliss, C. Strakosch, M. Lewis, V. Row, and R. Volpé, T lymphocyte sensitization and suppressor T lymphocyte defect in patients long after treatment for Graves' disease, Clin. Endocrinol. 18:61–72 (1983).
11. Benveniste, P., V. V. Row, and R. Volpé, Studies on the immunoregulation of thyroid autoantibody production in vitro, Clin. Exp. Immunol. 61:274–282 (1985).
12. Row, V. V., and R. Volpé, In vitro regulation of antithyroglobulin synthesis by lymphocytes of patients with Hashimoto's disease by an antigen-specific suppressor factor derived from cultures of normal human T lymphocytes, J. Clin. Lab. Immunol. 21:159–163 (1986).
13. Iitaka, M., J. Aguayo, V. V. Row, and R. Volpé, Studies of the effect of suppressor T cells in the induction of antithyroid microsomal antibody secreting cells in autoimmune thyroid disease. J. Clin. Endocrinol. Metab. 66:708–714 (1988).
14. Vento, S., J. E. Hegarty, G. F. Bottazzo, E. Macchia, R. Williams, and A. L. W. F. Eddlestone, Antigen specific suppressor cell function in autoimmune chronic active hepatitis, Lancet 1:1200–1204 (1984).
15. Vento, S., C. J. O'Brien, T. Condy, R. Williams, and A. L. W. F. Eddlestone, Is cellular immunity to the TSH receptor restricted to patients with Graves' disease? In The Thyroid and Autoimmunity (Drexhage, H. A., and Wiersinga, W. M., Eds.), Excerpta Medica International Congress Series 711, Elsevier, Amsterdam (1986), pp. 304–305.
16. Noma, T., J. Yata, Y. Shishiba, and B. Inatsuki, In vitro detection of antithyroglobulin antibody forming cells from the lymphocytes of chronic thyroiditis patients. An analysis of their regulation, Clin. Exp. Immunol. 49: 565–571 (1982).
17. Noma, T., Y. Kawano, T. Sasazuki, and J. Yata, Properties of suppressor T cell factor regulating antithyroglobulin antibody formation in the lymphocytes of chronic thyroiditis patients, Proceedings of the Sixth International Congress of Immunology, Toronto, 1986, July 6–11, Abstract No. 3.47.12 (Published by the National Research Council of Canada, Ottawa, NRCC, 25710 ISBN 0-660-53282-4.)
18. Tao, T. W., P. A. Gatenby, S. L. Leu, H. Pham, and J. P. Kriss, Helper and suppressor activities of lymphocyte subsets of antithyroglobulin products in vitro, J. Clin. Endocrinol. Metab. 61:520–524 (1985).
19. Mori, H., N. Hamada, and L. J. DeGroot, Studies on thyroglobin-specific suppressor T cell function in autoimmune thyroid disease, J. Clin. Endocrinol. Metab. 60:306–312 (1985).

20. Balasz, C. S., V. Stenzsky, L. Kozman, and N. R. Farid, Specific suppressor T cell function in a patient with Graves' disease and her healthy identical twin, Clin. Endocrinol. 20:683-693 (1984).
21. Volpé, R., M. W. Edmonds, P. V. Clarke, and V. V. Row, A viewpoint regarding the nature of the emergence of long acting thyroid stimulator of Graves' disease, Acta Endocrinol. panam. 1:155-170 (1970).
22. Volpé, R., M. W. Edmonds, L. Lamki, P. V. Clarke,and V. V. Row, The pathogenesis of Graves' disease. A disorder of delayed hypersensitivity? Mayo Clin. Proc. 47:824-834 (1972).
23. Wick, G., Concept of a multigenic basis for the pathogenesis of spontaneous autoimmune thyroiditis, Acta Endocrinol. (Copenh.) 115(Suppl. 281):63-69 (1987).
24. Wick, G., and J. Graf, Electron microscopic studies in chickens of the obese strain with spontaneous hereditary autoimmune thyroiditis, Lab. Invest. 27:400-411 (1972).
25. Kahn, L. D., and J. Dale, Virus-like particles in Hashimoto's disease and a variety of other tissues, Lab. Invest. 29:350-351 (1973).
26. Bottazzo, G. F., R. Mirakian, F. De Lazzari, T. Mauerhoff, I. Todd, and R. Pujol-Borrell, In Hormones and Immunity (Berczi, I., and Kovacs, K., Eds.), MTP Press, Norwell, Massachusetts (1987), pp. 296-311.
27. Bottazzo, G. F., R. Pujol-Borrell, T. Hanafusa, and M. Feldmann, Role of aberrant HLA-DR expression and antigen presentation in induction of endocrine autoimmunity, Lancet 2:1115-1119 (1983).
28. Belfiore, A., R. Pujol-Borrell, T. Mauerhoff, R. Mirakian, and G. F. Bottazzo, Effects of SV-40 transformation on HLA-expression by thyroid follicular cells, Ann d'Endocrinol. 47:17 (1986) (Abstr.).
29. Neufeld, B. S., M. Platzer, and T. F. Davies, Viral induction of thyroid cell MHC Class II gene expression, Proceedings of the American Thyroid Association, Washington, D.C., September 16-19 (1987), Abstract No. 34.
30. Londei, M., J. R. Lamb, G. F. Bottazzo, and M. Feldmann, Epithelial cells expressing aberrant MHC Class II determinants can present antigen to cloned human T cells, Nature 312:693-641 (1986).
31. Iwatani, Y., H. C. Gerstein, M. Iitaka, V. V. Row, and R. Volpé, Thyrocyte HLA-DR expression and interferon gamma production in autoimmune thyroid disease, J. Clin. Endocrinol. Metab. 63:695-708 (1986).
32. Mowat, W. M., Interferon and class II MHC antigen expression in autoimmunity, Lancet 2:283 (1985).
33. Grubeck-Loebenstein, B., M. Onvi, C. Greenall, K. Pirich, W. Waldhausl, and F. Feldmann, Stimulatory activities of antigen presenting cells in mixed leukocyte reactions in thyroid diseases, Acta Endocrinol. 115(Suppl. 281): 89-92 (1987).
34. Davies, T. F., Cocultures of human thyroid monolayer cells and autologous T cells: Impact of HLA Class II antigen expression, J. Clin. Endocrinol. Metab. 61:418-422 (1985).

35. Leclère, J., C. Faure, M. C. Bene, J. L. Thomas, J. L. Paul, and P. Hertemann, In situ immunological disorders in DeQuervain's thyroiditis. In Frontiers in Thyroidology (Medeiros Neto, G. and Gaitan, E., Eds.), vol. II, Plenum Press, New York (1986), pp. 1365–1368.
36. Leclère, J., M. D. Bene, A. Duprez, G. Faure, J. L. Thomas, J. M. Vitnaud, and C. Burlet, Behaviour of thyroid tissue from patient with Graves' disease in nude mice, J. Clin. Endocrinol. Metab. 59:175–177 (1984).
37. Usadel, K. H., J. Teuber, R. Paschke, M. Junker, and U. Schwedes, Transplantation of human endocrine tissue to nude mice: A suitable in vivo model for the study of pathomechanisms involved in autoimmune thyroid disease, Acta Endocrinol. 115(Suppl. 281):77–81 (1987).
38. Schumm-Draeger, P. M., K. H. Usadel, B. Bohm, H. J. C. Wenisch, R. Senekowitsch, C. R. Pickardt, and K. Schoffling, Thyrotoxic effects of high iodine doses on xenotransplanted autoimmune thyroid tissue in athymic nude mice, Acta Endocrinol. 115(Suppo. 281):118–124 (1987).
39. Bech, K., J. Nerup, and J. H. Larsen, *Yersinia enterocolitica* infection and thyroid diseases, Acta Endocrinol. (Copenh.) 84:87–92 (1977).
40. Bech, K., O. Clemmensen, J. H. Larsen, and J. Bendixen, Thyroid disease and *Yersinia*, Lancet 1:1060–1062 (1977).
41. Shenkman, L., and E. J. Bottone, Antibodies to *Yersinia enterocolitica* in thyroid disease, Ann. Intern. Med. 85:735–739 (1976).
42. Safran, M., T. L. Paul, E. Roti, and L. E. Braverman, Environmental factors affecting autoimmune thyroid disease. In Autoimmune Thyroid Disease (Wall, J. R., Ed.), Endocrinol. Metab. Clin. North Am. 16:327–342 (1987).
43. Wenzel, B. E., J. Heesmann, K. W. Wenzel, R. Gutekunst, and P. C. Scriba, Antibodies to plasmid-encoated proteins of enteropathic Yersinia in patients with autoimmune thyroid disease. Lancet 1:56 (1988).
44. Adams, D. D., Protection from autoimmune disease as the third function of the major histocompatibility gene complex, Lancet 2:245–249 (1987).
45. Knight, A., and D. D. Adams, Lack of allotypic variations in the autoantigen for the thyroid stimulating antibody, Clin. Exp. Immunol. 52:317–324 (1983).
46. Hamada, N., J. Yamakawa, A. Hinotani, Y. Okamoto, M. Ohno, H. Mori, J. Noh, K. Ito, and L. Portmann, Thyroid microsomal antigen in Graves' thyroid is not different from normal thyroid, Proceedings of the American Thyroid Association, Washington, D.C., September 16–21 (1987), Abstract No. 90.
47. von Westarp, C., A. J. S. Knox, V. V. Row, and R. Volpé, Comparison of thyroid antigens by the experimental production of precipitating antibodies to human thyroid fractions and the identification of an antibody which competes with long acting thyroid stimulation for thyroid binding, Acta Endocrinol. (Copenh.) 84:759–769 (1977).
48. Adams, D. D., Graves' disease. A paradigm for autoimmunity. In Thyroid Autoimmunity, (Pinchera, A., Ed.), Plenum Press, London, 1987, pp. 1–10.

49. Logtemberg, T., A. Kroon, F. H. J. Gmelig-Mayling, and R. E. Ballieux, Antigen and mitogen induced differentiation of circulating B cells in patients with autoimmune thyroid disease and normal individuals. In The Thyroid and Autoimmunity (Drexhage, H. A., and Wiersinga, W. M., Eds.), Excerpta Medica International Congress Series 711, Elsevier, Amsterdam, pp. 308–310.
50. Iwatani, Y., M. Iitaka, V. V. Row, and R. Volpé, Induction of thyroid autoantibody production: Synergistic effect of B cell mitogen combined with T cell mitogen, J. Clin. Endocrinol. Metab. 65:853–861 (1987).
51. Hara, Y., K. Satoh, T. Tanikawa, Y. Sakatsume, J. Ishii, and L. J. DeGroot, Spontaneous in vitro production of thyroglobulin specific helper factor in patients with autoimmune thyroid disease, J. Clin. Lab. Immunol. 22:107–112 (1987).
52. Jones, D. M., C. S. Teng, and R. Yeung, Evaluation of B cells, T helper cells and suppressor cell function in patients with Graves' disease before and after treatment with antithyroid drugs, Clin. Immunol. Immunopathol. 25:232–242 (1982).
53. DeBernardo, E., and T. F. Davies, Functional aspects of B cell autonomy in human thyroid disease, Life Sci. 32:139–152 (1983).
54. McGregor, A. M., A. M. Petersen, S. M. McLachlan, P. Rooke, B. Rees Smith, and R. Hall, Carbimazole and the autoimmune response in Graves' disease, N. Engl. J. Med. 303:302–307 (1982).
55. Totterman, T. H., F. A. Karlsson, M. Bengtsson, and I. Mendel-Hertvig, Induction of the circulating activated suppressor-like T cells by methimazole therapy for Graves' disease, N. Engl. J. Med. 316:15–22 (1987).
56. Volpé, R., Immunoregulation in autoimmune thyroid disease, N. Engl. J. Med. 316:44–46 (1987).
57. Volpé, R., A. Karlsson, R. Jansson, and P. A. Dahlberg, Thyrostatic drugs act through modulation of thyroid cell activity to induce remissions in Graves' disease, Acta Endocrinol. (Copenh.) 115(Suppl. 281):305–311 (1987).
58. Aguayo, J., P. Michaud, M. Iitaka, L. J. DeGroot, V. V. Row, and R. Volpé, Expression of thyroid peroxidase and thyroglobulin antigen released by cultured human thyrocytes. Effect of methimazole, Autoimmunity 2:133–146 (1988).
59. Chan, J. Y. C., and P. G. Walfish, Activated (Ia ¡) T lymphocytes and their subsets in autoimmune thyroid diseases: Analysis by dual laser flow microfluorocytometry, J. Clin. Endocrinol. Metab. 62:403–409 (1986).
60. Ludgate, M. E., A. M. McGregor, A. P. Weetman, S. Ratanachaiyavong, J. H. Lazarus, and G. H. Middleton, Analysis of T cell subsets in Graves' disease. Alteration associated with carbimazole, Br. Med. J. 228:526–530 (1984).
61. Karlsson, F. A., R. H. Totterman, and I. Mendel-Hertvig, Alterations in HLA-expressing T cell subsets during treatment of Graves' disease. In Fron-

tiers in Thyroidology, vol. II (Medeiros Neto, G., and Gaitan, E., Eds.), Plenum Press, New York (1985), pp. 1555-1557.

62. Londei, M., G. F. Bottazzo, and M. Feldmann, Human T cell clones from autoimmune thyroid glands: specific recognition of autologous thyroid cells, Science 228:85-89 (1985).
63. Kaulferssh, W., T. A. Waldmann, and J. R. Baker, Immunoglobulin and T cell gene rearrangements demonstrate that the immune response in autoimmune thyroid disease is polyclonal in nature, Proceedings of the 62nd Meeting of the American Thyroid Association, Washington, D.C., September 16-21 (1987), Abstract No. 89.
64. Beall, G. N., and S. R. Kruger, Production of human antithyroglobulin in vitro, II. Regulation by T cells, Clin. Immunol. Immunopathol. 16:498-503 (1980).
65. Dehee, D. H., and T. S. Edgington, Evidence for a B lymphocyte defect underlying the anti-X antierythrocyte autoantibody response of NZB mice, J. Immunol. 118:1859-1864 (1977).
66. Green, D. R., P. M. Flood, and R. K. Gershon, Immunoregulatory T cell pathways, Ann. Rev. Immunol. 1:439-452 (1983).
67. Smith, H. R., D. R. Green, P. A. Smathers, R. K. Gershon, E. S. Reveche, and A. D. Steinberg, Induction of autoimmunity in normal mice by thymectomy and administration of polyclonal B cell activators—Association with contrasuppressor function, Clin. Exp. Immunol. 51:579-585 (1983).
68. Morimoto, C., A. D. Sternberg, N. I. Letvin, M. Hagen, T. Takeuchi, J. Daley, H. Levine, and S. F. Schlossman, A defect of immunoregulatory T cell subsets in systemic lupus erythematosus patients demonstrated by anti-2H4 antibodies, J. Clin. Invest. 79:762-766 (1987).
69. Ludgate, M. E., S. Ratanachaiyavong, A. P. Weetman, R. Hall, and A. M. McGregor, Failure to demonstrate cell-mediated immune responses to thyroid antigens in Graves' disease using in vitro assays of lymphokine mediating migration inhibition, J. Clin. Endocrinol. Metab. 60:98-102 (1985).
70. Corazza, G. R., P. Sacheilli, M. Londei, M. Frisoni, and G. Gasparini, Gluten specific suppressor T cell function in coeliac disease, Gut, 27:392-398 (1986).
71. Ueki, Y., K. Eguchi, T. Fukuda, T. Otsuba, Y. Kawabe, G. Shimonura, M. Matsunaga, H. Tezuka, N. Ishikawa, K. Ito, and S. Nagataki, Dysfunction of suppressor T cells in thyroid glands from patients with Graves' disease, J. Clin. Endocrinol. Metab. 65:922-928 (1987).
72. Davies, T. F., and M. Platzer, The T cell suppressor defect in autoimmune thyroiditis: Evidence fo a high set 'immunostat,' Clin. Exp. Immunol. 63: 73-78 (1986).
73. Ahmann, A. J., and K. D. Burman, The role of T lymphocytes in autoimmune thyroid disease. In Autoimmune Thyroid Disease, (Wall, J. R., Ed.), Endocrinol. Metab. Clin. North Am. 16:287-326 (1987).
74. Rocklin, R. E., Modulation of cellular immune response in vivo and in vitro by histamine receptor bearing lymphocytes, J. Clin. Invest, 57:1051-1055 (1976).

75. Rocklin, R. E., D. Greineder, B. H. Littman, and K. L. Melman, Modulation of cellular immune function in vitro by histamine receptor bearing lymphocytes: mechanisms of action, Cell. Immunol. 37:162–168 (1978).
76. Torfs, C. P., M. C. King, V. Huey, J. Malmgren, and F. C. Grumet, Genetic interrelationship between insulin-dependent diabetes mellitus, the autoimmune thyroid diseases and rheumatoid arthritis, Am. J. Human Genet. 38: 170–187 (1986).
77. Volpé, R., and V. V. Row, Role of antigen specific suppressor T lymphocytes in the pathogenesis of autoimmune thyroid disease. In Autoimmunity and the Thyroid, (Walfish, P. G., Wall, J. R., and Volpé, R, Eds.), Academic Press, Orlando, Florida (1984), pp. 79–94.
78. Gerstein, H. D., R. Rastogi, Y. Iwatani, M. Iitaka, V. V. Row, and R. Volpé, The decrease in non-specific suppressor T lymphocytes in female hyperthyroid Graves' disease is secondary to the hyperthyroidism, Clin. Invest. Med. 10:377–344 (1987).
79. Van der Gaag, R. D., M. Von Blomberg-Van der Flier, E. Van der Plassche-Bores, M. Kokje-Kleingeld, and H. A. Drexhage, T suppressor cell defects in euthyroid non-endemic goitre, Acta Endocrinol. (Copenh.) 112:83–88 (1986).
80. Weetman, A. P., and A. M. McGregor, Autoimmune thyroid disease: Developments in our understanding, Endocrinol. Rev. 5:309–355 (1984).
81. Papac, M., J. Stein-Streilein, M. Zakaraija, J. M. McKenzie, F. Guffee, and M. A. Fletcher, Suppression of peripheral blood natural killer cell activity by excess thyroid hormone, J. Clin. Invest. 79:404–408 (1987).
82. Gray, J., and R. Hoffenberg, Thyrotoxicosis and stress, Q. J. Med. 54: 153–160 (1985).
83. Editorial. Emotional and immunity, Lancet 2:133–134 (1985).
84. Paschke, R., J. Tueber, U. Schwedes, and K. H. Usadel, Is remission of Graves' disease regulated by anti-idiotypic antibodies? Acta Endocrinol. 115(Suppl. 281):99–103 (1987).
85. Raines, K. B., J. R. Baker, Y. G. Lukes, L. Wartofsky, and K. D. Burman, Antithyrotrophin antibodies, Metabolism 61:217–222 (1985).
86. Zakarija, M., J. M. McKenzie, and W. H. Hoffman, Prediction and therapy of intrauterine and late-onset neonatal hyperthyroidism, J. Clin. Endocrinol. Metab. 62:368–371 (1986).
87. Aguayo, J., M. Iitaka, V. V. Row, and R. Volpé, Studies of HLA-DR expression on cultured human thyrocytes: effect of anti-thyroid drugs and other agents on interferon gamma induced HLA-DR expression. J. Clin. Endocrinol. Metab. 66:903–908 (1988).

Part III

Augmentation of Immune Response by H_2 Antagonists

9

In Vivo Effects of Cimetidine in Mice

WILLIAM B. ERSHLER *University of Wisconsin, Madison, Wisconsin*

I. INTRODUCTION

In experimental systems, histamine has been demonstrated to influence various immunologic responses, including those as fundamental as cytotoxicity (1,2). production of cytokines (3), and mitogen- and antigen-induced cell proliferation (1,4,5). It appears that histamine mediates such an influence by stimulating a subset of T cells that bear a specific receptor for the molecule (1,6). When examined by immunofluorescent technique those cells that are found to have histamine receptors also demonstrate cell surface antigens that are typical for T-suppressor cells (7).

Cimetidine is a histamine type II (H_2) antagonist that is widely used and is highly successful in the treatment of peptic ulcer disease (8,9). Despite the fact that histamine type II receptors are present on cells from a large number of tissues, adverse effects of cimetidine are few (10,11). The modulation of the immune response that might be induced by the inhibition of histamine-induced suppressor cell function has focused great interest on the compound among immunopharmacologists. In this chapter, selective data, derived from in vivo murine studies will be reviewed, particularly with reference to humoral and delayed-type hypersensitivity and to tumor rejection. This chapter was not intended to be comprehensive, but representative of a larger number of similar studies, and reflective of the potential clinical importance of cimetidine as an immunopharmacologic agent.

II. CIMETIDINE AND IMMUNITY-PROPOSED MECHANISMS

It is currently appreciated that there is a complex network of cellular interactions involved in the immune response. With the development of monoclonal antibody technology and associated fluorescence-activated cell sorter analysis, functionally distinct subsets of lymphocyte populations have been identified. One functional subset of T cells has been shown to be identified by antibody to the histamine type II receptor (1,2,7,12,13). Interaction of the ligand with this receptor induces the elaboration of a suppressor lymphokine that results in reduction of both T- and B-cell effector functions (14,15). For example, histamine-activated T-suppressor cells have been shown to suppress lymphocyte proliferation (4,5,16), lymphokine production (3,17), and immunoglobulin synthesis (18,19).

Insight into the mechanism whereby histamine activation mediates immune suppression was provided by Rocklin and colleagues (1,6,12,17,19-21). They found that lymph node cells from experimental animals, when cultured in the presence of histamine secrete a nondialyzable, soluble factor, that could mediate the effects of T-suppressor cells in vitro in a variety of immune assays. This factor produced by human lymphocytes has been further characterized (22,23), and it has been demonstrated that many of its effects may be mediated through monocyte production of prostaglandins and/or thromboxane B_2 (24).

Histamine-mediated immune suppression can be blocked by type II receptor antagonists (such as cimetidine), but not by type I receptor antagonists. Furthermore, not all T-suppressor cells are equally sensitive to histamine or the inhibitory effect of antihistamines. Griswold and colleagues (25) have demonstrated variable levels of cimetidine-induced inhibition of T cell-mediated suppression based upon both phenotype and function of the T-suppressor cell. In their model they examined three types of T suppressors;

1. Immune suppression mediated by ultraviolet (UV) light (mediated by $Ly1^+$-suppressor cells)
2. Suppressor cells that result in tolerance in animals injected with high doses of sheep red blood cells (SRBCs) (mediated by $Ly2^+$-suppressor cells)
3. Suppressor cells induced by dinitrobenzene sulfonic acid ($DNBSO_3$) (also mediated by $Lyt2^+$-suppressor cells)

These authors found that there was a relative difference in the capability of the antagonists (they tested cimetidine or oxymetidine) to inhibit these suppressor cells. For example, it took 20- to 200-fold greater doses to inhibit the UV-induced T-suppressor cells when compared to the $DNBSO_3$-induced T-suppressor cells. Yet, these histamine type II antagonists were ineffective in inhibiting those $Lyt2^+$ T-suppressor cells induced by high doses of SRBCs. It is therefore apparent that the variability in sensitivity to histamine type II antagonists is more complicated than indicated by simple T-cell phenotypes, and this work suggests that there is considerable heterogeneity in these immunoregulatory cells, and that histamine activation is probably only one of several inducers of T-suppressor activity.

III. MURINE MODELS—HUMORAL IMMUNITY

Histamine type II receptors are characteristically found on T-suppressor subsets, and type II receptor antagonists have been demonstrated to enhance in vitro immune responses (as discussed above), presumably on the basis of inhibition of histamine-stimulated T cell–mediated suppressor mechanisms. The possible importance of such immune modulation produced by the inhibitors of histamine at the type II receptor are highlighted by a series of experiments in which mice were treated with cimetidine and antibody response was measured. The appropriateness of this model is that for most protein antigens (such as tetanus toxoid, influenza hemagglutinin) successful, vigorous antibody response requires T-cell help, and is eventually down regulated by T-cell suppression (26,27). If T-suppressor cell function were diminished (such as by an inhibitor of histamine), one might expect to observe enhanced antibody response to vaccine.

That, in fact, is exactly what was observed in our laboratory (28). Young mice were treated with cimetidine or placebo daily (by intraperitoneal injection) and a number of immune parameters (including the specific antibody response to tetanus toxoid vaccine) were measured. There were four experimental groups. One group received low-dose cimetidine (25 mg/kg/day) and a second received a higher dose (100 mg/kg/day), whereas two control groups received an equivalent volume of saline (one control group received the tetanus vaccine and the second did not). The doses chosen were based upon published experience with the drug in rats (29), and represented what we predicted would be low and high therapeutic ranges without expected toxicity. No observable toxicity was recorded, and in each of the assays, increased responses were found in the cimetidine treatment groups. The mitogen-induced proliferative responses were interesting in that observed differences in splenic cell cultures were apparent even in those wells in which test lectin had not been added. That is, lymphocytes from those mice that received cimetidine had a higher level of deoxyribonucleic acid (DNA)

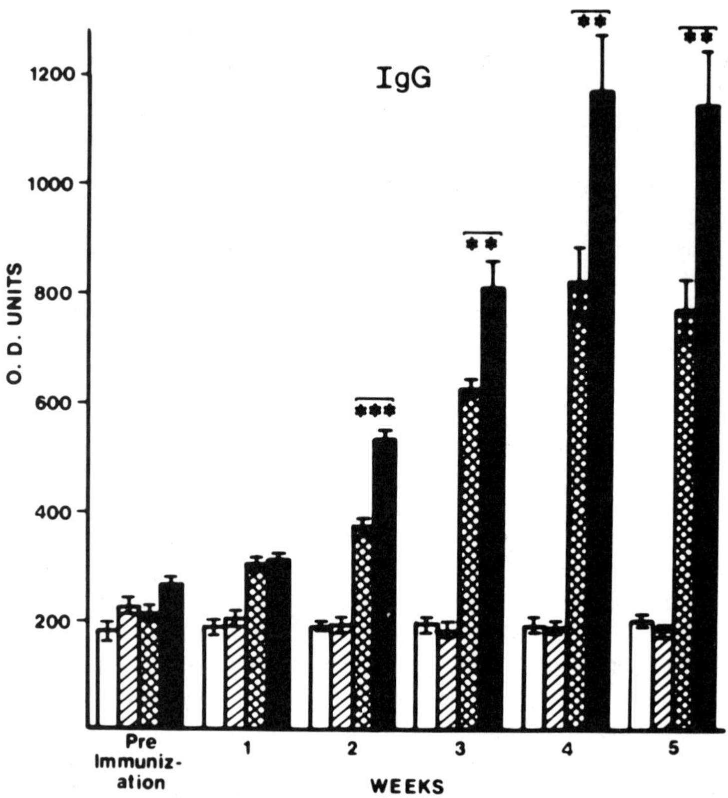

Figure 1 Antitetanus antibody (IgG) from control, nonimmunized mice (open bar), from CMD treated nonimmunized mice (hatched bar), from control, immunized mice (double hatched bar), and from cimetidine-treated immunized mice (solid bar). Antibody levels for each group were determined by ELISA, and the result was noted in arbitrary optical density units (OD units = measured optical density X 1000). For the immunized animlas, significantly more antitetanus IgG was measured 2 weeks after immunization, and each week thereafter (*$p < 0.05$, **$p < 0.02$, ***$p < 0.001$). (From Ref. 28, used with permission.)

synthesis without added mitogen, and the difference was magnified by the addition of the mitogens. Another observation was that those animals that had received low-dose cimetidine appeared to respond in these assays a bit better than the higher dose groups, which led us to believe that perhaps the cimetidine-histamine type II receptor interaction was more complex than we had predicted, or that we were observing a degree of an immunotoxic reaction in the high-dose group. That the latter was not the case was suggested by other of the assays. For example, the antibody response to the tetanus vaccine was clearly greater in the cimetidine group, and the best response were seen in the high-dose cimetidine group (as depicted in Fig. 1). By comparing the vaccine dilutions of sera from treatment and control groups, it was apparent that there was almost twice as much antibody present in the cimetidine group.

Resistance to bacterial or parasitic challenge has been classically considered primarily a humoral immune response; however there is no doubt that the cellular interactions are generally more complex than originally thought, and clearly both cellular and humoral components are involved. It is, therefore, reasonable to expect that modifier's of T-cell immunity would have some impact on the success of the vaccine (as above), or even more importantly on the resistance to subsequent challenge. Two studies have recently been published in which such observations were recorded. Zapata-Sirvent and colleagues (30) found that burn-injured mice, when subjected to needle puncture of the cecum had high mortality rates (~ 20% survival 10 days postburn), whereas normal mice subjected to cecal puncture had a survival rate of 64%. These authors found that it cimetidine was administered (10 mg/kg/day intraperitoneally) for the 10 days postburn, the survival pattern was similar to the normal mice (62%), and significantly greater than the control (burn) mice.

In a completely different system, Kelly and Colley (31) found fairly similar results with cimetidine administration to mice. Two different strains were examined with reference to their ability to become successfully immunized after exposure to radiation-attenuated *Schistosoma mansoni* cercariae. C57B1/6 mice were generally capable of becoming sensitized; however, CBA/J mice were not. Interestingly, when cimetidine (50 mg/kg/day) was administered in the drinking water for 7 days prior and 21 days after sensitization a significantly greater portion of the CBA/J were found to be resistant to subsequent challenge with viable organisms.

It is apparent, therefore, that under controlled circumstances in mice, antibody responses can be modified by cimetidine treatment, and that such treatments may also render a host more readily immunized (with vaccine) and even more resistant to primary challenge with pathogen (such as observed in the burned mice [30]).

IV. MEASURES OF FUNCTIONAL CELLULAR IMMUNITY IN CIMETIDINE-TREATED MICE

Mice treated with cimetidine have also been carefully scrutinized by those measures generally considered markers of cellular immunity. Utilizing both a burn-injury model (as above) and a trauma model, Hansbrough and colleagues have

Table 1 Effects of Cimetidine in vivo in Mice

Assay system	Ref.	Outcome
Humoral immunity and infectious challenge in cimetidine-treated mice		
Vaccine response	28	Mice injected with cimetidine had greater amounts of antitetanus antibody in response to tetanus toxoid vaccine.
Survival of burned mice after cecal puncture	30	Mice injected with cimetidine after burn injury and cecal puncture had a survival pattern comparable to normal mice (after burn) significantly greater than mice that receive burn and cecal puncture without cimetidine.
Resistance to *Schistisoma mansoni* after sesitization	31	Oral cimetidine prior to and after vaccination allowed resistance to subsequent challenge in CBA/H mice–A strain that is usually not resistant after vaccine.
Measures of functional cellular immunity in cimetidine treated mice		
Skin-graft survival	35	Mice fed oral cimetidine (30 mg/kg) had enhanced retention of syngeneic, cross-sexed skin grafts, but ultimately had the same percentage of long-term engraftment.
DNFB sensitization/ suppressor-cell model	37	Mice injected with cimetidine (10, 50, or 100 mg/kg) had abrogation of the suppressor cell–mediated inhibition of DNFB-induced inflammatory response.
Measures of antitumor responses in cimetidine-treated mice		
Lewis lung Ca (metastases, survival)	47	Mice fed oral cimetidine had fewer metastases and greater survival than controls.
EL-4 lymphoma (survival)	49,50	Mice fed oral cimetidine had greater survival than controls.
Cloudman melanoma	51,52	Mice tested with (tumor growth) histamine had accelerated tumor growth; immune-deficient mice treated with cimetidine had reduced growth.
C3H mammary carcinoma (survival)	53	Mice fed oral cimetidine had greater survival than controls.
Crocker 180 TG (tumor growth)	54	Mice treated sequentially with C-parvuum, cimetidine, interferon, and arginine butyrate had demonstrable tumor regression.

found that postburn (or trauma) T-lymphocyte subset distribution and delayed-type hypersensitivity responses are improved (i.e., approach normal) in mice that are treated with cimetidine (30,32–34). In contrast, Goldberg et al. (35) found that skin-graft survival could be prolonged by cimetidine treatment. In the A/J strain of mice, male-to-female skin grafts are rejected by approximately 50% of recipients. Rejection occurs presumably on the basis of immune responses elicited against the H-Y antigen, since in other strains antibody to this antigen has been demonstrated in recipients of cross-sex skin grafts (36). In cohorts of female mice that received 30 mg/kg/day of cimetidine in their drinking water, there were a greater percentage of animals with viable skin grafts, and this difference in graft survival was apparent for approximately 3 months. After that time, skin-graft survival was nearly identical in the cimetidine-treated and control groups. If cimetidine mediates its effects solely by inhibition of T-suppressor cells, these observations would suggest that the mechanism of cross-sex skin-graft rejection are more complex than the simple model of an in vivo DTH. Based upon earlier work, it would have been predicted that DTH (and presumably skin-graft rejection) would have been enhanced by the inhibition of cells bearing histamine type II receptors. Presumably, other components of the inflammatory response were inhibited by cimetidine treatment, as suggested by the authors.

Clearly, inhibition of suppressor-cell function has been demonstrated by in vivo treatment with cimetidine. For example, Jin and colleagues (37) found that one dose of cimetidine treatment was successful in inhibiting suppressor cell-mediated tolerance to 1-fluoro-2,4-dinitrobenzene (DNFB). In this model, BALB/c mice were injected with cimetidine (varying doses from 10 to 100 mg/kg) or saline (control) prior to or at the time of injection of 5×10^7 DNFB-coupled syngeneic lymphocytes. Seven days later, a single cell suspension of splenic and lymph node lymphocytes from these sensitized mice were injected into naive syngeneic hosts and immediately and 24 hr later (days 0 and 1), 0.5% DNFB solution (4:1, acetone:olive oil) was applied to the abdominal skin. On day 5, these mice were challenged with the same solution applied to the dorsum of each ear, and 1 day later, ear thickness was measured. Animals that had not received the prior sensitization of DNFB lymphocytes (and no cimetidine or saline injection), but were sensitized with DNFB on days 0, 1, and 5 had marked ear swelling, whereas those that had been sensitized but had not received cimetidine (controls) had minimal swelling; observations that are typical for this type of assay, and considered to reflect in vivo DTH and the effect of suppressor-cell function engendered by prior sensitization, respectively (38, 39). In this work, cimetidine was clearly shown to undermine those mediators of inhibition of DTH. That is, in a dose- and schedule-dependent way, those mice that received lymphocytes from sensitized, but cimetidine-treated mice, had an inflammatory response upon DNFB sensitization of the ear comparable to animals that had not received splenic lymphocytes at all (positive controls); and as mentioned, those animals that received the splenic cell injections but no cimetidine had virtually no measurable inflammation. As was observed earlier in a different model (28), it was apparent that the lower dose of cimetidine (50 mg/kg) was associated with maximal response, and the higher dose (100 mg/kg) with less. Also, it is probably of some importance to note that of the various schedules tested, cimetidine injection 2 days prior and on the day of primary sensitization with DNFB lymphocytes was optimal in producing the response when compared to administration 1 or 3 days after the injection. These experiments provided a clear demonstration that in vivo cimetidine treatment had predictable biologic activity consistent with the construct of inhibition histamine type II receptor-bearing T-cuppressor cells. Certainly, the results are consistent with the multitude of studies of the effects of cimetidine in vitro, including those in which cimetidine treatment (in vitro) augmented graft-versus-host reactions in a xenogeneic model (40), and also those studies in which skin testing with recall-type antigens has been shown in people to be enhanced by cimetidine administration (41,42).

V. CANCER MODELS IN MICE

As with the majority of immunomodulatory molecules that have had demonstrated in vitro and in vivo activities similar to those described above, the experimentation inevitably involves tumor models, with the hopeful expectation of demonstrating antitumor activity. This is particularly relevant with cimetidine because of the increasingly prevalent reports of murine tumor systems which seem to be influenced by T-suppressor cells. For example, with certain experimental tumors such as the methylchlolanthrene-induced fibrosarcomas, the spleens of tumor-bearing mice harbor cells that specifically undermine antitumor immunity. It has been demonstrated in such systems that in mice that were rendered resistant by inoculation with irradiated tumor cells, the immunity that was clearly demonstrable in control animals was abrogated by the syngeneic transfusion of spleen cells from tumor-bearing mice (43,44). Furthermore, the cells capable of producing such an effect were shown to be suppressor cells of T lineage (45,46). It was a reasonable hypothesis, therefore, to expect that selective inhibitors of suppressor-cell function might actually be associated with antitumor response.

In that light, Osband and coworkers (47) studied mice that were treated continuously with cimetidine in their drinking water (0.2, 2.0, or 10.0 mg/ml) and were subjected to inoculation of Lewis lung carcinoma (3LL) in the foot pad. When the primary tumor grew to a certain size (7.5 mm), the foot was surgically amputated. The number of suppressor cells (defined as those that demonstrated cell surface histamine type II receptors increased severalfold in the spleens of tumor-bearing mice. This increase was associated with coincident increased measurable suppressor-cell function in vitro (in a phytohemagglutinin lymphocyte activation assay with cells preincubated with histamine). Animals in the cimetidine treatment group had less in vitro suppression, and more importantly, had fewer pulmonary metastases and greater survival. Although there are several problems inherent in the model (e.g., those associated with the use of a tumor line such as 3LL [48]; the use of cimetidine in drinking water without accurate dosing), the results were intriguing, and this study has served as a catalyst for similar studies in mice, and even clinical trials (as discussed below).

In murine studies that were occurring at about the same time, Gifford et al. (49,50) also provided exciting results. These investigators added cimetidine to drinking water at several calculated doses (15, 40, 100, and 200 mg/kg/day based upon observed water intake). They inoculated C57Bl/6 mice with EL-4, a chemically induced, syngeneic lymphoma, and found a dose-dependent increase in survival in the cimetidine treatment group. This protective effect of cimetidine appeared greater in those experiments involving young mice (2 months) when compared to middle-aged mice (8 months). Animals that survived the initial tumor were later rechallenged and were found not to be immune (i.e., despite the previous exposure, there was no observed resistance upon subsequent rechallenge, albeit at a higher inoculum of tumor). Retreatment with cimetidine coincident with the rechallenge, however, was associated with increased duration of survival. Although not definitively involving T-suppressor mechanisms, these results support the general contention that under well-defined circumstances the immunomodulatory activity of cimetidine may have practical antineoplastic correlates.

Utilizing another murine tumor line (Cloudman melanoma), Nordland and colleagues also explored the potential importance for selective immune manipulation by pharmacologic agents (51,52). They had previously demonstrated that the dose of tumor antigen was the critical determinant in which way the immunoregulatory balance would lean (i.e., T helper or T suppressor), and tumor growth was influenced accordingly (51). These investigators went further to show that histamine treatment enhanced tumor growth, whereas treatment with cimetidine was inhibitory (52).

Other investigators have reported similar results with cimetidine in murine tumor models. Thus, Penhaligon and colleagues (53) demonstrated a greater survival duration and cure rate in a metastases model involving C3H mice with a syngeneic mammary carcinoma tumor line. In these experiments, mice were fed cimetidine in their drinking water at a dose of 10 mg/ml. Cerutti and Chany (54) proceeded one step further to include cimetidine in a multi-immunopharmacologic approach to treatment of tumor (Crocker 180-TG)-inoculated mice. This approach involved sequential treatment with C-Parvuum, cimetidine interferon, and arginine butyrate, and the authors were able to demonstrate significant improvement and minimal toxicity with such an approach.

The translation of these promising findings from the highly artificial circumstance of inbred strains of mice with highly antigenic tumors to the clinical situation in which tumors are frequently without demonstrable tumor antigens and patients are clearly heterogeneous with respect to their underlying medical conditions and their ability to muster immunologic responses (either effector or suppressor) has been disappointing. Certainly, occasional anecdotal reports, or even trials, have indicated a possible improvement with cimetidine treatment (especially in patients with melanoma or renal cell carcinoma) (55); for the most part, the lack of more widespread clinical use of cimetidine as an immunomodulatory agent in cancer patients no doubt reflects the lack of definite activity when systematically analyzed in clinical trial. For example, in an unpublished series that we conducted (W. B. Ershler, J. A. Stewart, J. D. Robert, and C. F. Myers), of 30 patients with advanced solid tumor malignancy on no other anticancer drugs), we observed one patient who had a transient (3 months) reduction in metastatic renal cell carcinoma. In that trial in which patients received 300 mg of cimetidine twice daily, no observable toxicity was noticed; however there was also no detectable differences in certain in vitro parameters (T-cell number, mitogen-induced blastogenesis). The results of this trial and the lack of published clinical trials indicating efficacy leave us to conclude that the utility of cimetidine in the clinical sphere as an anticancer approach should remain investigational. This certainly is not meant to belittle the important observations from the murine systems, but to point out that the defined role for the type of immunomodulation that can be achieved by cimetidine in such patients has yet to be declared.

VI. CONCLUSIONS

Cimetidine is a molecule of intense biologic and therapeutic interest. As the prototype histamine type II antagonist, its clinical utility has been established in the treatment of peptic ulcer disease. Because of the known importance of histamine as a regulator of immune functions, especially of those cells bearing histamine type II receptors, exploration of its immunomodulatory effects has been both logical and fruitful. In this chapter, the effects of the drug administered in vivo (by a variety of routes, doses, and schedules) upon certain selected "immune" functions has been reviewed. By no means comprehensive, this chapter is a sampling of the investigations in which cimetidine was administered to the intact animal, and hopefully reflects both what is known and unknown about the important immunomodulatory effects that can be achieved by drugs in this class. Certainly, as the systems become more complex, the interactions and the involvement of other influences on immune function cloud the picture, and the awareness of these make the demonstrable activity of cimetidine in the whole animal impressive observations. In subsequent chapters in this volume, a more dissected approach to the analysis of the specific role for cimetidine as an immunopharmacologic agent will be detailed.

REFERENCES

1. Rocklin, R. E., Modulation of cellular immune responses in vivo and in vitro by histamine receptor-bearing lymphocytes, J. Clin. Invest. 57:1051–1058 (1976).
2. Schwartz, A., P. W. Askenase, and R. K. Gershon, Histamine inhibition of the *in vitro* induction of cytotoxic T-cell responses, Immunopharmacol. 2: 179–190 (1980).
3. Dohlsten, M., H. O. Sjogren, and R. Carlsson, Histamine inhibits interferon γ production via suppression of interleukin-2 synthesis, Cell. Immunol. 101: 493–501 (1986).
4. Thomas, Y., R. Huchet, and D. Grandjon, Histamine-induced suppressor cells of lymphocyte mitogenic response, Cell. Immunol. 59:268–275 (1981).
5. Suzuki, S., and R. Huchet, Mechanism of histamine induced inhibition of lymphocyte response to mitogens in mice, Cell. Immunol. 62:396–405 (1981).
6. Rocklin, R. E., J. Beard, S. Gupta, R. A. Good, and K. L. Melmon, Characterization of the human blood lymphocytes that produce a histamine-induced suppressor factor (HSF), Cell. Immunol. 51:226–237 (1980).
7. Damle, N. K., and S. Gupta, OKT8+ T cells mediate histamine-induced suppressor T cell function, IRCS J. Med. Sci. 9:911–912 (1981).
8. Richardson, C. T., Effect of h-2 receptor antagonists on gastric acid secretion and serum gastrin concentration: A review, Gastroenterology 74:366–370 (1978).
9. Finklestein, W., and K. J. Isselbacher, Drug therapy: Cimetidine, N. Engl. J. Med. 299:992–996 (1978).
10. Cimetidine Tagamet: Update on adverse effects, Med. Lett—Drugs and Therapeutics 20:77–78 (1977).
11. Bauman, J., J. Elenbass, and S. C. Hamburger, Cimetidine: A review, JAMWA 35:5–12 (1980).
12. Rocklin, R. E., Histamine-induced suppressor factor (HSF) effect on migration inhibitory factor (MIF) production and proliferation, J. Immunol. 118: 1734–1738 (1977).
13. Plaut, M., L. M. Lichtenstein, E. Gillespie, and C. S. Henney, Studies on the mechanism of lymphocyte mediated cytolysis. IV. Specificity of the histamine receptor on effector cells, J. Immunol. 111:389–394 (1973).

14. Rocklin, R. E., D. K. Greineder, and K. L. Melmon, Histamine induced suppressor factor (HSF): Further studies on the nature of the stimulus and the cell which produces it, Cell. Immunol. 44:404–415 (1979).
15. Rocklin, R. E., and A. Haberek-Davidson, Histamine activates suppressor cells in vitro using a coculture technique, J. Clin. Immunol. 1:73–79 (1981).
16. Wang, S. R., and B. Zweiman, Histamine suppression of human lymphocyte responses to mitogens, Cell. Immunol. 36:28–36 (1978).
17. Rocklin, R. E., Histamine-induced suppressor factor (HSF): Effect on migration inhibitory factor (MIF) production and proliferation, J. Immunol. 118:1734–1738 (1977).
18. Shearer, G. M., K. L. Melmon, Y. Weinstein, and M. Sela, Regulation of antibody response by cells expressing histamine receptors, J. Exp. Med. 136: 1302–1307 (1972).
19. Nair, M. P. N., and S. A. Schwartz, Effect of histamine and histamine antagonists on natural and antibody-dependent cellular cytotoxicity on human lymphocytes *in vitro*, Cell. Immunol. 81:45–60 (1983).
20. Rocklin, R. E., A. L. Scheffer, D. K. Greineder, and K. L. Melmon, Generation of antigen specific suppressor cells during allergy desensitization, N. Engl. J. Med. 302:1213–1219 (1980).
21. Rocklin, R. E., D. Greineder, B. H. Littman, and K. L. Melmon, Modulation of cellular immune function in vitro by histamine receptor bearing lymphocytes: Mechanism of action, Cell. Immunol. 37:162–173 (1978).
22. Garovoy, M. R., M. A. Reddish, and R. E. Rocklin, Histamine-induced suppressor factor (HSF): Inhibition of helper T cell generation and function, J. Immunol. 130:357–361 (1983).
23. Plaut, M., and L. M. Lichtenstein, Histamine and immune responses. In Pharmacology of Histamine Receptors (Ganellin, C. R., and Patsons, M. G., Eds.), London, Wright and Sons (1982), p. 392.
24. Rocklin, R. E., I. Kiselis, D. J. Beer, P. Rossi, F. Maggi, and J. A. Ballanti, Augmentation of prostaglandin and thromboxane production in vitro by monocytes exposed to histamine-induced suppressor factor (HSF), Cell. Immunol. 77:92–98 (1983).
25. Griswold, D. E., S. Alessi, A. M. Badger, G. Poste, and N. Hanna, Differential sensitivity of T suppressor cell expression to inhibition by histamine type 2 receptor antagonists, J. Immunol. 137:1811–1815 (1986).
26. Willcox, H. N. A., Thymus dependence of the antibody response to tetanus toxoid in mice, Clin. Exp. Immunol. 22:341–347 (1975).
27. Virelizier, J.-L., R. Postlethwaite, G. C. Schild, and A. C. Allison, Antibody responses to antigenic determinants of influenza hemagglutinin. 1. Thymus dependence of antibody formation and thymus indepencence of immunological memory, J. Exp. Med. 140:1559–1570 (1974).
28. Ershler, W. B., M. P. Hacker, B. J. Burroughs, A. L. Moore, and C. F. Myers, Cimetidine and the immune response. 1. In vivo augmentation of nonspecific and specific immune response, Clin. Immunol. Immunopathol. 26: 10–17 (1983).

29. Brimblecombe, R. W., W. A. M. Duncan, G. J. Durant, J. C. Emmett, C. R. Ganellin, and M. E. Parsons, Cimetidine–a non-thiourea H_2-receptor antagonist, J. Int. Med. Res. 3:86–92 (1975).
30. Zapata-Sirvent, R. L., J. F. Hansbrough, E. M. Bender, E. J. Bartle, A. Mansour, and W. H. Carter, Postburn immunosuppression in an animal model. IV. Improved resistance to septic challenge with immunomodulatory drugs, Surgery 95:290–295 (1984).
31. Kelly, E. A., and D. G. Colley, Effects of immunomanipulations on resistance induced by irradiated Schistisoma mansoni cercarial sensitization of C57BL/6 and CBA/J mice, Am. J. Med. Hyg. 35:803–811 (1986).
32. Hansbrough, J. F., Peterson, V. M., R. L. Zapata-Sirvent, and H. Claman, Restoration of cell-mediated immunity by immunomodulatory drugs, Surgery 95:290–295 (1984).
33. Zapata-Sirvent, R. L., and J. F. Harsbrough, Postburn immunosuppression in an animal model. III. Maintenance of normal splenic helper and suppressor lymphocyte subpopulations by immunomodulatory drugs, Surgery 97: 721–727 (1985).
34. Zapata-Sirvent, R. L., J. F. Harsbrough, and E. J. Bartle, Prevention of post traumatic alterations in lymphocyte subpopulations in mice by immunomodulatory drugs, Arch. Surg. 121:116–122 (1986).
35. Goldberg, E. H., J. S. Goodwin, S. E. Arritt, and R. C. Williams, Prolongation of male skin graft survival by female mice treated with cimetidine, Transplantation 28:422–433 (1979).
36. Goldberg, E. H., E. A. Boyse, M. Scheid, and D. Bennett, Production of H-Y antibody by female mice that fail to reject male skin, Nature 238:55–57 (1972).
37. Jin, Z., A. Kumar, R. P. Cleveland, D. L. Murray, and D. B. Kaufman, Inhibition of suppressor cell function by Cimetidine in a murine model, Clin. Immunol. Immunopathol. 38:350–356 (1986).
38. Miller, S. D., and H. N. Claman, The induction of hapten-specific T-cell tolerance by using hapten-modified lymphoid cells. I. Characteristics of tolerance induction, J. Immunol. 117:1519–1526 (1976).
39. Claman, H. N., S. D. Miller, M. S. Sy, and J. W. Moorehead, Suppressive mechanisms involving sensitization and tolerance in contact allergy, Immunol. Rev. 50:105–132 (1980).
40. Mavligit, G. M., D. B. Calvo, Y. Z. Patt, and E. M. Hersh, Immune restoration and/or augmentation of local xenogeneic graft versus host reaction by Cimetidine in vitro, J. Immunol. 126:2272–2274 (1981).
41. Avella, J., J. E. Madsen, H. J. Binder, and P. W. Askenase, Effects of histamine H2-receptor antagonists on delayed hypersensitivity, Lancet 1:624–626 (1978).
42. Richtsmeier, W. J., and D. Eisele, In vivo anergy reversal with Cimetidine in patients with cancer, Arch. Otolaryngol. Head Neck Surg. 112:1074–1077 (1986).

43. Fujimoto, S., M. I. Greene, and A. H. Sehon, Regulation of the immune response to tumor antigens. I. Immune suppressor cells in tumor bearing hosts, J. Immunol. 116:791–799 (1976).
44. Isakov, N., S. Segal, N. Hollander, and M. Feldman, An immunoregulatory factor associated with spleen cells from tumor bearing animals. I. Effects on tumro growth and antibody production, Int. J. Cancer 22:465–470 (1978).
45. Fujimoto, S., M. I. Greene, and A. H. Sehon, Regulation of the immune response to tumor antigens. II. The nature of the immunosuppressor cells in tumor bearing hosts, J. Immunol. 116:800–806 (1976).
46. Greene, M. L., M. E. Dorf, M. Pierres, and B. Benacerraf, Reduction of syngeneic tumor growth by an I-J alloantiserum, Proc. Nat. Acad. Sci. U.S.A. 74:5118–5121 (1977).
47. Osband, M. E., D. Hamilton, Y.-J. Shen, E. Cohen, M. Shlesinger, P. Lavin, A. Brown, and R. McCaffrey, Successful tumor immunotherapy with Cimetidine in mice, Lancet 1:636–638 (1981).
48. Hewitt, H. B., A critical examination of the foundations of immunotherapy for cancer, Clin. Radiol. 30:361–369 (1979).
49. Gifford, R. R. M., R. M. Ferguson, and B. V. Voss, Cimetidine reduction of tumor formation in mice, Lancet 1:638–640 (1981).
50. Gifford, R. R. M., B. V. Voss, and R. M. Ferguson, Cimetidine protection against lethal tumor challenge in mice, Surgery 90:344–351 (1981).
51. Nordlund, J. J., A. E. Ackles, and R. K. Gershon, Quantitative factors which determine the effect of the immune response on growth of Cloudman melanoma in DBA/2 mice, Cell. Immunol. 56:258–272 (1980).
52. Nordlund, J. J., and P. W. Askenase, The effect of histamine, antihistamines, and a mast cell stabilizer in the growth of Cloudman melanoma cells in DBA/2 mice, J. Invest. Dermatol. 81:28–31 (1983).
53. Penhaligon, M., J. Anthoons, D. Pilkington, R. A. Wolstencroft, T. Bates, and A. H. Nias, Anti-metastatic effect of Cimetidine on mice bearing a C3H mouse mammary adenocarcinoma: Survival abd lymphocyte function studies, Clin. Exp. Metast. 2:37–53 (1984).
54. Cerutti, I., and C. Chany, Importance of coordinated immune stimulation in experimental anti-tumor treatment, Int. J. Immunopharmacol. 7:783–787 (1985).
55. Flodgren, P., S. Borgstrom, P. E. Jonsson, C. Lindstrom, and H. O. Sjogren, Metastatic malignant melanoma: Regression induced by combined treatment with interferon [HuIFN-alpha(Le)] and Cimetidine, Int. J. Cancer 32:657–665 (1983).

10

Superficial Fungal Diseases

JOSEPH L. JORIZZO and TINA B. SMITH *Bowman Gray School of Medicine of Wake Forest University, Winston-Salem, North Carolina*

I. INTRODUCTION

The early experimental work in guinea pigs by Rocklin and associates (1) which demonstrated that histamine inhibits cell-mediated immunity (CMI) (i.e., CMI was assessed by skin-test reactivity, migration inhibitory factor (MIF), and lymphocyte proliferation) is summarized elsewhere in this text. Rocklin also demonstrated in guinea pigs that histamine-induced suppression of CMI was completely reversed by pretreatment with histamine type II (H_2) receptor antagonists such as metiamide (1). Rosenberg and associates (2) first applied Rocklin's concept that the use of histamine type II blockers could be effective in allowing the cutaneous expression of CMI to a clinical situation. They were using dinitrochlorobenzene (DNCB) to treat patients with alopecia areata. Several of these patients developed an acquired tolerance to DNCB, which would have rendered the treatment ineffective. Rosenberg and associates gave these tolerant patients oral cimetidine 300 mg four times daily and restored the CMI response to DNCB in their patients (2,3).

At this same time period, we had studied a family consisting of eight members in three generations (age 10 months to 53 years) affected with chronic mucocutaneous candidiasis (4). Chronic mucocutaneous candidiasis (CMC) is an uncommon, therapy-resistant superficial candidosis of skin, hair, nails, and mucous membranes that is often associated with abnormalities of CMI ranging from mild antigen-specific abnormalities to life-threatening immune deficiency (5). Chronic mucocutaneous candidiosis had earlier been proposed as an excellent model for the study of CMI by Kirkpatrick (6). Evaluation of our family of patients with CMC had shown an impairment of the CMI response to *Candida* antigen as measured by negative results to the following tests to *Candida* antigen: intradermal skin tests, in vitro lymphocyte transformation, and lymphokine (leukocyte migration inhibitory factor [LIF]) production (4). The investigation of cimetidine as an immunomodulator in these patients offered the dual advantage of providing an opportunity to add clinical support to the concept that histamine type II receptor blockade could allow for the expression of CMI, and of providing a relatively safe, available immune enhancer to use in selected patients with CMC (7).

Clinical and immunopathological aspects of CMC will be reviewed in detail. Our 1980 study of cimetidine therapy in CMC willbe reviewed. The clinical problem of therapy-resistant extensive dermatophytosis will be presented. An update of cimetidine therapy for CMC and for therapy-resistant dermatophytosis will be offered in an anecdotal fashion because systematic assessment of this therapy in these conditions has not been reported since our 1980 study. This may be due in part to the clinical success of a new therapy, oral ketoconazole, in this patient population (8). Of related interest, however, was our inability to detect immune-enhancing properties for ibuprofen, an inhibitor of other (i.e., not histamine) autacoids, the prostaglandins, also assessed in patients with CMC (9).

II. CHRONIC MUCOCUTANEOUS CANDIDIASIS

A. Clinicopathologic Aspects

Chronic mucocutaneous candidiosis differs from routine superficial candidal infection of the skin, nails, and oral and genital mucosae by the persistance of the infection, the progression to granulomatous candidosis, and by the resistance of the infection to therapy (10,11). Mucosal surfaces respond to the chronic inflammation induced by the candidal organisms by becoming hypertrophic. Fissuring is a common complication. Cutaneous lesions may take on a verrucous appearance owing to dramatic hyperkeratosis. Nail plate invasion by candidal organisms is not a feature of simple candidal paronychia. Chronic mucocutaneous candidiasis patients have nails which demonstrate nail plate invasion by candidal organisms as a rule. Thus, the presence of direct invasion of the nail plate by yeast with resultant hypertrophic dystrophy is very suggestive of a diagnosis of CMC.

Chronic mucocutaneous candidiasis is not characterized by internal dissemination of *Candida* species as is seen with candidal sepsis. Esophageal and the more recently described laryngeal involvement are not common (12).

Dermatophytosis, which is extensive and therapy resistant, is a frequent associated superficial fungal infection in patients with CMC (13). As with candidal infection in patients with CMC, dermatophytosis may involve any cutaneous site, hair, and nails. Lesions may also be hyperkeratotic.

Histopathologic features of the hyperkeratotic ("granulomatous") lesions of CMC include: hyperkeratosis and parakeratosis and a dense chronic inflammatory cell infiltrate in the dermis. Plasma cells and occasional multinucleated giant cells may be present in addition to lymphocytes (6). Despite the dermal inflammation, organisms remain almost exclusively confined to the keratinizing layers of the epidermis. Scanning electron microscopic studies reveal penetration of pseudohyphae through holes in keratinizing cells (14).

B. Immunologic Aspects

Patients with CMC are unable to contain mucocutaneous spread of superficial fungal infections; however, systemic dissemination of candidal infection is not a feature of CMC. Host defense mechanisms which protect against systemic dissemination of candidal organisms have been recently reviewed (15-17). These mechanisms are presumed to be intact in patients with CMC. The stratum corneum is an effective physical barrier against all candidal species except *C. albicans* and *C. stellatoidea*. External factors may alter the barrier (e.g., maceration) and epithelial defense mechanisms such as desquamation can not always compensate. The next line of defense may involve the alternative complement pathway, which can be directly activated by candidal cell wall products. The inflammatory cells attracted by complement components (e.g., C4a) can help contain the invading yeast organisms. Serum factors, especially iron-free transferrin, are potent inhibitors of candidal dissemination. The exact mechanism of action is unknown, but may relate to removal of iron needed for growth of the organisms.

1. Severe Immunodeficiency

Chronic mucocutaneous candidiasis can occur as a minor component of the severe multiple infections seen in patients with several life-threatening immunodeficiency syndromes. Unfortunately, patients with these syndromes often die in infancy from disseminated viral, fungal, bacterial, or other infections. Immunodeficiency syndromes which particularly predispose the patient to CMC include: DiGeorge's syndrome (congenital thymic aplasia), Nezelof-Allibone syndrome (thymic alymphoplasia), severe comboned immunodeficiency, variable immunodeficiency, and hyperimmunoglobulin E syndromes (e.g., Job's syndrome, Buckley's syndrome) (19-21). Chronic mucocutaneous candidiasis can also be a feature of iatrogenic immunosuppression and of AIDS (autoimmune deficiency syndrome). The association of CMC with severe immunodeficiency syndromes reinforces the concept that CMC is not a single disease entity, but rather a symptom complex associated with multiple predisposing abnormalities, particularly of cellular immunity.

2. Nonlethal Immunodeficiency

A deficit in our understanding ofthe pathogenesis of CMC results from the absence of reports of complete immunologic evaluation performed on large numbers of patients. Most reports described small patient groups who have been evaluated by one or a small group of tests. Kirkpatrick has been a leader in the evaluation of patients with CMC. He has reviewed a number of immunologic deficits which can occur in patients with CMC, and Littman and associates have reported that up to one-third of patients with CMC have no demonstrable immunologic defect even when evaluated extensively using modern immunodiagnostic techniques (6,11,21). Lehner and associates have also reviewed the immunodeficiencies seen in these patients, as have others (22,23).

Of the two-thirds to three-quarters of CMC patients with a demonstrable immune deficit, the majority have either complete anergy or at least anergy to *Candida* antigen as demonstrated by testing with a panel of intradermal skin tests, and in the past, dinitrochlorobenzene sensitization. In vitro testing allows for separation of these patients into three groups: lymphocyte transformation (LT) positive and macrophage inhibitory factor (MIF) positive, LT positive and MIF negative, and LT negative and MIF negative (21,22,24). A number of other nonlethal immune defects have been reported in small groups of patients with CMC. A partial listing of these includes: various serum factors which inhibit lymphocyte transformation or leukocyte killing of *Candida*, deficient serum or salivary immunoglobulin A (IgA), defective manocyte chemotaxis or killing of *Candida*, abnormal complement function, and abnormal macrophage function (23).

a. Medical Associations

Several subgroups of CMC exist in which distinct medical associations are prominent features of the symptom complex. The *Candida*-endocrinopathy syndrome is often inherited as an autosomal recessive condition characterized by childhood onset of CMC followed by significant autoimmune polyglandular (parathyroid, thyroid, adrenal, and diabetes mellitus) endocrine disease (6). In addition to auto-antibodies against endocrine tissue, antibodies may also be found against melanocytes in patients with associated vitiligo (25). Therapy for the endocrine disorders does not affect the CMC and vice versa.

The association of CMC with thymoma has been well described in a subgroup of patients with adult onset of both conditions. Some of these patients have had myeloperoxidase deficiency. Myasthenia gravis and hematologic abnormalities are also a feature as seen in this subgroup of patients (26).

A fascinating subgroup of CMC patients are those with decreased iron absorption. These patients show correction of their CMC and of their in vitro lymphocyte function abnormalities with parenteral iron therapy (27).

Additional random associations of CMC with other medical abnormalities have been reported. Malabsorption and chronic active hepatitis have been described. Dental enamel dysplasia may result from poor oral hygiene owing to inflammation from chronic oral candidiasis. The keratoconjunctivitis that has been described in these patients is generally not responsive to therapy of the candidiasis and is poorly characterized (28).

b. Therapy

Resistance to therapy is a diagnostic criterion of CMC. Topical anticandidal therapies with agents such as imidazoles, nystatin, and topical amphotericin B are at best palliative. Associated dermatophyte infections do not respond to oral griseofulvin. Prior to the introduction of oral ketoconazole therapy, successful treatment of CMC was best accomplished with potent antifungal agents, such as low-dose amphotericin B, to induce clinical remission. However, owing to the chronic nature of the immune defects associated with CMC, relapse within 12 months of the cessation of antifungal therapy necessitated immunotherapy to prevent the recurrence of infection (5). Various other systemic therapies proved undesirable owing to the rapid development of resistant organisms (flucytosine), side effects such as liver enzyme induction, nausea, neutropenia, and mental disturbances (clotrimazole), or the necessity of hospitalization (low-dose amphotericin B). These therapies have largely been replaced by oral ketoconazole therapy (5). Systemic imidazole therapy will be discussed after the review of cimetidine therapy.

Despite the heterogeneity of symptom complexes associated with CMC, the uniform presence of what is proposed to be a primary or secondary deficiency in cell-mediated immunity has prompted the study of therapy with immune enhancers. The suggested role for these agents is that of prolonging clinical remission previously achieved with potent systemic antifungal agents (5). Littman and associates demonstrated the conversion of negative *Candida* skin test responses to positive responses, along with the induction of lymphokine (migration inhibitory factor) production in response to *Candida* antigen following treatment with transfer factor, a cell-free dialyzable extract of leukocytes which has the capacity to transfer delayed hypersensitivity reactions to anergic persons (22). Discouraging results of therapeutic trials with thymic extracts in immune deficiency are attributed to the lack of understanding of the precise action of these extracts and to the likelihood that these extracts exert their actions on postthymic cells, thus rendering them ineffective without a suitable substrate population to enhance. Thymus transplantation has been advocated as a procedure best utilized for treatment of mile T-cell defects, including CMC, which is unresponsive to ketoconazole. The use of posttransplantation immunosuppression has been shown to prolong the duration of clinical remission in CMC (30).

III. CIMETIDINE IN CMC

Cimetidine, a histamine type II receptor antagonist, has been shown to reproducibly reverse certain defects in the immune response to *Candida* antigen in patients with CMC. Four adult patients with dominantly inherited CMC, manifested by chronic, therapy-resistant candidal infections of nails, skin, and mucous membranes, were studied to establish a possible role for cimetidine as an immunomodulator. Baseline determinations of in vivo and in vitro cell-mediated immunity to *Candida* antigen as measured by intradermal skin tests, lymphocyte transformation, and LIF production to *Candida* antigen revealed anergy in all four patients. The patients were given a 4-week course of cimetidine, 300 mg by mouth four times daily. Following treatment, all four patients developed positive intradermal skin test reactions to *Candida* antigen as indicated by greater than 15 nm of induration, whereas two of four patients experienced conversion to production of LIF to *Candida* antigen. Therapy was discontinued for 4 weeks with subsequent skin test and lymphokine production responses reverting to baseline negative values. An additional 4 weeks of cimetidine treatment was instituted, and all four patients again manifested strongly positive skin test reactions and LIF production to *Candida* antiben (Fig. 1). Lymphocyte transformation was not affected by cimetidine treatment. During the short duration of the study, cimetidine alone had no effect on the clinical manifestations of candidiasis. One patient with associated extensive tinea corporis, previously refractory to therapy, cleared with administration of oral griseofulvin (which was started after the formal study) during cimetidine therapy. There was no evidence of side effects attributed to cimetidine therapy (7).

A possible mechanism of action of cimetidine as an immunomodulator in patients with CMC, based on Rocklin's work, is cimetidine blockage of histamine type II receptors on suppressor T cells which modulate lymphokine production and skin test reactivity (1,7). The blockage of histamine type II receptors could be expressed by the inhibition of a soluble, histamine-induced suppressor factor acting to prevent LIF factor production and skin test reactivity.

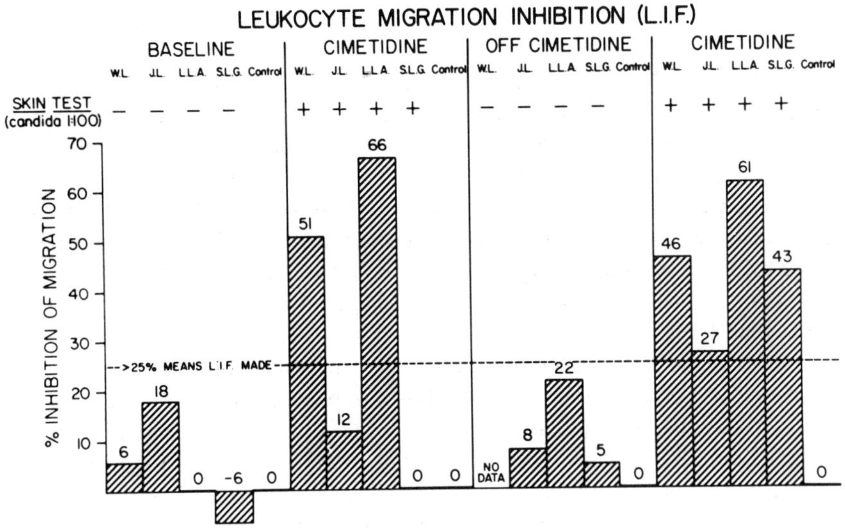

Figure 1 Intradermal skin test and LIF responses to *Candida* antigen by cimetidine patients on and off cimetidine therapy.

The lack of effect on lymphocyte transformation, despite improvement in lymphokine production and skin test reactivity, is in accordance with studies utilizing other immunomodulators. The effects of cimetidine were interpreted as nonspecific with conversion of the streptokinase/streptodornase skin test in addition to the *Candida* skin test, suggesting the possibility of application of the immunomodulator to other situations characterized by impaired CMI (7).

The demonstration of cimetidine as an immune enhancer in CMC through histamine type II receptor antagonism led to the study of the role of prostaglandins in the regulation of immune response and of the potential for cellular immune enhancement by inhibitors of prostaglandin synthesis in CMC patients. Laboratory evidence exists for depression of various parameters of cell-mediated immunity by prostaglandins PGE_1 or PGE_2 in animal systems with reversal of inhibition by the prostaglandin synthetase blocker indomethacin, and in vivo confirmation of these findings has been achieved with Hodgkins' disease patients who have shown reversal of depressed lymphocyte response to mitogen following oral indomethacin treatment (9). In a recent study evaluating four patients with CMC as a model to study the specific cellular immune-enhancing potential of ibuprofen, the prostaglandin synthetase inhibitor failed to demonstrate any consistent effect during 4-week on and off cycles (400 mg/kg four times daily for adults; 6 mg/kg four times daily for children). Ibuprofen did not consistently enhance cellular immunity to *Candida* antigen as assessed by delayed-type hypersensitivity skin test responses and lymphocyte transformation to *Candida* antigen. An absence of effect on T-cell subsets and on the production of the lymphokine, human immune interferon, in response to staphylococcal enterotoxin A was observed. Progression of CMC in two patients during ibuprofen therapy lends clinical support to the lack of efficacy of ibuprofen as an immune enhancer in CMC. In two patients who were studied 8-10 weeks following discontinuation of oral ketoconazole therapy, clinical recurrence of CMC was not prevented by oral ibuprofen therapy (9). This finding is in contrast to the capacity of cimetidine to maintain systemic antifungal agent-induced remissions for greater than 1 year (7,23).

Ketoconazole, an orally active antifungal agent structurally related to miconazole and clotrimazole, has been shown to be safe and effective in the treatment of patients with oral thrush, vulvovaginal candidiasis, candiduria, systemic *Candida*, and CMC (31). The drug has been found to be useful for both initial and long-term maintenance therapy of mucocutaneous lesions due to infection by sensitive strains of *Candida* in patients with CMC (33). In most cases, concurrent dermatophytoses resolve along with chronic candidal infections, although increased doses may be required (8). In one study in which long-term results of ketoconazole were studied, 13 patients were followed for up to 3 years, with all patients responding well. Clinical and mycologic clearing occurred in 1-2 months for oral lesions, 2 months for skin lesions, 3-4 months for paronychiae, and 4-14 months for nail plate lesions (32). The main limitation in therapy with ketoconazole involves the recurrence of candidal infection when oral therapy is decreased or discontinued. Maintenance therapy may be required indefinitely with dosage recommendations ranging from full-dose maintenance to biweekly or triweekly dosage schedules (31,33). Because of lower toxicity associated with ketoconazole than with amphotericin B the drug has been designated as preferable for patients with primary immunodeficiencies requiring treated repeated treatment courses and long-term maintenance courses of antifungal therapy (33). It is important to distinguish between the transient and more frequent laboratory abnormality of asymptomatic increase in liver function values as opposed to the symptomatic hepatitislike reactions which occur in 1/10,000 to 1/15,000 patients treated with ketoconazole (32).

The theoretic possibility of the emergence of candidal organisms resistant to ketoconazole must also be considered (33). In patients relapsing following 2 years of continuous therapy, it was impossible to determine whether the acquisition of resistant organisms from the environment was responsible or whether the patients' own organisms gradually developed resistance to the drug (8,32). The importance of following fungal cultures of involved areas has been stressed, since concurrent infection with dermatophytes occurs in 20% of patients with CMC, and failure to recognize the etiology of resistant lesions may lead to unsatisfactory treatment responses (8). Owing to the overrepresentation of pernicious anemia, a marker of achlorhydria, in patients with CMC, it is important to monitor plasma concentrations of ketoconazole in cases apparently refractory to treatment, since a failure to respond may be secondary to defective intestinal absorption (32).

Despite excellent clinical responses observed following therapy with oral ketoconazole, researchers have been unable to document significant changes in immunologic status that could be attributed to ketoconazole therapy (33). In a study of immune functions in eight patients with CMC, clinical improvement following 6 months of ketoconazole therapy (200 mg daily) was not associated with the amelioration of cutaneous delayed hypersensitivity to *Candida* antigen or of in vitro lymphocyte responses to *Candida* antigen to T-cell mitogens. Profound clinical improvement following therapy was likely due to a marked decrease in antigen load. These results suggest that the defect in cell-mediated immunity occurring in CMC patients is heterogeneous, and they support a primary disturbance of cellular immune function in CMC (34).

Itraconazole, a new agent which is poorly absorbed following oral administration, is much more potent in vitro than ketoconazole and possesses a broader spectrum of activity. In a small, uncontrolled trial of the drug, both patients with CMC demonstrated clinical improvement. One 27-year-old male with familial CMC received 100 mg daily for 5 months with marked but incomplete improvement, and then following 6 additional months on an increased dose of 299 mg daily experienced continuing resolution to nearly complete clearance. A 27-year-old male with AIDS who had *Candida albicans* isolated from mucosal and cutaneous lesions experienced clearing of thrush in 1 month, cutaneous lesions in 3–4 months, and esophagitis in 6 weeks while receiving itraconazole 100 mg daily. There were no adverse reactions attributed to the drug in any of 12 patients studied. The improvement of CMC in both the familial case and the AIDS-associated case demonstrates efficacy in these patients, and suggests a role for itraconazole in treatment and in prophylaxis for the immunocompromised host. An additional benefit of prophylactic therapy with itraconazole in the immunocompromised host, which is not achievable with ketoconazole, is the suppression of *Torrilopsis glabrata* colonization in addition to that of *Candida*. Large-scale clinical trials are necessary for comparison of itraconazole to other drugs in the treatment of CMC (35).

The clinical symptom complex of CMC represents the expression of a variety of heterogeneous immune defects which are lifelong, and which represent an immunodeficient state requiring reconstitution of cellular immunity for definitive cure (33). The study of cimetidine as an immunomodulator has provided clinical support to the existence of histamine type II receptors on lymphocytes which modulate cell-mediated immune functions.

The role of prostaglandins is less certain with the failure of the prostaglandin synthetase inhibitor ibuprofen to induce significant change parameters of CMI to *Candida* antigen. Ketoconazole, which has been demonstrated to effectively induce remission in CMC, has inhibited the study of autacoid inhibitors such as cimetidine in the treatment of CMC. Because long-term maintenance therapy with ketoconazole is usually necessary in CMC patients owing to the frequency of recurrent infection, a role for cimetidine as maintenance therapy for CMC patients in remission should continue to be explored. While clinical trials with increasing duration of follow-up have helped to define expectations of therapy for CMC, further elucidation of the pathogenesis of the disease complex will be necessary to further define the immune defects involved so that they may be specifically targeted for treatment.

IV. OTHER SUPERFICIAL FUNGAL INFECTIONS

Dematophytosis is a very common form of superficial fungal infection. Tinea capitis, corporis, manum, barbae, cruris, pedis, andunguium result from infection with fungi from the genera *Trichophyton, Microsporum*, and *Epidermophyton*. The organisms live in the keratinizing layers of skin, hair, and nails. Most infections with these agents respond promptly to therapy with topical imidazoles or other antifungal creams or to systemic griseofulvin therapy (36). A significant problem exists with chronic therapy (i.e., griseofulvin-resistant dermatophytosis). The predominant offending organism is *Trichophyton rubrum*. This organism is a "parasite" which has evolved to such a degree that it produces little clinical inflammation and is barely perceptible to the host cellular immune system. In one study, only 11% of patients with chronic dermatophyte infections showed delayed hypersensitivity responses to intradermal trichophytin despite obvious clinical disease (37). One study suggested that the anergy to trichophytin antigen in atopic individuals could relate to a strong immediate hypersensitivity reaction to the antigen with resultant neutralization of the antigen and a false negative skin test (38). In vitro tests, however, suggest that true impairment of CMI to trichophyton antigen exists in some patients with chronic dermatophytosis (39,40).

Therapy with oral ketoconazole, possibly with low-dose and or intermittent-maintenance therapy, has become the accepted mode of treatment for patients with chronic, therapy-resistant dermatophytosis (41,42,43). The timing of the emergence of oral ketoconazole therapy has surely been the major factor in limiting investigation of oral cimetidine, an immune enhancer for the treatment of chronic, therapy-resistant dermatophytosis. Anecdotal reports of cimetidine therapy for this indication exist (44,45), and no controlled studies correlating clinical response with skin tests and in vitro studies of lymphocyte transformation and lymphokine production to trichophytin antigen exist. A role may well be established by future studies for cimetidine in maintaining a ketoconazole-induced remission in patients with chronic, therapy-resistant dematophytosis.

REFERENCES

1. Rocklin, R. E., Modulation of cellular-immune responses *in vivo* and *in vitro* by histamine receptor-bearing lymphocytes, J. Clin. Invest. 57:1051–1058 (1976).
2. Daman, L. A., and E. W. Rosenberg, Acquired tolerance to dinitrochlorobenzene reversed by cimetidine, Lancet 2:1087 (Letter) (1977).
3. Breullard, F., and E. Szapiro, Cimetidine in acquired tolerance to dinitrochlorobenzene, Lancet 1:726 (Letter) (1978).
4. Sams, W. M., Jr., J. L. Jorizzo, R. Snyderman, B. V. Vegasothy, F. E. Ward, M. Weiner, J. G. Wilson, W. S. Yount, and S. B. Willard, Chronic mucocutaneous candidiasis: Immunologic studies in three generations of a single family, Am. J. Med. 67:948–959 (1979).
5. Jorizzo, J. L., Chronic mucocutaneous candidosis: An update, Arch. Dermatol. 118:963–965 (1982).
6. Kirkpatrick, C. H., R. R. Rich, and J. E. Bennett, Chronic muco-cutaneous candidiasis: Model building in cellular immunity, Ann. Intern. Med. 74: 955–978 (1971).
7. Jorizzo, J. L., W. M. Sams, Jr., B. V. Jegasothy, and A. J. Olansky, Cimetidine as an immunomodulator: Chronic mucocutaneous candidiasis as a model, Ann. Intern. Med. 92:192–195 (1980).
8. Horsburgh, C. R., and C. H. Kirkpatrick, Longterm therapy of chronic mucocutaneous candidiasis with ketoconazole: Experience with twenty-one patients, Am. J. Med.74:23–29 (1983).
9. Jorizzo, J. L., R. M. Goldblum, J. C. Daniels, M. P. Langford, H. B. Rudloff, Y. Ichikawa, and E. B. Gonzalez, Evaluation of immune-enhancing effects of ibuprofen in an immunodeficiency model, Int. J. Dermatol. 24:183–187 (1985).
10. Jorizzo, J. L., The spectrum of mucosal and cutaneous candidosis, Dermatol. Clin. 2:1:19–27 (1984).
11. Kirkpatrick, C. H., and P. G. Sohnle, Chronic mucocutaneous candidiasis. In Immunodermatology (D. Satai and R. A. Good, Eds.), Plenum Press, New York (1981), pp. 495–514.
12. Dudley, P., R. Lobayashi, H. M. Rosenblatt, W. J. Byrne, M. E. Ament, and E. R. Stiehm, Candida laryngitis in chronic mucocutaneous candidiasis: Its association with Candida esophagitis, Ann. Otol. Rhenol. Laryngol. 89:574–575 (1980).
13. Shama, S. K., and C. H. Kirkpatrick, Dermatophytosis in patients with chronic mucocutaneous candidiasis, J. Am. Acad. Dermatol. 2:285–294 (1980).

14. Wilborn, W. H., and L. P. Montes, Scanning electron microscopy of oral lesions in chronic mucocutaneous candidiasis, J.A.M.A. 244:2294–2297 (1980).
15. Edwards, J. E., Jr., R. I. Lehrer, E. R. Stiehm, T. J. Fischer, and L. S. Young, Severe candidal infections: Clinical perspective, immune defense mechanisms and current concepts of therapy, Ann. Intern. Med. 89:91-106 (1978).
16. Ray, T. L., and K. D. Wnepper, Recent advances in cutaneous candidiasis, Int. J. Dermatol. 17:683–690 (1978).
17. Rogers, T. L., and E. Balesh, Immunity to Candida albicans, Microbial. Rev. 44:660–682 (1980).
18. Ray, T. L., and K. D. Wupper, Experimental cutaneous candidiasis in rodents: Role of the stratum corneum barrier and serum complement as a mediator of a protective inflammatory response, Arch. Dermatol. 114:538–543 (1978).
19. Gosseye, S., and C. Nezelof, T System immunodeficiences in infancy and childhood, Pathol. Res. Pract. 171:142–158 (1981).
20. Rosen, F. S., Cooper, M. D., and R. J. P. Wedgwood, The primary immunodeficiencies, N. Engl. J. Med. 311:235–242, 300–310 (1984).
21. Wolfson, J. S., A. J. Sober, and R. H. Rubin, Dermatologic manifestations of infection in the compromised host, Ann. Rev. Med. 34:205–217 (1983).
22. Littman, B. H., R. E. Rocklin, R. Parkman, and J. R. David, Transfer factor treatment of chronic mucocutaneous to Candida antigen, Clin. Immunol. Immunopathol. 9:97–110 (1978).
23. Lehner, T., J. M. A. Wilton, and L. Ivanyi, Immunodeficiencies in chronic mucocutaneous candidosis, J. Immunol. 22:775–787 (1972).
24. Jorizzo, J. L., Chronic mucocutaneous candidosis: An update, Arch. Dermatol. 118:963–965 (1982).
25. Valdimarsson, H., J. M. Higgs, R. S. Wells, M. Yamamura, J. R. Hobbs, and P. J. L. Hoh, Immune abnormalities associated with chronic muco-cutaneous candidiasis, Cell. Immunol. 6:348–361 (1973).
26. Howanitz, N., J. L. Nordlund, A. B. Lerner, and J. C. Bystryn, Autoantibodies to melanocytes: Occurrence in patients with vitiligo and chronic mucocutaneous candidiasis. Arch. Dermatl. 117:705–708 (1981).
27. Kirkpatrick, C. H., and D. B. Windhorst, Mucocutaneous candidiasis and thymoma, Am. J. Med. 66:939–945 (1979).
28. Higgs, J. M., and R. S. Wells, Chronic mucocutaneous candidiasis: Associated abnormalities of iron metabolism, Br. J. Dermatol. 86(Suppl.):88–102 (1972).
29. Wagman, R. D., J. J. Kazdan, S. W. Kooh, and D. Fraser, Keratitis associated with the multiple endocrine deficiency autoimmune disease, and candidiasis syndrome, Am. J. Ophthalmol. 103:569–575 (1987).
30. Hong, R., Reconstitution of T-cell deficiency by thymic hormone or thymus transplantation therapy, Clin. Immunol. Immunopathol. 40:136–141 (1986).

31. Montagnani, A., M. Negosanti, and A. Patrizi, Ketoconazole treatment of chronic mucocutaneous candidiasis, Drugs. Exp. Clin. Res. XII:409–412 (1986).
32. Mobacken, H., and S. Moberg, Ketoconazole treatment of 13 patients with chronic mucocutaneous candidiasis, Dermatologica 173:229–236 (1986).
33. Rosenblatt, H. M., and E. R. Stiehm, Therapy of chronic mucocutaneous candidiasis, Am. J. Med. 74:20–22 (1983).
34. Mobacken, H., L. Lindholm, and S. Moberg, Immunological studies in chronic mucocutaneous candidiasis before and after ketoconazole treatment, Acta Derm. Venereol. (Stockh.) 67:257–260 (1987).
35. Phillips, P., R. Fetchick, I. Weisman, S. Foshee, and J. R. Graybill, Tolerance to and efficacy of itraconazole in treatment of systemic mycoses: Preliminary results. Rev. Infect. Dis. 9(Suppl. 1):587–593 (1987).
36. Lesher, J. L., and J. G. Smith, Antifungal agents in dermatology, J. Am. Acad. Dermatol. 17:383–394 (1987).
37. Hay, R. J., Chronic dermatophyte infections: I. Clinical and mycological features, Br. J. Dermatol. 106:1–7 (1982).
38. Hunziker, N., and R. Brun, Lack of delayed reacation in presence of cell-mediated immunity in trichophytin hypersensitivity, Arch. Dermatol. 116:1266–1268 (1980).
39. Ahmed, A. R., Immunology of human dermatophyte infections. Arch. Dermatol. 118:521–525 (1982).
40. Hay, R. J., and G. Shennan, Chronic dermatophyte infections. II: Antibody and cell-mediated immune responses, Br. J. Dermatol. 106:191–198 (1982).
41. Robertson, M. H., P. Rich, F. Parker, and J. M. Hanifin, Ketoconazole in griseofulvin-resistent dermatophytosis, J. Am. Acad. Dermatol. 6:224–229 (1982).
42. Cox, F. W., R. L. Stiller, D. A. South, and D. A. Stevens, Oral ketoconazole for dermatophyte infections, J. Am. Acad. Dermatol. 6:455–462 (1982).
43. Lesher, J. L., and J. G. Smith, Jr., Antifungal agents in dermatology, J. Am. Acad. Dermatol. 17:383–394 (1987).
44. Pressar, S. E., and H. Blank, Cimetidine: Adjunct in treatment of tinea capitis, Lancet 1:108–109 (Letter) (1981).
45. Jorizzo, J. L., E. B. Smith, and J. C. Henry, Griseofulvin-resistant dermatophytosis, Arch. Dermatol. 118:2–3 (Letter) (1982).

11

Primary Immune Deficiency Diseases

MARK BALLOW* and WILLIAM B. WHITE *University of Connecticut Health Center, School of Medicine, Farmington, Connecticut*

I. INTRODUCTION

A number of primary and secondary immune deficiency disorders have been associated with changes in immunoregulatory function, particularly increased suppressor-cell activity. These changes produce modulations of both humoral and cell-mediated immune responses in these diseases. Abnormalities in immunoregulation have been reported in a wide range of disorders that include both primary immune deficiency disease and secondary or acquired immunodeficiency disorders; e.g., chronic parasitic infection (1), Hodgkin's disease (2,3), and acute thermal injury (4). One of the first groups of primary immune deficiencies to be analyzed for abnormalities of immunoregulation was common variable hypogammaglobulinemia (5). This is a very heterogeneous group of immune disorders characterized by hypogammaglobulinemia and an increased incidence of infection with variability in the degree of hypogammaglobulinemia, times of onset, patterns of clinical manifestations, and immune dysfunction (6). Using a polyclonal B-cell activator such as pokeweed mitogen (PWM), a number of studies have focused on the differentiation of B cells into plasma cells and abnormalities of immunoregulation.

**Present affiliation*: The Children's Hospital of Buffalo and State University of New York at Buffalo, Buffalo, New York

II. SUPPRESSOR-CELL ACTIVITY IN PATIENTS WITH PRIMARY IMMUNODEFICIENCY

Waldmann and colleagues (5) were one of the first groups to present data on abnormalities of suppressor-cell function in patients with primary immune deficiency disorders. Patients with common variable hypogammaglobulinemia fail to secrete immunoglobulins in vitro of all the immunoglobulin isotypes in response to PWM. In order to determine whether the failure of immunoglobulin synthesis in patients with common variable hypogammaglobulinemia was due solely to an intrinsic B-cell defect, or whether it was due to the presence of suppressor cells, Waldmann and colleagues (7) cocultured lymphocytes from normal subjects with the peripheral blood lymphocytes of patients. In nine of 13 patients with common variable hypogammaglobulinemia, the synthesis of all classes of immunoglobulins in vitro was reduced by a factor of 85-100 %. When the peripheral blood mononuclear cells were separated into T cells and B cells, the purified T cells upon coculture with normal B cells suppressed immunoglobulin synthesis. Coculture of lymphocytes from normal, unrelated individuals did not result in significant inhibition of immunoglobulin synthesis. Similar observations have been made by Broom et al. (8) and Siegel et al. (9).

Other studies have examined whether other types of B-cell immunodeficiency disorders have abnormalities of immunoregulation. Waldmann et al. (10) reported that patients with benign thymomas and associated hypogammaglobulinemia have an increased suppressor activity when the patient's lymphocytes were cocultured with normal control lymphocytes in the presence of PWM. Thus, like the patients with common variable hypogammaglobulinemia, patients with thymoma and hypogammaglobulinemia may also have an associated increased suppressor T-cell activity.

While patients with infantile X-linked agammaglobulinemia (Bruton's disease) have a defect in the differentiation of pre-B cells into mature B cells, Waldmann et al. (11), Siegel et al. (9), and Schwartz et al. (12) have demonstrated that some patients with Bruton's disease may also have an increase in circulating suppressor T cells which inhibit the maturational process of B cells into plasma cells. Of interest, a secondary development of T-cell suppressors has been observed in an animal model of immune deficiency by Blaese and cowokers (13). These investigators demonstrated that agammaglobulinemia could be adoptively transferred to normal chickens by thymic cells obtained from adult agammaglobulinemic birds which had previously been made agammaglobulinemic by surgical bursectomy and irradiation at the time of hatching. Although not the initiating factor in the hypogammaglobulinemia or agammaglobulinemia, the suppression by T cells may nevertheless contribute to the perpetuation and diminished synthesis of immunoglobulins in vivo. Similar secondary events undoubtedly occur in patients with infantile X-linked agammaglobulinemia.

Of interest from the diagnostic perspective in patients with underlying primary immune deficiency are the potential immunoregulatory changes induced by therapy with immune serum globulin. Studies by Durandy et al. (14) and more recently by White et al. (15) have demonstrated that the administration of intramuscular gamma globulin (14) or intravenous immune serum globulin (15) can markedly increase suppressor-cell activity.

It was of interest to determine whether the increased suppressor T-cell activity for B-cell maturation in patients with common variable hypogammaglobulinemia and thymoma with hypogammaglobulinemia was either a primary or secondary event. In one subset of patients with common variable hypogammaglobulinemia, Waldmann and coworkers (7,10,11) showed that the increased suppressor activity may play a primary role in the pathogenesis of the hypogammaglobulinemia. In three patients, the B-cell/macrophage fraction (in the presence of appropriate T-cell help after removal of autologous T cells) synthesized significant quantities of immunoglobulin M (IgM) in vitro when cultured with PWM. However, when the autologous T cells were cocultured with normal B cells, immunoglobulin synthesis was suppressed, whereas the patient's B-cell/macrophage fraction did not suppress immunoglobulin synthesis of normal lymphocytes in coculture. Thus, in this small subset of patients, T-suppressor cell activity played a primary immunoregulatory role.

In summary, the studies by Waldmann and coworkers (5,10,11), Siegal et al. (9), Williams and coworkers (16,17), and more recently, our laboratory (18) have demonstrated that common variable hypogammaglobulinemia is a heterogeneous group of immune deficiency disorders with a variety of pathophysiologic defects. Most of the patients appear to have a primary B-cell defect that either exists alone or together with increased suppressor T-cell activity. However, a subset of patients exists in which the abnormality of immunoglobulin synthesis is not due to an intrinsic B-cell differentiation defect, but instead is due to a regulatory disorder of increased suppressor T-cell function which inhibits B-cell maturation into plasma cells and antibody synthesis. In these patients, suppressor T cells may play a more primary role in the pathogenesis of the hypogammaglobulinemia.

A. Modification of Suppressor-cell Activity

Several laboratories have investigated the manipulation of this suppressor T-cell population. The suppressor activity could be abrogated by antithymocyte serum and complement lysis (7,11). In addition, the suppressor activity of the T-cell fraction on B-cell immunoglobulin synthesis was corticosteroid sensitive. When suppressor T cells from patients with common variable hypogammaglobulinemia were treated with hydrocortisone succinate and cocultured with normal cells, immunoglobulin synthesis occurred in the presence of PWM. Other studies by

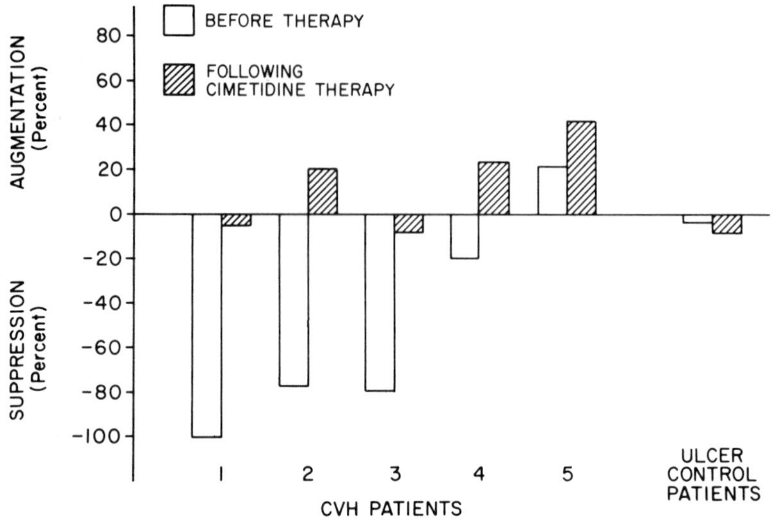

Figure 1 The effect of 1 month of cimetidine therapy on suppressor cell activity in five patients with common variable hypogammaglobulinemia. (From Ref. 18, used with permission.)

Morito et al. (16) and studies in our laboratory (15) have demonstrated that this suppressor T-cell population is also irradiation sensitive.

A number of studies have examined approaches to manipulate this increased suppressor activity in hopes of clinically using these approaches in correcting, at least in part, the hypogammaglobulinemia. Several investigators have demonstrated that a subset of T-suppressor cells bear a receptor for histamine (discussed elsewhere in this book). Histamine can influence a variety of lymphocyte functions such as the proliferative response to mitogens and alloantigens (19,20), antibody synthesis (21), lymphocyte-mediated cytotoxicity (22-24), and the production of lymphokines (25). From these investigations, it is believed that the observed immunosuppression is mediated through the interaction of type II histamine receptors on T-suppressor cells. Furthermore, the activation of T cells bearing histamine type II receptors is responsible for the histamine-induced immunosuppression observed in a number of animal model systems (26). In support of this concept is the finding that pharmacological agents which block the histamine type II receptor but not the type I receptor abrogates suppressor cell activity in vitro. Many of these studies have been reviewed elsewhere in this book.

It was these studies together with the observations by Waldmann (5,9-11) and others (9,16,17) of the increased functional suppressor T-cell activity in patients with common variable hypogammaglobulinemia that led to investigations in our laboratory of the effects of a histamine type II receptor blocker, cimetidine, in patients with common variable hypogammaglobulinemia (18). Five adult patients, ranging from 25-62 years of age, with common variable hypogammaglobulinemia were studied. Replacement gamma globulin therapy was discontinued 6 weeks before the patients entered the study and was withheld until completion of the project. Baseline determinations of T- and B-cell function and quantitative suppressor-cell activity were made prior to the initiation of cimetidine therapy at 1200 mg/day in four divided doses. At baseline, three of the five patients demonstrated increased suppressor-cell activity as shown by the diminished immunoglobulin secretion in cocultures of control normal B cells with patient's T cells (Fig. 1). After 1 month of cimetidine therapy there was a marked reduction of suppressor-cell activity in these three patients (Fig. 1). Patients four and five, who did not demonstrate prior increased suppressor activity, and three control patients with peptic ulcer disease showed no changes in functional suppression or immunoglobulin secretion after 1 month of cimetidine therapy. In four of the five patients, neither immunoglobulin secretion in vitro in response to PWM nor the serum immunoglobulin levels changed significantly during or after therapy.

In one patient, in whom we had the opportunity to follow longitudinally, baseline studies demonstrated some immunoglobulin synthesis (both IgG and IgM) in vitro when the T cells were removed from the patient's B-cell fraction and normal control T cells were added as a source of help (Fig. 2). These studies suggested that if one could remove the suppressor T cells or abrogate the suppressor activity, there was residual B-cell function in this patient which enabled the B cells to differentiate into plasma cells to secrete immunoglobulins. As shown in Figure 3, on treatment of this patient with cimetidine, the in vitro IgG synthesis in response to PWM rose to almost 4000 ng/ml and the serum IgG level increased from a level of 19 to 212 mg/dl. Suppressor activity decreased simultaneously from a level of 98 - 4% after 1 month of cimetidine therapy. Upon discontinuing the cimetidine therapy, increased suppressor activity returned approximately 3 months after stopping the drug. Cimetidine therapy was resumed again for 2 months whereupon the in vitro polyclonal response to PWM increased again with IgG synthesis reaching almost 800 ng/ml. The serum IgG level rose to similar levels as observed previously. This patient did well during cimetidine therapy with only three mild upper respiratory tract infections dur-

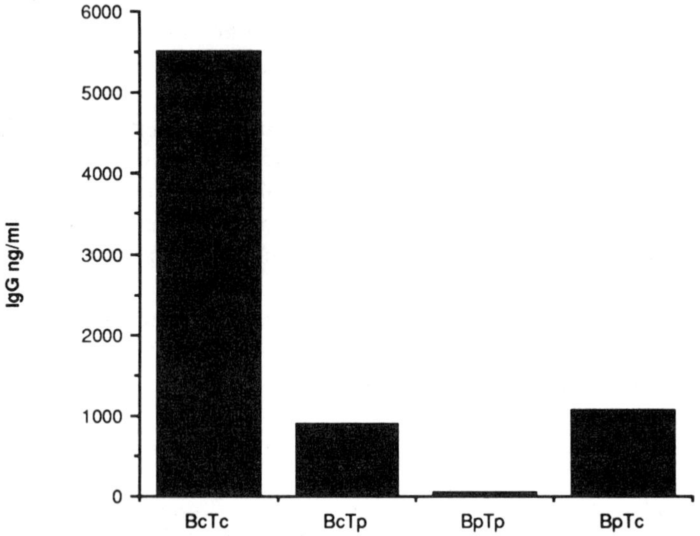

Figure 2 Baseline immunologic data (recombination cell analyses) in a patient with common variable hypogammaglobulinemia. Marked suppressor-cell activity is demonstrated; by removing this T-cell fraction and adding T cells from a normal subject, in vitro production of immunoglobulin occurred, although still diminished compared to control B cells.

ing the last 18 months of study. Unfortunately, he moved out of the area and was lost to follow-up.

This subset of patients as described by Waldmann and associates accounts for a very small proportion of patients with common variable hypogammaglobulinemia. Only one such patient has been found in our group of approximately 30 patients studied over the past 5 years with common variable hypogammaglobulinemia. All of the remaining patients demonstrated some intrinsic B-cell defect even on the addition of normal helper T-cell fractions after removal of patient's T cells. One must also be careful, as we have recently demonstrated (15), that the increased suppressor T-cell activity in these patients is not secondary to the replacement gammaglobulin therapy. Therefore, discontinuation of gamma globulin therapy even by itself could lead to the resolution of the increased suppressor T-cell activity. Nevertheless, the use of cimetidine therapy to abrogate increased suppressor T-cell activity may be useful in certain select patients with common variable hypogammaglobulinemia.

Efremidis and colleagues (27) described their experience in a patient with common variable hypogammaglobulinemia who was treated with cimetidine therapy because of recurrent peptic ulcers. Of interest, a vasculitis rash cleared within 72 hr of starting cimetidine therapy. Lymphokine migration inhibitory

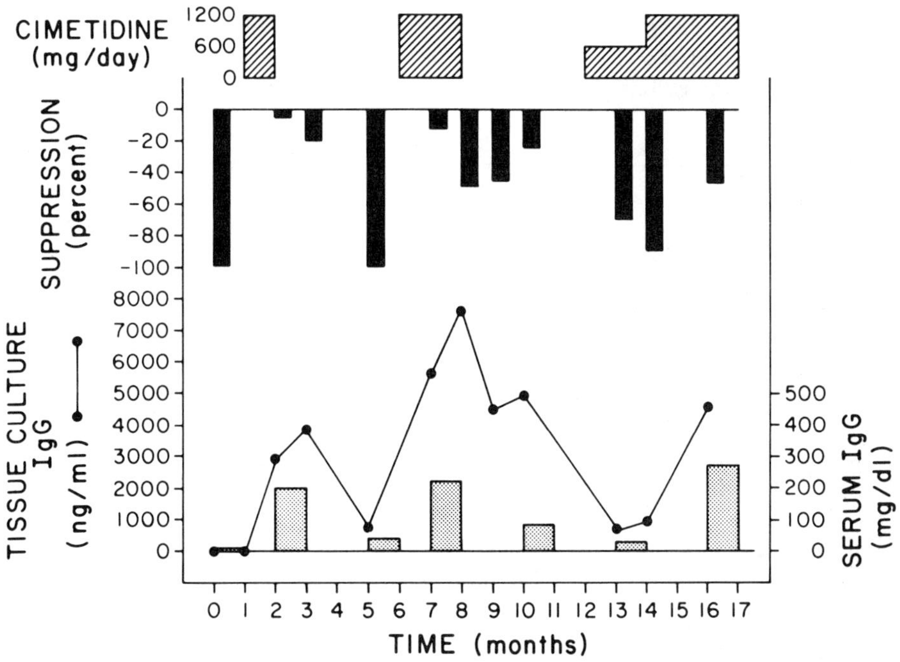

Figure 3 Cimetidine modulation of functional suppressor activity and immunoglobulin G production in a patient with common variable hypogammaglobulinemia.

factor production was greatly enhanced. Within 4 weeks of initiation of cimetidine therapy, the serum immunoglobulins increased. Discontinuation of the cimetidine resulted in the reappearance of the vasculitic rash. Administration of a histamine type I angatonist did not abolish the skin rash when given for 1 week. In another preliminary study, Brockmeyer et al. (28) reported that the administration of cimetidine at 1200 mg/day in two patients with acquired immune deficiency produced a decrease in the proportion of suppressor (CD8 positive) lymphocytes in the peripheral blood and a substantial increase in the T-4/T-8 ratio. It is of interest that we observed a similar change in the proportion of CD8 positive lymphocytes in the peripheral blood of our patients with common variable hypogammaglobulinemia (18).

In contrast, in a rare familial immune deficiency syndrome associated with congenital liver disease originally described by Mellis and Bale (29), familial hepatic veno-occlusive disease, Etzioni et al. (30) did not observe any changes in the proportions of CD8+ cells or in the impaired PWM-induced immunoglobulin synthesis in vitro with a therapeutic trial of cimetidine. However, a rather

Table 1 Leukocyte Migration Inhibition (LIF) and Delayed Skin Hypersensitivity (DHS) in Patients with Chronic Mucotaneous Candidiasis Treated with Cimetidine

Patient		1	2	3	4
Baseline	LIF(%)	6[a]	18	0	−6
	DHS	N[b]	N	N	N
1 Month cimetidine therapy[c]	LIF(%)	51	12	66	0
	DHS	+	+	+	+
Drug rest[d]	LIF(%)	ND	8	22	5
	DHS	N	N	N	N
1 Month cimetidine therapy	LIF(%)	46	27	61	43
	DHS	+	+	+	+

[a]LIF greater than 25% is a positive test.
[b]Negative.
[c]1200 mg pday in divided doses of cimetidine.
[d]4 weeks.
ND, not done.
Source: Adapted from Ref. 31, used with permission.

low dose of cimetidine was given (200 mg/day), and the patient had underlying liver disease which may have altered the metabolism of the cimetidine. Furthermore, the in vitro B-cell immunoglobulin synthesis of T- and B cell-separated fractions showed poor immunoglobulin synthesis by the patient's B-cell fraction in the presence of normal control T cells, suggesting a significant intrinsic B-cell defect in the differention of B cells to immunoglobulin-secreting plasma cells.

Jorizzo et al. (31) studied the effects of cimetidine in four adult patients with chronic mucocutaneous candidiasis. These patients suffered from chronic, often therapy-resistant, candidal infections of the mucus membranes, skin, and nails. These patients demonstrated an immune defect in cell-mediated immune responses to *Candida* as measured by negative intradermal skin activity, in vitro lymphocyte transformation responses, and lymphokine production (32,33). Immunomodulatory agents such as transfer factor have been shown to partially correct or improve the clinical manifestations of patients with chronic mucocutaneous candidiasis (34). In this study by Jorizzo et al. (31), cimetidine (300 mg/tid) was administered for two 4-week periods with a rest period in between. As Table 1 shows, all four patients converted their *Candida* skin test reactivity to positive after cimetidine therapy. When the cimetidine was discontinued for 4 weeks repeat skin testing showed negative responses, but returned to strongly positive after reinstitution of cimetidine. The leukocyte migration inhibitory factor production also improved dramatically after each course of cimetidine therapy in response to *Candida* antigen. However, the lymphocyte proliferative responses to *Candida* antigen was not affected by cimetidine therapy, and there was no effect on the clinical manifestations of the candidiasis in these patients. Although cimetidine appeared to restore skin test reactivity and leukocyte migration inhibitory factor production in patients with chronic mucocutaneous candidiasis, there was no effect on the lymphocyte proliferative responses to *Candida*. The latter observations may be related to the absence of a clinical response.

III. CONCLUSIONS

In view of the variability of both the suppression and in vitro immunoglobulin secretion seen in patients with common variable hypogammaglobulinemia, the long-term effects of reversing suppressor-cell activity with histamine type II antagonists are not clear. However, in one well-studied patient who had the appropriate combination of immune defects, oral therapy with cimetidine reversed the suppressor-cell activity, increased immunoglobulin G synthesis, and kept the patient virtually free from bacterial infections for almost 2 years. These findings along with the preliminary data from the Duke group (31) showing short-term improvement in immunologic parameters in patients with chronic mucucutaneous candidiasis support further work along these lines of inquiry. Further studies with cimetidine as well as other histamine type II antagonists (e.g., ranitidine, famotidine) appear warranted in selected patient populations with immune deficiency disorders.

REFERENCES

1. Coulis, P. A., R. M. Lewert, and F. W. Fitch, Splenic suppressor cells and cell-mediated cytotoxicity in murine schistoscomiasis, J. Immunol. 120: 1074 (1987).
2. Hillinger, S. M., and G. P. Herzig, Impaired cell mediated immunity in Hodgkin's disease mediated by suppressor lymphocytes and monocytes. J. Clin. Invest. 61:1620 (1978).
3. Goodwin, J. S., P. R. Messner, A. D. Bankhurt, G. T. Peake, J. Saiki, and R. C. Williams, Jr., Prostaglandin-producing suppressor cells in Hodgkin's disease. N. Engl. J. Med. 297:963 (1977).
4. Miller, C. L., and C. C. Baker, Changes in lymphocyte activity after thermal injury. The role of suppressor cells, J. Clin. Invest. 63:202 (1979).
5. Waldmann, T. A., S. Broder, R. M. Blaese, W. Strober, Role of suppressor T cells in pathogenesis of common variable hypogammaglobulinemia. Lancet 2:609 (1974).

6. Buckley, R. M., Humoral Immunodeficiency, Clin. Immunol. Immunopathol. 40:13–24 (1986).
7. Waldmann, T. A., S. Broder, M. Durm et al., T cell suppression of pokeweed mitogen induced immunoglobulin production. In Mitogens in Immunobiology (Oppenheim, J. J., and Rosenstreich, D. L., Eds.), Academic Press, New York, (1976), p. 509.
8. Broom, B. C., E. G. De La Concha, A. D. B. Webster, G. L. Janossy and G. L. Asherson, Intracellular immunoglobulin production in vitro by lymphocytes from patients with hypogammaglobulinemia and their effect on normal lymphocytes, Clin. Exp. Immunol. 23:73 (1976).
9. Siegal, F. P., M. Siegal, and R. A. Good, Role of helper, suppressor, and B-cell defects in the pathogenesis of the hypogammaglobulinemias, N. Engl. J. Med. 299:172–178 (1978).
10. Waldmann, T. A., S. Broder, M. Durm, M. Blackman, R. Krakam and B. Meade, Suppressor T cells in the pathogenesis of hypogammaglobulinemia associated with thymoma, Trans. Assoc. Am. Physicians 88:120 (1976).
11. Waldmann, T. A., S. Broder, R. Krakauer, R. P. MacDermott, M. Durm, C. Goldman, and B. Meade, The role of suppressor cells in the pathogenesis of common variable hypogammaglobulinemia and the immunodeficiency associated with myeloma, Fed. Proc. 35:2067–2072 (1976).
12. Schwartz, S. A., Y. S. Choi, L. Shou, and R. A. Good, Modulatory effects on immunoglobulin synthesis and secretion by lymphocytes from immunodeficient patients, J. Clin. Invest. 59:1176–1187 (1977).
13. Blaese, R. M., P. L. Weiden, I. Koski, and N. Dooley, Infectious agammaglobulinemia: Transmission of immunodeficiency with grafts of agammaglobulinemic cells, J. Exp. Med. 140:1097 (1974).
14. Durandy, A., A. Fischer, and C. Griscelli, Dysfunctions of pokeweed mitogen-stimulated T and B lymphocyte responses induced by gammaglobulin therapy, J. Clin. Invest. 67:867–877 (1981).
15. White, W. B., C. R. Desbonnet, and M. Ballow, Immunoregulatory effects of intravenous immune serum globulin therapy in common variable hypogammaglobulinemia, Am. J. Med. 84:431–436 (1987).
16. Morito, T., D. Bankhurst, and R. C. Williams, Jr., Studies of T- and B-cell interactions in adult patients with combined immunodeficiency, J. Clin. Invest. 65:422–431 (1980).
17. Rodriquez, M. A., A. D. Bankhurst, and R. C. Williams, Jr., Characterization of the suppressor activity in lymphocytes from patients with common variable hypogammaglobulinemia: Evidence for an associated primary B-cell defect, Clin. Immunol. Immunopathol. 29:35–50 (1983).
18. White, W. B., and M. Ballow, Modulation of suppressor-cell activity by cimetidine in patients with common variable hypogammaglobulinemia, N. Engl. J. Med. 312:198–202 (1985).
19. Thomas, Y., R. Huchet, and D. Granjon, Histamine-induced suppressor cells of lymphocyte mitogenic response, Cell. Immunol. 59:268–275 (1981).

20. Badger, A. M., J. Young, and G. Poste, Inhibition of phytohaemmaglutinin-induced proliferation of human peripheral blood lymphocytes by histamine and histamine H_1 and H_2 agonists, Clin. Exp. Immunol. 51:178–184 (1983).
21. Shearer, G. M., K. L. Melmon, Y. Weinstein, M. Sela, Regulation of antibody response by cells expressing histamine receptors, J. Exp. Med. 136: 1302–1307 (1972).
22. Plaut, J., L. M. Lichtenstein, E. Gillespie, and C. S. Henney, Studies on the mechanisms of lymphocyte-mediated cytolysis. IV. Specificity of the histamine receptor on effector T cells, J. Immunol. 111:389–394 (1973).
23. Schwartz, A., P. W. Askenase, and R. K. Gershon, Histamine inhibition of the in vitro induction of cytotoxic T-cell responses, Immunopharmacology 2:179–190 (1980).
24. Nair, M. P. N., and S. A. Schwartz, Effect of histamine and histamine antagonists on natural and antibody-dependent cellular cytotoxicity of human lymphocytes in vitro, Cell. Immunol. 81:45–60 (1983).
25. Rocklin, R. E., Modulation of cellular-immune responses in vivo and in vitro by histamine receptor-bearing lymphocytes, J. Clin. Invest. 57:1051–1058 (1976).
26. Griswold, D. E., S. Alessi, A. M. Badger, G. Poste, and N. Hanna, Inhibition of T suppressor cell expression by histamine type 2 (H_2) receptor antagonists, J. Immunol. 132:3054–3057 (1984).
27. Efremidis, A. P., Z. Giannopoulous, and A. Tourkantonis, Cimetidine and hypogammaglobulinemia, N. Engl. J. Med. 313:265 (1985) (correspondence).
28. Brockmeyer, N., E. E. Ohnhaus, E. Kruezelder, and E. Kuwert, Cimetidine and hypogammaglobulinemia, N.Engl. J. Med. 313:265–266 (1985) (correspondence).
29. Mellis, C., and P. M. Bale, Familial hepatic veno-occlusive disease with probable immune deficiency, J. Pediatr, 88:236–242 (1976).
30. Etzioni, A., A. Benderly, E. Rosenthal, V. Shehadah, L. Auslander, N. Lahat, and S. Pollack, Defective humoral and cellular immune functions associated with veno-occlusive disease of the liver, J. Pediatr. 110:549–554.
31. Jorizzo, J. L., W. M. Sams, Jr., B. V. Jegasothy, and A. J. Olansky, Cimetidine as an immunomodulator: Chronic mucocutaneous candidiasis as a model, Ann. Int. Med. 92:192–195 (1980).
32. Kirkpatrick, C. H., R. R. Rich, and J. E. Bennett, Chronic mucocutaneous candidiasis: Model-building in cellular immunity, Ann. Int. Med. 74:955–978 (1971).
33. Kirkpatrick, C. H., R. R. Rich, and T. K. Smith, Effect of transfer factor on lymphocyte function in anergic patients, J. Clin. Invest, 51:2948–2958 (1972).
34. Kirkpatrick, C. H., and T. K. Smith, Chronic mucocutaneous candidiasis: Immunologic and antibiotic therapy, Ann. Int. Med. 80:310–320 (1974).

12

Surgery, Anesthesia, and Trauma

JOHN F. HANSBROUGH and MICHELE A. GADD *University of California, San Diego Medical Center, San Diego, California*

I. INTRODUCTION

Over the last 15 years, a large body of research has focused on the role of injury in inducing a state of suppressed immunity. Immune suppression undoubtedly contributes to infectious complications which often follow severe injury. Infections which trigger a vicious cycle leading to to multiple organ failure and death are the most frequent cause of death, not only of surgical and injured patients (6), but of other groups of critically ill patients. Recent evidence indicates that immune down regulation may follow not only severe injury but may also be a sequela of elective surgical procedures and even anesthesia (7-15).

A great deal of evidence has now implicated suppressor cells in the development of immune suppression after injury (16-20). Particularly since some of the immunosuppressive effects of histamine are believed to be mediated through interactions with histamine type II (H_2) receptors, and T-suppressor cells (T_S) appear to be the principal immunologic target for histamine type II agonists (21, 22), it seems logical to investigate histamine and immune responses following injury.

Histamine has been shown to play roles in several pathophysiologic alterations following shock and trauma (23-26). Histamine has been implicated in some of the vascular-permeability increases after thermal injury (26,27), although arachidonic acid metabolites also appear to play important roles (28). Two primary mechanisms have been suggested as contributing to histamine release following thermal injury: increased spontaneous degranulation of heat-stimulated mast cells (29), and complement-mediated degranulation triggered at the site of injury by heat-modified tissue proteins (30). In addition, neutrophils have been shown to release a factor capable of stimulating histamine release from mastlike cells (31). Cimetidine (but not ranitidine, another histamine type II antagonist, or mepyramine, a type I antagonist) has been shown to significantly block early postburn edema formation (26,32), thus suggesting the participation of tissue histamine in physiologic events following injury.

However, surprisingly little work has been carried out to examine the immunologic effects of histamine antagonist agents following burn and nonburn injury. This chapter will cover the limited amount of work which has been reported by our laboratory and by others regarding the effects of histamine antagonist drugs on the immune response in experimental and clinical models of injury as well as after surgical procedures and anesthesia.

II. IMMUNE RESPONSES AFTER INJURY

The nature and occurrence of multiple immune-suppressive effects after injury has been studied extensively in the last 20 years (5,33). However, the occurrence of many immune defects does not correlate well with subsequent infectious morbidity and death (34). Anergy has been perhaps the most frequently studied aspect of immunity in surgical and traumatized patients, and the relationship of anergy to infections in the postsurgical and injured patients seems clear (2,9,35). However, the cause-effect relationship between anergy and infections needs to be clarified. One of the goals of our own work on the immune-suppressive effects of injury has been to identify events which initiate the immune-suppressive cycle after injury, and to examine relationships among the various arms of immunity after injury.

Much experimental work in this field suggests that of all types of trauma, burn injury presents the most severely immune-suppressive effect on the host (33); this is generally supported by clinical experiences. Most of our own work has centered on the immune-suppressive sequelae of thermal injury, but supporting work from our laboratory has examined the immune response after other types of injury and after anesthesia. Perhaps certain critical immune-suppressive events are common to different types of injury and stress; release of histamine at the tissue level may prove to be such a common, contributory event.

As noted above, one of the important challenges which remains is the demonstration of a causal relationship between clinical anergy and bacterial infections. Infections which occur in anergic patients are usually bacterial, normally handled by the humoral or inflammatory host defense systems, and are not thought to be handled directly by the cell-mediated immune system. Although chemotactic, phagocytic, and bactericidal infections in anergic patients may also be depressed (36-39), and inhibitors of these functions have been identified in anergic patients (40,41), clear cause-effect relationships between the inflammatory and cell-mediated immune systems have only begun to be shown (42–44). Our studies, for example, have shown a marked inability of neutrophils from burned animals and from burned humans to generate high-energy oxygen compounds following stimulation (oxidative burst) (45), and others have shown similar results in injured patients (34). Defective neutrophil oxidative burst activity has been shown to correlate with defective intracellular microbicidal capacity. It remains to be demonstrated whether defects in T-cell functions and neutrophil functions, which are separable easy to demonstrate after injury, have any cause-effect relationships.

In contrast to these suppressed immune functions, there is evidence that antibody responses in anergic surgical patients are intact (46). We have presented evidence which indicates that general immunoglobulin production in severely burned humans is markedly increased (47), and have demonstrated that nonspecific antibody production and specific antibody responses in anergic, burned mice are supranormal (48). Thus, the focus of studies on immunoenhancement after injury should probably reside in the evaluation of T-lymphocyte and neutrophil functions and their possible interrelationships.

III. HISTAMINE AND INJURY

If histamine antagonists have important immunologic effects after injury, it must be implied that histamine is liberated at sufficient levels after injury to affect immune responses. Histamine is localized largely in mast cells and basophils, and histamine content in intracellular granules may exceed 0.3 M (49). In the absence of cell activation, histamine turns over slowly or not at all; in the presence of tissue injury induced by surgical procedures or injury, it is very likely that histamine is secreted locally and achieves high local concentrations. Because of its small size and diffusability, histamine is readily dispersed from local sites, helping to limit its regional action to a relative brief period; however, high transient local concentrations of histamine may be sufficient to trigger an effective immunologic response after injury.

Clearly, as evidenced by other contributors to this volume, histamine has important immunologic effects, including interaction of histamine type II (H_2) agonists with suppressor cells (21,22), and the possible conversion of T-helper cells to T-suppressor cells, which has been reported to be irreversible (50,51). Histamine may have other more indirect effects on immunity after injury. Histamine at the local site may directly affect leukocyte migration (49,52-54). The accumulation of neutrophils in particular may lead to further immunologic effects. For example, neutrophils accumulating in large numbers in local tissue areas after injury of inflammation may increase local concentration of other immunoactive compounds, including hydrogen peroxide, which is strongly inhibitory for some T-cell functions (55), and which has been suggested as one of the mediators of immune suppression after injury (56,57). Indeed, evidence has been presented suggesting that circulating neutrophils are activated following burn injury, as evidenced by increased expression of the complement receptors CR1 and CR3, probably mediated by C5a (58). Complement activation may be an important event after injury (59,60) and subsequent infections (61,62), and C3a, C4a, and C5a all have histamine-releasing effects. C5a is also able to induce a respiratory burst in neutrophils (63), which could contribute to increased secretion and increased local tissue levels of active oxygen intermediates, including hydrogen peroxide (discussed above). We have shown that vitamin E, which functions as an antioxidant, has some immune protective effects after thermal injury in mice (64).

Some effects of histamine may be exerted in part via other mediators. For example, in human lung tissue, histamine increases prostaglandins E_2 (PGE_2) and $F_2\alpha$ ($PGF_2\alpha$) synthesis (65). Since prostaglandins have been shown to play an important role in immunosuppression (66,67), and particularly after injury (68-70), this sequence of events may play an important role leading to immunosuppression after injury. For example, direct T-suppressor activation of monocytes PGE_2 secretion has been demonstrated (71). Thus, histamine may contribute indirectly to the multiple immunologic events which occur after injury, including the propagation of a vicious cycle of cell-mediated interactions, which eventually lead to immune depression and increased host susceptibility to infections.

IV. HISTAMINE TYPE II ANTAGONISTS AND IMMUNITY AFTER BURN INJURY

Burn injury presents probably one of the most severely immunosuppressive effects known to the individual. Multiple components of immunity are suppressed after thermal injury, including various aspects of the inflammatory responses, some humoral responses, and cell-mediated immunity (CMI).

Since several groups have shown that suppressed cell-mediated immunity after burn injury is associated with sepsis and increased mortality (16,17), we began our studies of postburn immune suppression by studying contact sensitivity in a murine model of burn injury. We utilized an assay which employs the sensitization of animals with topically applied 2,4-dinitrofluorobenzene (DNFB)

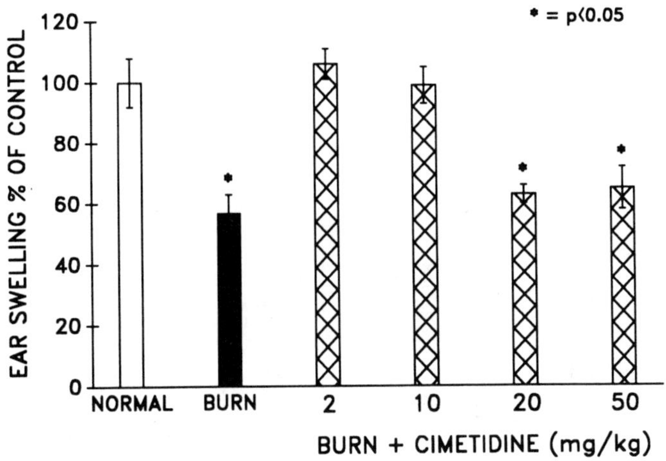

Figure 1 Contact sensitization of mice was depressed when DNFB was applied to the abdominal skin 10 days after burn injury, reflected by decreased swelling of the ears following subsequent antigen challenge. Contact sensitivity was maintained at "normal" levels when burned mice were treated with daily intraperitoneal injections of cimetidine after burn injury, in doses of 2 and 10 mg/kg/day; higher doses were ineffective.

on 2 successive days, followed 5 days later by ear challenge using the same agent. The immune reaction was quantitated by measuring with a micrometer the ear thickness before and 24 hr after DNFB ear challenge. This assay has been shown to reproducibly measure cell-mediated immune function, and reactivity can be conferred on naive mice by transfer of T cells from sensitized mice, but not with macrophages (72).

With this experimental system we have shown that cell-mediated immunity is markedly depressed after burn injury. An important result of these studies has been the demonstration that the onset of immune depression after burn injury is progressive; the ability of mice to respond to contact sensitization is normal in the first week after injury, and maximal suppression does not appear until the second postburn week (73). By 3 weeks, immunity as measured by the contact sensitivity response has returned to normal.

Using this assay we have shown that CMI is improved in burned mice following daily administration of appropriate doses of either cimetidine or ranitidine (Fig. 1) (74-77). In sensitized, burned mice DNFB-dependent ear swelling was reduced to 52% of normal ($p < 0.001$). Daily administration of cimetidine by intraperitoneal injection in doses of 2 and 10 mg/kg resulted in complete restoration of CMI, reflected by return of ear swelling to 106 and 98% of normal

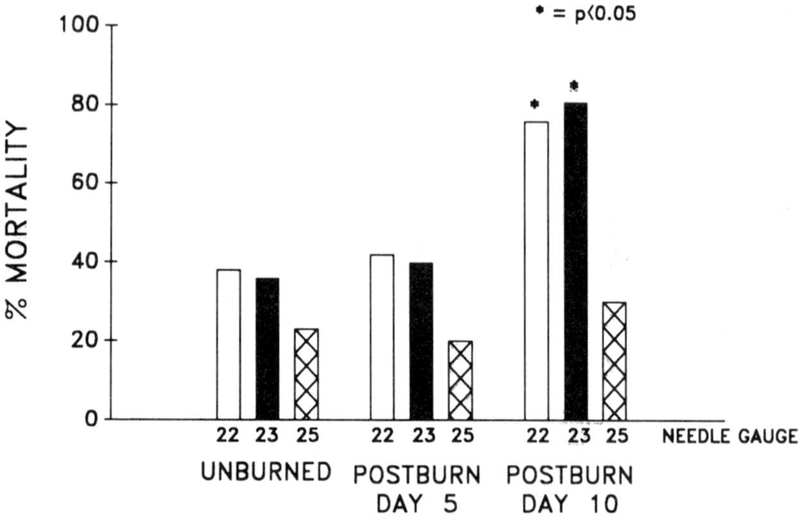

Figure 2 The cecal ligation and puncture (CLP) model presents an intra-abdominal septic challenge to the animal (20); the degree of contamination (and subsequent mortality) is controlled by the size of the needle used for through-and-through puncture. Mortality is measured for 4 days after challenge; few animals die after this time period, and animals which expire have a fulminant peritonitis. This illustration indicates unpublished data from our laboratory; mortality was markedly increased in burned mice when septic challenge was performed on the tenth day after injury.

levels, respectively. Higher doses of cimetidine (20 and 50 mg/kg/day) did not improve CMI. Ranitidine doses of 2 and 10 mg/kg/day were also completely immunorestorative ($p < 0.0005$), whereas 0.2 mg/kg/day was not effective in restoring CMI. In contrast, daily administration of diphenhydramine, a histamine type I receptor antagonist, did not improve CMI when it was administered in various dosages to burned animals.

We have also studied the ability of cimetidine to improve resistance to infection after burn injury. We utilized an experimental model of intra-abdominal sepsis which had been previously developed by several other groups (78,79). This model utilizes the ligation of the base of the cecum in mice to produce a closed obstruction, accompanied by through-and-through cecal puncture with a needle. This model appears to be a reasonable analog of surgical sepsis, with blood cultures positive for multiple enteric organisms as early as 1 hr after the procedure. Death is closely associated with the size of the needle used for cecal puncture, indicating that the degree of fecal contamination in the abdominal

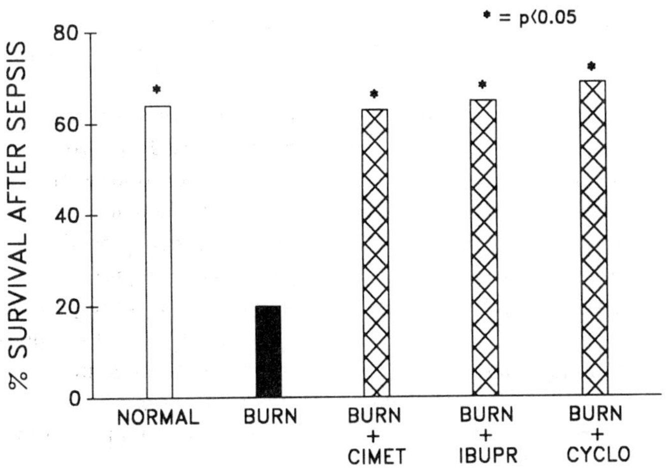

Figure 3 Survival of burned mice after septic challenge was improved (not different from survival of normal mice) when animals received specific drug therapy following injury. All three drugs (cimetidine, ibuprofen, and cyclophosphamide) may have effects on suppressor cells, but other mechanisms of action are quite possible.

cavity is the determining factor in producing lethal sepsis. The cecal ligation and puncture model obviates the necessity of culturing and titrating bacterial strains in the laboratory, and greatly simplifies studies to measure overall host resistance to infectious challenge.

Using the cecal ligation-puncture (CLP) model, we have shown that resistance to sepsis is depressed after murine burn injury when an appropriately sized needle is utilized for the cecal puncture (Fig. 2); an important characteristic of postburn immune suppression is shown in this illustration. Resistance to sepsis is not decreased when CLP is performed 5 days after burn injury, but mortality is markedly increased when CLP is performed on the tenth postburn day. This substantiates our data regarding contact sensitization after burn injury (above), which also demonstrated a delayed (10-14 day) onset of immune suppression after burn injury (73).

When cimetidine was administered daily to mice after burn injury by intraperitoneal injection, survival was markedly improved when CLP was performed on the tenth postburn day (80) (Fig. 3). Figure 3 also shows that survival was improved when animals received ibuprofen or cyclophosphamide in the postburn period, indicating that the drugs may act through a common pathway (possibly related to suppressor-cell proliferation or function). This will be discussed more fully in the following section. In a model of musculoskeletal trauma in mice (81), we demonstrated that the same three drugs are able to improve survival after CLP.

The mode of action of the histamine type II antagonists in improving postburn immunity remains unclear. Histamine, probably released by host mast cells and basophils in response to burn injury, may activate suppressor lymphocytes bearing surface histamine type II receptors. Extremely low concentrations of histamine cause the release from suppressor lymphocytes of histamine-induced suppressor factor (HSF), a lymphokine which suppresses the production of migration inhibitory factor (MIF) and proliferative responses to antigens (21,82,83). A number of studies have implicated suppressor lymphocytes in the profound immune depression which follows severe burn injury; for example, immune depression can be transferred to normal animals by harvesting of suppressor lymphocyte populations from normal mice and reinfusion of the cells into normal animals (18).

The dose-effect responses with cimetidine are interesting. In our studies, treatment of burned mice with low doses of cimetidine (2 and 10 mg/kg/day) improved CMI, whereas higher doses (20 and 50 mg/kg/day) were not beneficial. This dosage dependency may indicate a biphasic mode of action of cimetidine; at low doses suppressor cells may be preferentially inhibited, whereas at higher dosage a more global inhibitory effect seems to occur, perhaps reflecting the effect of the drug on helper cell populations. Khan et al. have shown that suppressor T cells are more responsive than helper cells to histamine; the Leu 2^+ subset included all histamine-inducible suppressor cells, and after treatment with histamine type II these cells inhibited both phytohemagglutinin (PHA)-induced T-cell proliferation and pokeweed mitogen-induced B-cell differentiation (84,85).

Depression of CMI after burn injury appears to be antigen nonspecific. In order to further examine the immunologic effects of histamine type II antagonists on suppressor-cell activity in the mouse, our group in collaboration with Drs. Claman and Mekori at the University of Colorado studied antigen-specific immune suppression using a murine tolerance model; this model has been shown to involve both clone inhibition and induction of T-suppressor cells (86). Dinitrobenzene sulfonic acid (DNBS) administered for 7 days before DNFB sensitization induced significant inhibition of CMI. Cimetidine treatment begun several hours before the animals were made tolerant did not cause any significant change in CMI (87). Similarly, in a transfer model of antigen-specific tolerance, we found that cimetidine and ranitidine had no effect; and finally, using a supraoptimal dose of antigen for sensitization, which activates specific suppressor cells (88), cimetidine also had no effect. In contrast to our studies, Griswold et al. (89) found that both cimetidine and ranitidine inhibited specific T-suppressor cell activity in a similar model of DNBS-induced tolerance to

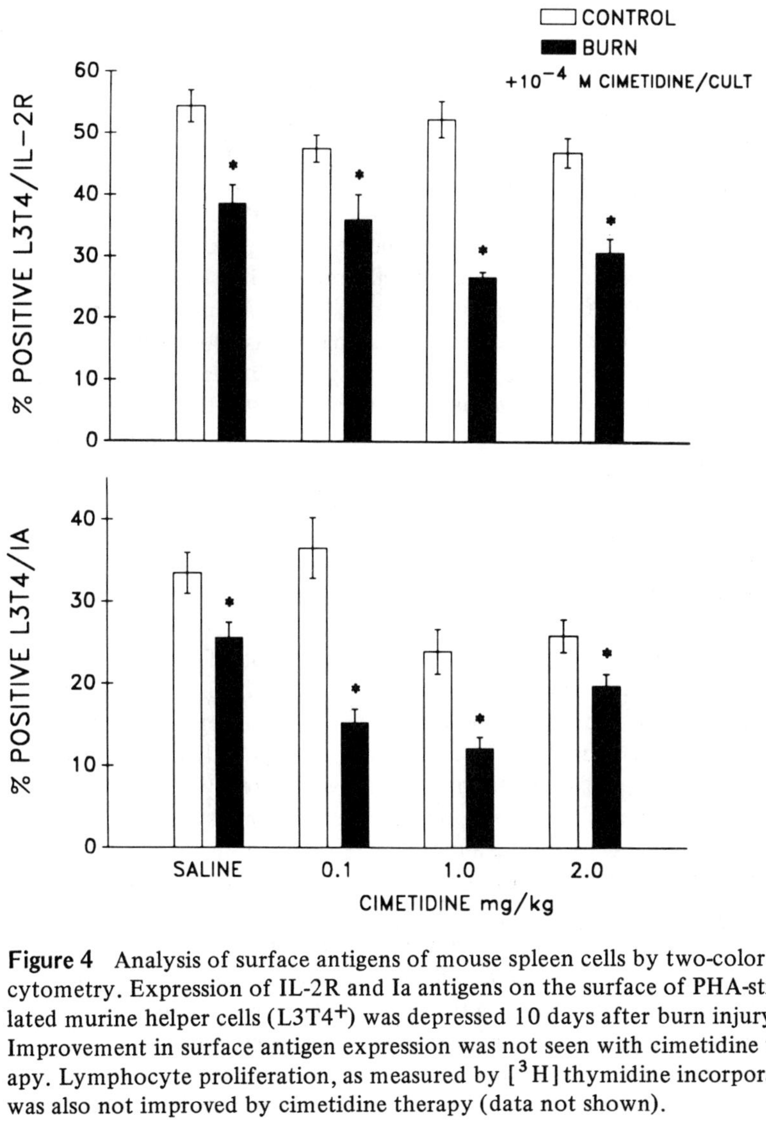

Figure 4 Analysis of surface antigens of mouse spleen cells by two-color flow cytometry. Expression of IL-2R and Ia antigens on the surface of PHA-stimulated murine helper cells (L3T4$^+$) was depressed 10 days after burn injury. Improvement in surface antigen expression was not seen with cimetidine therapy. Lymphocyte proliferation, as measured by [^{3}H]thymidine incorporation, was also not improved by cimetidine therapy (data not shown).

DNFB in mice. Jin et al., in similar models (90), also found that cimetidine inhibited suppressor-cell activity. Reasons for the discrepancies in these results are unclear, but may relate to drug dosages and administration regimens.

It has been difficult to demonstrate by in vitro tests that histamine type II antagonist drugs can improve immunity after burn injury. We found that the marked suppression of lymphocyte proliferation which occurred subsequent to burn injury was not improved by daily cimetidine administration (76). A major reason for the difficulty in evaluating immunomodulating therapy by in vitro tests may lie in the necessity for removing cells from the host immunologic environment; many in vivo immunoregulatory pathways are undoubtedly interrupted, including potential effects of circulating and tissue mediators. In more recent work, in attempts to identify more specific in vitro immune defects after injury which may be amenable to further investigations, we have studied the expression of surface antigens on lymphocytes during mitogen activation. T-cell activation in vitro has been shown to involve the expression of particular surface antigens at various phases of the stimulatory processes (91). Interleukin (IL-2) receptor (IL-2R) expression, for example, occurs early following stimulation and well before cellular deoxyribonucleic (DNA) synthesis, whereas surface Ia antigen expression occurs during or after DNA synthesis (91,92).

The inability of T-cell populations to activate and proliferate may be a fundamental defect after some types of injury. Impaired T-cell activation capacity has been reported in burned patients (93), and immature circulating T lymphocytes have been identified in injured patients (94). Relative to histamine, histamine-induced suppressor factor has been shown to greatly depress Ia expression by stimulated lymphocytes (95). We have identified marked, reproducible defects in mitogen-induced surface antigen expression in burn-derived lymphocytes from both mice and humans, thus demonstrating blocks in critical early steps in T-cell activation (96). In parallel studies, however, we have been unable to show that cimetidine can improve in vitro lymphocyte activation processes. As shown in Figure 4, coexpression of helper-associated antigen (L3T4) and either IL-2 receptor or Ia antigen on the surface of stimulated lymphocytes remained markedly depressed during the culture period, even in the face of cimetidine administration on a daily basis after burn injury and with cimetidine continued in the culture medium (10^{-4} M concentration) (unpublished data). In data not shown here, we have found that postburn mitogen-induced lymphocyte activation and proliferation is not improved by adding exogenous IL-2 to the culture medium. Since some T-cell suppressive effects secondary to histamine-induced suppressor factor have been reported to be reversed with exogenous IL-2 (97), this indicates that postinjury immune suppression is multifactorial and complex, and that improvement of contact sensitivity in the injured animals does not signal complete abrogation of immune suppression by the therapeutic agents.

V. HISTAMINE TYPE II ANTAGONISTS AFTER NONBURN TRAUMA

Although burn injury probably presents the most significant immune suppressive challenge to the host, blunt and penetrating nonburn trauma, in proportion to the severity of injury and the patient's age, clearly produces a state of altered host resistance to infection (34,36,39,98).

Animal models of traumatic injury have been developed which appear to reflect clinically important immunologic events. In section IV above, animal models of controlled burn injury were described. A useful model of musculoskeletal trauma has also been described in mice; under anesthesia, the hind limb is crushed, fractured, and amputated (20). Survival of the amputated mice after injury is nearly 100%, and the animals appear healthy; however, a period of immune depression ensues, which was shown to involve the development of suppressor-cell populations, which appeared to be monocytes/macrophages on close examination (20). Immune suppression has been observed as early as 2 hr after the injury.

Using this murine model, we have shown that in vitro lymphocyte proliferation and expression of lymphocyte surface activation antigens after mitogen stimulation are slightly depressed in the first several days after injury. The immunologic suppression appears to occur early after injury, in contrast to the response seen in the burned animal in which immune depression is a progressive event, occurring in the second postburn week. In this model of musculoskeletal trauma, we have not detected the later depression of contact sensitivity which characterizes the murine burn injury model. Early (but not late) immune depression was noted in the initial work by Mannick's group describing this experimental model (20), in which suppression of lymphocyte function was seen on the first and second days after injury with rapid subsequent resolution. Although Mannick identified a suppressor monocyte/macrophage in these studies, the net result was T-cell down regulation.

These injured animals are also highly susceptible to intra-abdominal septic challenge if the infectious challenge is performed within several days of the injury. Using the cecal ligation and puncture model described previously, we showed that mortality was 36.3% in normal mice after CLP, but mortality rose to 63.8% when CLP was performed on the day following hind-limb amputation. Administration of cimetidine immediately after the injury lowered the mortality to 31.2% (81). Ibuprofen and low-dose cyclophosphamide also led to increased survival in this challenge model, suggesting that the drugs might all have effects on the induction of suppressor cells by injury. This information offers further hope that histamine type II antagonist therapy can improve immune functions in severely injured patients. However, much more investigation is necessary to determine the mechanisms of action and ways to monitor immune parameters after treatment, since "escape" from environmental influences makes the evaluation of in vitro assays of immune functions difficult in treated individuals.

VI. HISTAMINE TYPE II ANTAGONISTS, IMMUNE DEPRESSION, ANESTHESIA, AND SURGERY

Increasing evidence suggests that suppressed immunity may accompany major surgical procedures and may lead to increased infectious complications (1,9,14, 15,99,100). In a recent review of 2202 patients, an association was shown between failure of skin reactivity to five antigens and susceptibility to serious intracavitary abscesses or septicemia after extensive surgical treatment (3). Thirty-three percent of anergic patients became septic, and 31% died. Of the patients who were reactive on admission, 8% became septic and 4% died. It has also been suggested that postsurgical immune suppression may contribute to postoperative dissemination of carcinoma (10,101).

It has also been demonstrated that anergy developing during the perioperative course or during the hospital admission is a strong predictor of postoperative morbidity. In the study quoted above (3), of the 295 patients who were reactive upon admission and remained reactive, 12% became septic and 2% died. Ninety-eight of the patients were reactive upon admission and deteriorated to an anergic state during hospitalization; 44% developed sepsis and 40% died. Therefore, it would seem valuable to identify mechanisms leading to immune suppression developing *during* or as a result of a surgical procedure, and to attempt to block immune suppressive processes.

There is little data available concerning the effect of histamine type II antagonist drugs on the immune response following surgery. We have shown in preliminary studies that cimetidine administered to patients in the perioperative period can prevent postoperative alterations in lymphocyte phenotypes in the circulating blood (8,102). Uncomplicated, elective cholecystectomy led to postoperative decreases in helper/inducer T cells and increases in T-suppressor/cytotoxic populations. In a parallel group of patients, cimetidine administered in the perioperative period prevented these changes in circulating T-cell phenotypes. However, those early studies were performed using fluorescent microscopy to enumerate T-cell populations after labeling with monoclonal antibodies. Future studies using flow cytometry will be important, since the results obtained using the two techniques will differ because of the greatly increased sensitivity afforded by flow cytometry.

The immunologic effects of anesthesia must be separated from those of

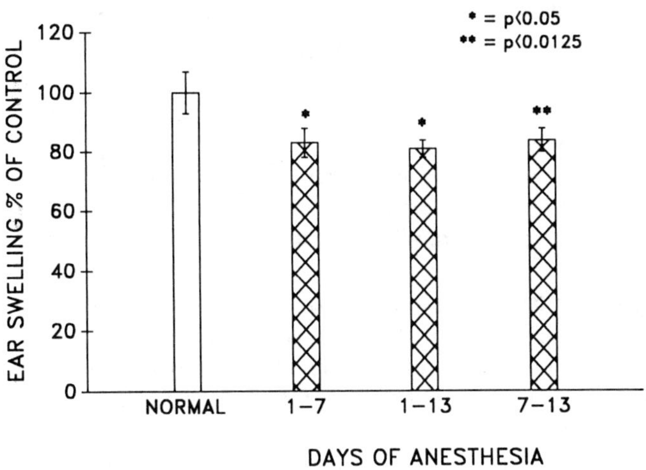

Figure 5 Contact sensitization of mice by DNFB was slightly (but statistically) depressed when mice were anesthetized for 30 min each day with penthrane, for the days indicated. All animals were sensitized with DNFB on days 14 and 15, and ear challenge occurred 5 days later.

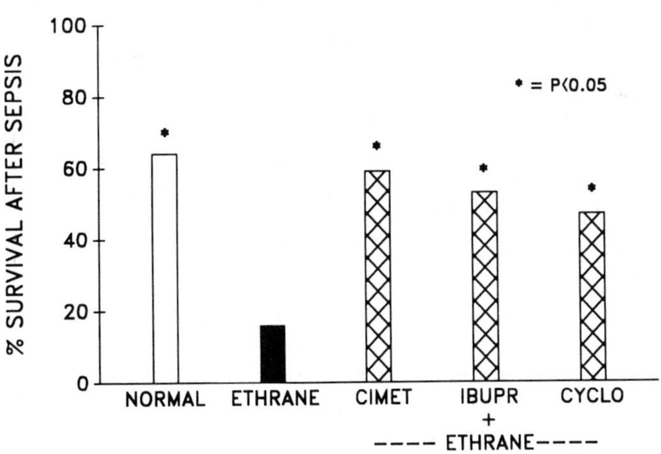

Figure 6 Mice were anesthetized with ethrane for a period of 2 hr. Twenty-four hours later they received a septic challenge with cecal ligation and puncture; survival was markedly depressed in the anesthesized animals. Treatment of the animals with the indicated drugs on the day of anesthesia improved septic survival.

surgery; however, information available concerning the immune suppressive effect of anesthesia, separable from the effects of surgery, are limited and somewhat contradictory in many areas (103). Since there is clear evidence that many anesthetic agents may lead to clinically significant histamine release in patients (104,105), it seems reasonable from this information alone to consider the immunologic effects of anesthetics. Since anesthetic-induced histamine release is dependent in part upon the particular anesthetic agent utilized, it will be necessary to study a variety of anesthetic drugs for their immune suppressive potential.

In murine studies, our laboratory has demonstrated that anesthesia with various agents, in the absence of associated surgery, is immune suppressive. A 2-hr period of inhalational (isoflurane, enflurane, and halothane) or intravenous (ketamine, pentobarbital) anesthesia resulted in lowering of the T-cell helper to suppressor ratio as well as markedly decreased resistance to septic challenge (cecal ligation and puncture) when challenge occurred 24 hr after the anesthetic (7). Others have reported decreased resistance to infectious challenge following anesthesia in animals (11,12), and depression of microbicidal capacity of neutrophils (13). In unpublished studies, we showed that repeated anesthesia led to slight but statistically significant depression in the ability of mice to respond to topically applied DNFB (Fig. 5).

In additional, previously unpublished studies, we showed that cimetidine as well as two other immunopotentiating drugs (ibuprofen, a prostaglandin blocker, and low-dose cyclophosphamide, an inhibitor of suppressor-cell proliferation [106]) administered to mice during the perianesthetic period improved the ability of anesthetized mice to survive after subsequent septic challenge (Fig. 6); the data in this illustration (as well as the septic survival data from mice after burn and musculoskeletal trauma discussed in sections IV and V above) indicate that a common mechanism might be involved in the lowered resistance to sepsis which appears to occur after multiple types of injury and stress. We suspect that suppressor T cells may be activated after stress and tissue injury by histamine release; suppressor cells might then produce soluble mediators, including HSF. It has been shown that suppressor cells and HSF can stimulate monocytes to produce prostaglandins (70,83,107), which in turn exert an immune suppressive effect, including perhaps further stimulation of suppressor cells and inhibition of helper cells (66,67,71). Thus, it might be logical to expect that several drugs with diverse properties might be able to interrupt the cycle of cellular events after injury which result in down regulation of immune responses. Since PGE_2 seems to be the most popular candidate in most studies for mediating immune-suppressive effects after injury (68-70), it will be important to define the relationship between the various messengers and intermediaries in the study of injured cells.

VII. HISTAMINE TYPE II ANTAGONISTS AND TRAUMA-INDUCED IMMUNE SUPPRESSION: THE FUTURE

More detailed studies are required to work out the mechanisms of action of histamine antagonists after injury as well as to determine optimum drug dosages and dosage intervals. For example, in our murine studies we found that cimetidine must be continued throughout the duration of the postburn period prior to antigenic sensitization in order to achieve improvement in cell-mediated immunity (74).

Pitfalls in assay techniques must also be realized. For example, in studies of lymphocyte reactivity in burned mice receiving prostaglandin-blocking drugs, we found that indomethacin not only had to be administered throughout the postburn period, but also had to be included in the lymphocyte culture medium if substantial benefit in lymphocyte proliferation was to be seen (108). We suspect that monocyte PGE_2 production, which probably plays a critical role in postburn immunosuppression (68-70), is inhibited in vivo by cyclooxygenase blockade, but that when cells are placed in culture there is rapid escape unless pharmacologic blockade is continued in vitro. Since histamine-induced suppressor factor secreted by suppressor T cells may play a pivotal role after injury in stimulating PGE_2 secretion by monocytes, this observation has relevance to the study of histamine type II antagonists as well. This finding makes it difficult to utilize many routine in vitro tests to determine the true in vivo effect of immune-modulating therapy in the injured host. Since PGE_2 seems to clearly play an important role in postinjury immune suppression, it would be helpful if studies could demonstrate that the HSF-PGE_2 circuit plays an immunologically significant role after injury.

The abdominal sepsis challenge models have provided useful information, and suggest that overall host resistance to infection can be manipulated at least experimentally. However, more specific immunologic tests will be required to prove specific actions of drugs, since most immunoactive drugs have multiple proven or potential modes of action. It will be crucial to examine the effects of immune-modulating agents on neutrophil functions, since neutrophil dysfunction probably plays a key role in the injured host. We have developed more specific tests of immune functions which can be applied to small animals, including tests for neutrophil phagocytosis and neutrophil oxygen metabolism (45,47, 108). These neutrophil functions are depressed after murine burn injury, and to a lesser degree after nonburn trauma. Both histamine antagonists and prostaglandin-blocking drugs have hemodynamic and other consequences, and these effects may have more potential benefit to the injured host than the immunologic effects.

It must be considered that immune suppression after injury may play a protective role to the host. An overwhelming, systemic inflammatory response to dead tissue or to a wound, for example, might well result in widespread damage to the injured victim. Inflammatory and autoimmune reactions with immediate and long-term tissue and organ damage might follow a vigorous local and systemic immune response to intracellular proteins and membrane structures, which are undoubtedly presented to the immunologic environment following widespread cell destruction and lysis. Similarly, neutrophils which are nonspecifically activated after injury (58) may mediate widespread organ damage (109). Thus, immune depression may have an important protective role after injury, and attempts to reverse these processes must proceed cautiously.

On the other hand, immunomodulating therapy may have undesirable side effects unrelated to immunologic effects. The side effects of histamine type II antagonist agents may pose problems particularly in critically ill patients, and changes in drug clearance and metabolism in these patients may make it difficult to maintain effective and safe drug levels. The ulcerogenic effects of the cyclooxygenase-blocking agents are of course well known, however, and it will undoubtedly be safer if we would be able to interrupt undesirable arachidonic acid pathways with the histamine type II antagonists rather than the nonsteroidal anti-inflammatory agents.

Finally, there are obviously differences in immune regulatory mechanisms between animals and humans. Immune-modulating therapy must proceed only if we are armed with timely and accurate tests to continuously and frequently monitor immune status in the patient being treated. In most clinical settings, this close followup is not presently available.

REFERENCES

1. Keane, R. M., W. Birmingham, C. M. Shatney, R. A. Winchurch, and A. M. Munster, Prediction of sepsis in the multitraumatic patient by assays of lymphocyte responsiveness, Surg. Gynecol. Obstet. 156:163–167 (1983).
2. Meakins, J. L., J. B. Pietsch, O. Birbenick, O. R. Kelly, H. Rode, J. Gordon, and L. D. MacLean, Delayed hypersensitivity: Indicator of acquired failure of host defenses in sepsis and trauma, Ann. Surg. 186:241–250 (1977).
3. Christou, N. V., Host-defense mechanisms in surgical patients: A correlative study of the delayed hypersensitivity skin-test response, granulocyte function and sepsis, Can. J. Surg. 28:39–49 (1985).
4. Christou, N. V., A. P. H. McLean, and J. L. Meakins, Host defense in blunt trauma; interrelationships between kinetics of anergy and depressed neutrophil function, nutritional status and sepsis, J. Trauma 20:833–841 (1980).
5. Miller, S. E., C. L. Miller, and D. D. Trunkey, The immune consequences of trauma, Surg. Clin. North Am. 62:167–182 (1982).
6. Baker, C. C., L. Oppenheimer, B. Stephens, F. R. Lewis, and D. D. Trunkey, Epidemiology of trauma deaths, Am. J. Surg. 140:144–150 (1980).

7. Hansbrough, J. F., R. L. Zapata-Sirvent, E. J. Bartle, J. L. Anderson, L. Elliott, M. A. Mansour, and W. H. Carter, Alteration of splenic lymphocyte populations and increased mortality from sepsis following anesthesia in mice, Anesthesiology 63:267–273 (1985).
8. Hansbrough, J. F., E. M. Bender, R. L. Zapata-Sirvent, and J. Anderson, Altered helper and suppressor lymphocyte populations in surgical patients: A measure of postoperative immunosuppression, Am. J. Surg. 148:303–307 (1984).
9. Christou, N. V., and J. L. Meakins, Delayed hypersensitivity in surgical patients: a mechanism for anergy, Surgery 86:78–85 (1979).
10. Lundy, J., E. J. Lovett, S. Hamilton, and P. Conran, Halothane, surgery, immunosuppression and pulmonary metastases, Cancer 41:827–830 (1978).
11. Bruce, D. L., Effect of halothane anesthesia on experimental Salmonella peritonitis in mice, J. Surg. Res. 7:180–185 (1967).
12. Duncan, P. G., B. F. Cullen, and N. N. Pearsall, Anesthesia and the modification of response to infection in mice, Anesth. Analg. 55:776–781 (1976).
13. Welch, W. D., Effect of enflurane, isoflurane, and nitrous oxide on the microbial activity of human polymorphonuclear leukocytes. Anesthesiology 61:188–192 (1984).
14. Mealy, K., C. O'Farrelly, R. Stephens, and C. Feighery, Impaired neutrophil function during anesthesia and surgeryis due to serum factors, J. Surg. Res. 43:393–397 (1987).
15. Howard, R. J., Effects of burn injury, mechanical trauma and operation on immune defenses, Surg. Clinics North Am. 59:199–211 (1980).
16. Miller, C. L., and C. Baker, Changes in lymphocyte activity after thermal injury. The role of suppressor cells, J. Clin. Invest. 63:202–210 (1979).
17. Wolfe, J. H. N., A. B. Saporoschetz, A. E. Young, N. E. O'Connor, and J. A. Mannick, Suppressive serum, suppressor lymphocytes, and death from burns, Ann. Surg. 193:513–520 (1981).
18. Kupper, T. S., C. C. Baker, T. A. Ferguson, and D. R. Green, A burn induced Ly-2 suppressor cell lowers resistance to bacterial infection, J. Surg. Res. 38:606–612 (1985).
19. Green, D. R., Wang, N., and H. Zheng, A suppressor-inducer factor produced by burn trauma-associated T cells, J. Burn Care Rehab. 8:521-526 (1987).
20. Wang, B. S., E. H. Heacock, A. V. O. Wu, and J. A. Mannick, Generation of suppressor cells in mice after surgical trauma, J. Clin. Invest, 66:200–209 (1980).
21. Rocklin, R. E., J. Beard, S. Gupta, R. A. Good, and K. L. Melmon, Characterization of the human blood lymphocytes that produce a histamine induced suppressor factor, Cell. Immunol. 51:226–237 (1980).
22. Rocklin, R. E., D. K. Greineder, and K. L. Melmon, Histamine-induced suppressor factor: Further studies on the nature of the stimulus and the cell which produces it, Cell. Immunol. 44:404–415 (1979).

23. Altura, B. M., Reticuloendothelial system (RES) phagocytic depression in shock is ameliorated by H_1-receptor antihistamines, Eur. J. Pharmacol. 59: 165–172 (1979).
24. Altura, B. M., Reticuloendothelial system function and histamine release in shock and trauma: Relationship to microcirculation, Klin. Wochenschr. 60: 882–890 (1982).
25. Altura, B. M., and S. Halevy, Beneficial and detrimental actions of histamine H_1- and H_2-receptor antagonists in circulatory shock, Proc. Natl. Acad. Sci. U.S.A. 75:2941–2944 (1978).
26. Boykin, J. V., E. Eriksson, M. M. Sholley, and R. N. Pittman, Cold-water treatment of scald injury and inhibition of histamine-mediated burn edema, J. Surg. Res. 31:111–123 (1981).
27. Casley-Smith, J. R., and J. Window, Quantitative morphological correlation of alterations in capillary permeability, following histamine and moderate burning, in the mouse diaphragm; and the effects of benzopyrones, Microvasc. Res. 11:279–305 (1976).
28. Alexander, F., M. Mathieson, K. H. T. Teoh, W. V. Huval, S. Lelcuk, C. R. Valeri, D. Shepro, and H. B. Hechtman, Arachidonic acid metabolites mediate early burn edema, J. Trauma 25:709–712 (1984).
29. Fredholm, B., and O. Hagermark, Studies on histamine-release from skin and from peritoneal mast cells of the rat induced by heat. Acta Derm. Venereol. (Stockh.) 50:273–277 (1970).
30. Arturson, G., Microvascular permeability to macromolecules in thermal injury, Acta Physiol. Scand. 463 (Suppl.):111–122 (1979).
31. White, M. V., and M. A. Kaliner, Neutrophils and mast cells I. Human neutrophil-derived histamine-releasing activity, J. Immunol. 139:1624–1630 (1987).
32. Boykin, J. V., S. L. Crute, and B. W. Haynes, Jr., Cimetidine therapy for burn shock: a quantitative assessment, J. Trauma 25:864–870 (1985).
33. Ninnemann, J. L., Immunologic defenses against infection: Alterations following thermal injuries, J. Burn Care Rehab. 3:355–366 (1982).
34. Polk, H. C., C. D. George, S. R. Wellhausen, K. Cost, P. R. Davidson, M. P. Regan, and A. P. Borzotta, A systematic study of host defenses in badly injured patients, Ann. Surg. 204:282–299 (1986).
35. MacLean, L. D., Delayed type hypersensitivity testing in surgical patients, Surg. Gynecol. Obstet. 166:285–293 (1988).
36. Christou, N. V., A. P. H. McLean, and J. L. Meakins, Host defense in blunt trauma; interrelationships between kinetics of anergy and depressed neutrophil function, nutritional status and sepsis, J. Trauma 20:833–841 (1980).
37. Superina, R. A., N. V. Christou, and J. L. Meakins, Failure of neutrophil delivery into skin windows in anergic surgical patients, Surg. Forum 31:68–70 (1980).
38. Christou, N. V., and J. L. Meakins, Phagocytic and bactericidal functions of polymorphonuclear neutrophils from anergic surgical patients, Can. J. Surg. 25:444–448 (1982).

39. Meakins, J. L., A. P. H. McLean, R. Kelly, O. Bubenik, J. B. Pietsch, and L. D. MacLean, Delayed hypersensitivity and neutrophil chemotaxis: Effect of trauma, J. Trauma 18:240–247 (1978).
40. Christou, N. V., and J. L. Meakins, Partial analysis and purification of polymorphonuclear neutrophil chemotactic inhibitors in serum from anergic patients, Arch. Surg. 118:156–160 (1983).
41. Van Epps, D. E., D. L. Palmer, and R. C. Williams, Characterization of serum inhibitors of neutrophil chemotaxis associated with anergy. J. Immunol. 113:189–200 (1974).
42. Djeu, J. Y., and D. K. Blanchard, Regulation of human polymorphonuclear neutrophil (PMN) activity against Candida albicans by large granular lymphocytes via release of a PMN-activating factor, J. Immunol. 139:2761–2767 (1987).
43. Murray, H. W., B. Y. Rubin, H. Masur, and R. B. Roberts, Impaired production of lymphokines and immune (gamma) interferon in the acquired immunodeficiency syndrome, N. Engl. J. Med. 310:883–889 (1984).
44. Weisbart, R. H., A. J. Lusis, and A. Kacena, Neutrophil migration inhibition factor from T lymphocytes (NIF-T): partial purification by antibody affinity chromatography and further characterization, Clin. Immunol. Immunopathol. 22:408–418 (1982).
45. Gadd, M. A., and J. F. Hansbrough, The effect of thermal injury on murine neutrophil oxidative metabolism, J. Burn Care Rehab., in press.
46. Nohr, C. W., N. V. Christou, H. Rode, J. Gordon, and J. L. Meakins, In vivo and in vitro humoral immunity in surgical patients, Ann. Surg. 200:373–380 (1984).
47. Hansbrough, J. F., L. M. Miller, T. O. Field, and M. A. Gadd, Review of clinical experience and pharmacokinetics with the use of intravenous gamma globulin in burn patients, Pediatr. Infect. Dis., in press.
48. Gadd, M. A., J. F. Hansbrough, T. O. Field, and C. Soderberg, Antibody formation and clearance after thermal injury in the mouse, J. Surg. Res., in press.
49. Plaut, M., and L. M. Lichtenstein, Cellular and chemical basis of the allergic inflammation response: Component parts and control mechanisms. In Allergy: Principles and Practice (Middleton, E., Reed, C. E., and Ellis, E. F., Eds.), Mosby, St. Louis (1978), pp. 115–138.
50. Polmar, S. H., and R. E. Birch, Regulation of Fc receptor expression on T-lymphocyte subsets mediated by adenosine and histamine receptors. In Immunoregulation and Autoimmunity (Krakauer, R. S., and Cathcart, M. K., Eds.), Elsevier/North Holland, New York (1980), pp. 11–20.
51. Birch, R. E., and S. H. Polmar, Induction of F_{cgamma} receptors on a subpopulation of human T lymphocytes by adenosine and impromide, an H_2-histamine agonist, Cell. Immunol. 57:455–467 (1981).
52. Plaut, M., Histamine, H_1 and H_2 antihistamines and immediate hypersensitivity reactions, J. Allergy Clin. Immunol. 63:371–375 (1979).

53. Rocklin, R. E., Modulation of cellular-immune responses in vivo and in vitro by histamine receptor-bearing lymphocytes, J. Clin. Invest. 57:1051–1058 (1976).
54. Gallin, J. I., A. M. Weinstein, E. B. Cramer, and A. P. Kaplan, Histamine modulation of human eosinophile locomotion *in vitro* and *in vivo*. In The Eosinophil in Health and Disease (Mahmond, A. A., and Austen, K. F., Eds.), Grune & Stratton, New York (1980), pp. 185–206.
55. Staite, N. D., R. P. Messner, and D. C. Zoschke, Inhibition of human T lymphocyte E rossette formation by neutrophils and hydrogen peroxide. Differential sensitivity between helper and suppressor T lymphocytes, J. Immunol. 139:2424–2430 (1987).
56. Patterson, D. A., R. Rapoport, M. A. K. Patterson, B. M. Freed, and N. Lempert, Hydrogen peroxide-mediated inhibition of T-cell response to mitogens is a result of direct action on T cells, Arch, Surg. 123:300–304 (1988).
57. Freed, B. M., R. Rapoport, and N. Lempert, Inhibition of early events in the human T-lymphocyte response to mitogens and alloantigens by hydrogen peroxide, Arch. Surg. 122:99–104 (1987).
58. Moore, F. D., Jr., C. Davis, M. Rodrick, J. A. Mannick, and D. T. Fearon, Neutrophil activation in thermal injury as assessed by increased expression of complement receptors, N. Engl. J. Med. 314:948–953 (1986).
59. Heideman, M., B. Kaijser, and L. Gelin, Complement activation and hematologic, hemodynamic, and respiratory reactions early after soft tissue injury, J. Trauma 18:696–700, 1978.
60. Kapur, M. M., P. Jain, and M. Gidh, The effect of trauma on serum C3 activation and its correlation with injury severity score in man, J. Trauma 26: 464–466 (1986).
61. Schirmer, W. J., J. M. Schirmer, G. B. Naff, and D. E. Fry, Complement activation in peritonitis: Association with hepatic and renal perfusion abnormalities, Am. Surg. 53:683–687 (1987).
62. Fearon, D. T., S. Ruddy, P. H. Schur, and W. R. McCabe, Activation of the properdin pathway of complement in patients with gram-negative bacteremia, N. Engl. J. Med. 292:937–940 (1975).
63. Goldstein, I. M., D. Roos, H. B. Kaplan, and G. Weissman, Complement and immunoglobulins stimulate superoxide production by human leukocytes independent of phagocytosis, J. Clin. Invest. 56:1155–1163 (1975).
64. Rundus, C., V. Peterson, R. Zapata-Sirvent, J. Hansbrough, and W. Robinson, Vit E improves cell-mediated immunity in the burned mouse: A preliminary study, Burns 11:11–15 (1984).
65. Platshon, L., and M. Kaliner, The effects of the immunologic release of histamine upon human lung cyclic nucleotide levels and prostaglandin generation, J. Clin. Invest. 62:1113–1121 (1978).
66. Stenson, W. F., and C. W. Parker, Prostaglandin, macrophages and immunity, J. Immunol. 125:1–5 (1980).
67. Fulton, A. M., and J. G. Levy, The possible role of prostaglandins in mediating immune suppression by nonspecific T-suppressor cells, Cell. Immunol. 52:29–37 (1980).

68. Faist, E., A. Mewes, C. C. Baker, T. Strasser, S. S. Alkan, P. Rieber, and G. Heberer, Prostaglandin E_2 (PGE_2)-dependent suppression of interleukin a (IL-2) production in patients with major trauma, J. Trauma 27:837–848 (1987).
69. Ninnemann, J. L., A. E. Stockland, and J. Condie, Induction of prostaglandin synthesis-dependent suppressor cells with endotoxin: Occurrence in patients with thermal injuries, J. Clin. Immunol. 3:142–150 (1983).
70. Miller-Graziano, C. L., M. Fink, J. Y. Wu, G. Szabo, and K. Kodys, Mechanisms of altered monocyte prostaglandin E_2 production in severely injured patients, Arch. Surg. 123:293–299 (1988).
71. Koster, F. T., J. C. Williams, and J. S. Goodwin, Cellular immunity in Q fever: Modulation of responsiveness by a suppressor T cell-monocyte circuit, J. Immunol. 135:1067–1072 (1985).
72. Claman, H. N., S. D. Miller, P. J. Conlon, and J. W. Moorhead, Control of experimental contact sensitivity, Adv. Immunol. 30:121–157 (1980).
73. Hansbrough, J. F., V. Peterson, E. Kortz, and J. Piacentine, Postburn immunosuppression in an animal model. Monocyte dysfunction induced by burned tissue, Surgery 93:415–427 (1983).
74. Hansbrough, J. F., R. L. Zapata-Sirvent, E. M. Bender, and V. Peterson, Prevention of suppressed cell-mediated immunity in burned mice with histamine-2 receptor antagonist drugs, J. Surg. Res. 39:150–156 (1985).
75. Hansbrough, J. F., R. L. Zapata-Sirvent, and V. M. Peterson, Immunomodulation following burn injury, Surg. Clinics North Am. 67:69–92 (1987).
76. Hansbrough, J. F., V. Peterson, R. L. Zapata-Sirvent, and H. N. Claman, Postburn immunosuppression in an animal model. II. Restoration of cell-mediated immunity by immunomodulating drgus, Surgery 95:290–295 (1984).
77. Bender, E. M., J. F. Hansbrough, R. L. Zapata-Sirvent, and H. N. Claman, Restoration of immunity in burned mice by cimetidine, J. Trauma 25:131–137 (1985).
78. Baker, C. C., I. H. Chaudry, H. O. Gaines, and A. E. Baue, Evaluation of factors affecting mortality rate after sepsis in a murine cecal ligation and puncture model, Surgery 94:331–335 (1983).
79. Wichterman, K. A., A. E. Baue, and I. H. Chaudry, Sepsis and septic shock—A review of laboratory models and a proposal, J. Surg. Res. 29:189–201 (1980).
80. Zapata-Sirvent, R. L., J. F. Hansbrough, M. A. Mansour, E. J. Bartle, and W. H. Carter, Postburn immunosuppression in an animal model. IV. Improved resistance to septic challenge with immunomodulating drugs, Surgery 99: 53–99 (1986).
81. Hansbrough, J. F., R. L. Zapata-Sirvent, S. R. Shackford, D. B. Hoyt, and W. H. Carter, Immunomodulating drugs increase resistance to sepsis in traumatized mice, J. Trauma 26:625–230 (1986).
82. Beer, D. J., and R. E. Rocklin, Histamine-induced suppressor-cell activity, J. Allergy Clin. Immunol. 73:439–452 (1984).

83. Beer, D. J., L. J. Rosenwasser, C. A. Dinarello, and R. E. Rocklin. Cellular interactions in the generation and expression of histamine-induced suppressor activity, Cell. Immunol. 69:101–112 (1982).
84. Khan, M. M., P. Sansoni, E. G. Engleman, and K. L. Melmon, Pharmacologic effects of autacoids on subsets of T cells, J. Clin. Invest. 75:1578–1583 (1985).
85. Sansoni, P., E. D. Silverman, M. M. Khan, K. L. Melmon, and E. G. Engleman, Immunoregulatory T cells in man: Histamine induced suppressor T cells are derived from a Leu 2 (T8+) subpopulation distinct from that which gives rise to cytotoxic T cells, J. Clin. Invest. 75:650–656 (1985).
86. Miller, S. D., M. S. Sy, and H. N. Claman, The induction of hapten-specific T cell tolerance using hapten modified lymphoidmembranes, Eur. J. Immunol. 7:165–170 (1977).
87. Mekori, Y. A., E. M. Bender, R. L. Zapata-Sirvent, J. F. Hansbrough, and H. N. Claman, The effect of histamine receptor antagonists on specific and nonspecific suppression of experimental contact sensitivity, J. Allergy Clin. Immunol. 76:90–96 (1985).
88. Sy, M. S., S. D. Miller, and H. N. Claman, Immune suppression with supra-optimal doses of antigen in contact sensitivity. I. Demonstration of suppressor cells and their sensitivity to cyclophosphamide, J. Immunol. 119:240–244 (1977).
89. Griswold, D. E., A. Salvatore, A. M. Badger, G. Poste, and N. Hanna, Inhibition of T suppressor cell expression by histamine type 2 receptor antagonists, J. Immunol. 132:3054–3057 (1984).
90. Jin, Z., A. Kumar, R. P. Cleveland, D. L. Murray, and D. B. Kaufman, Inhibition of suppressor cell function by cimetidine in a murine model, Clin. Immunol. Immunopathol. 38:350–356 (1986).
91. Cotner, T., J. M. Williams, L. Christenson, H. M. Shapiro, T. B. Strom, and J. Strominger, Simultaneous flow cytometric analysis of human T cell activation. Antigen expression and DNA content, J. Exp. Med. 157:461–472 (1983).
92. Cantrell, D., and K. A. Smith, Transient expression of interleukin 2 receptors. Consequences for T cell growth, J. Exp. Med. 158:1895-1911(1983)
93. Teodorczyk-Injeyan, J. A., B. G. Sparkes, G. B. Mills, W. J. Peters, and R. E. Falk, Impairment of T cell activation in burn patients: A possible mechanism of thermal injury-induced immunosuppression, Clin. Exp. Immunol. 65:570–581 (1986).
94. Wood, J. J., J. B. O'Mahony, M. L. Rodrick, and J. A. Mannick, Immature T lymphocytes after injury characterized by morphology and phenotypic markers, Ann. Surg. 206:564–571 (1987).
95. Garovoy, M. R., M. A. Reddish, and R. E. Rocklin, Histamine-induced suppressor factor (HSF): Inhibition of helper T cell generation and function, J. Immunol. 130:257–261 (1983).
96. Gadd, M. A., and J. F. Hansbrough, Defective T-cell surface antigen expression following mitogen stimulation: An index of lymphocyte dysfunction after controlled murine injury, submitted, Ann. Surg.

97. Nair, M. P. N., J. M. Cilik, and S. A. Schwartz, Histamine-induced suppressor factor inhibition of NK cells: Reversal with interferon and interleukin 2, J. Immunol. 136:2456–2462 (1986).
98. Lanser, M. E., M. Patrizio, G. Brown, B. Coleman, and J. H. Siegel, Serum-mediated depression of neutrophil chemiluminescence following blunt trauma, Ann. Surg. 202:111–118 (1985).
99. Riddle, P. R., and M. C. Berenbaum, Postoperative depression of the lymphocyte response to phytohaemagglutinin, Lancet 1:746–748 (1967).
100. Park, S. K., J. I. Brody, H. A. Wallace, and W. S. Blakemore, Immunosuppressive effect of surgery, Lancet 1:53–55 (1971).
101. Lundy, J., E. J. Lovett, S. Hamilton, and P. Conran, Immune impairment and metastatic tumor growth, Cancer 43:945–951 (1979).
102. Hansbrough, J. F., R. L. Zapata-Sirvent, and E. M. Bender, Prevention of alterations in postoperative lymphocyte subpopulations by cimetidine and ibuprofen, Am. J. Surg. 151:249–255 (1986).
103. Thomson, D. A., Anesthesia and the immune system, J. Burn Care Rehab., 8:483–487 (1987).
104. Lorenz, W., and A. Doenicke, Anaphylactoid reactions and histamine release by barbiturate induction agents: Clinical relevance and patho-mechanism, Anesthesiology 63:351–352 (1985).
105. Ahnefeld, F. W., A. Doenicke, and W. Lorenz, Histamines and antihistamines in anesthesia and surgery, Klin. Wochenschr. 60:871–1062 (1982).
106. Mitsuoka, A., M. Baba, and S. Morikawa, Enhancement of delayed hypersensitivity by depletion of suppressor T-cells with cyclophosphamide in mice, Nature 262:77–78 (1976).
107. Beer, D. J., S. M. Matloff, and R. E. Rocklin, The influence of histamine on immune and inflammatory responses, Adv. Immunol. 35:209–268 (1984).
108. Hansbrough, J. F., and M. A. Gadd, Immunomodulation after burn and trauma in an animal model. In Proceedings of the First International Congress on the Immune Consequences of Trauma, Shock and Sepsis, Munich, March 1988 (Faist, E., Ed.), Springer Verlag, Berlin, in press.
109. Hohn, D. C., A. J. Meyers, S. T. Gherini, A. Beckmann, R. E. Markison, and A. M. Churg, Production of acute pulmonary injury by leukocytes and activated complement, Surgery 88:48–58 (1980).

13
Burn Shock

JOSEPH V. BOYKIN, JR.* *Medical College of Virginia, Richmond, Virginia*
NANCY H. MANSON *University of Virginia, Charlottesville, Virginia*

I. INTRODUCTION

If severely burned patients can survive the initial inhalation injury and subsequent microbial infections, they are still susceptible to the development of burn shock, cardiovascular collapse, and death. Inhalation injury and microbial infections are among the leading causes of death early after burn (1,2). With endogenous defense systems profoundly compromised, patients are particularly vulnerable to microbial infections. In the initial phases postinjury, there are declines in circulating concentrations of immunoglobulins, fibronectin, and complement plus a depression in cell-mediated immune responses (2).

The dramatic changes in the inflammatory response and in the immune system following thermal injury contribute to microvascular damage, resulting in loss of intravascular fluid volume, burn shock, and subsequent cardiovascular collapse (Fig. 1). For example, complement activation, specifically an increase in C5a, initiates neutrophil generation of oxygen-derived radicals (3). Oxygen free radicals induce lipid peroxidation which increases the capillary membrane

**Current affiliation*: The Institute for Plastic and Reconstructive Surgery, Richmond, Virginia.

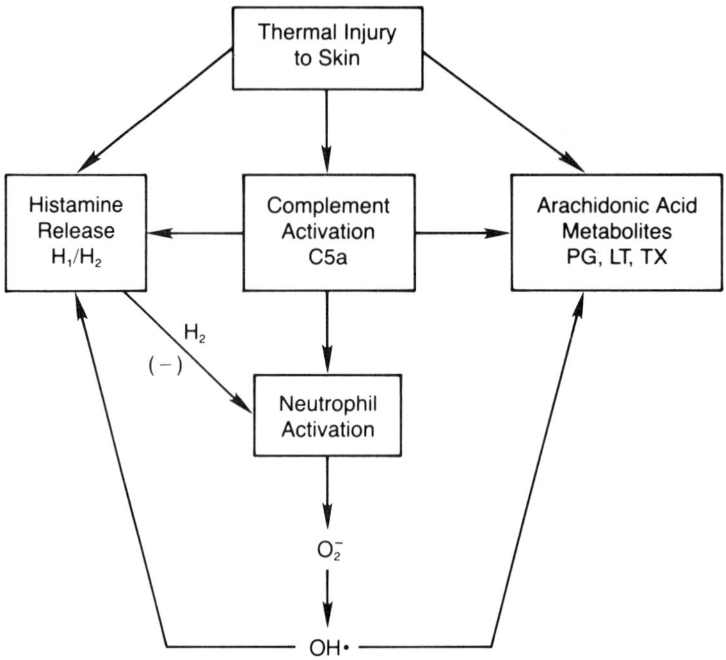

Figure 1 Suggested mediators of thermal injury. Thermal injury initiates the release of vasoactive factors which in addition to direct effects on the vasculature interact with each other.

permeability contributing to loss of intravascular fluid volume (4). Neutrophil chemotaxis in response to C5a contributes to the transient neutropenia develop-following burn. In rats, depletion of complement or neutrophils will prevent lung injury developing after burn (5). A major goal of therapeutic intervention following severe thermal injury is to protect the integrity of the microvasculature, thereby preventing hypovolemia, shock, and collapse of the cardiovascular system.

Complement activation is one of several suggested mediators of hypovolemia. Vasoactive agents released in the early phases of postinjury such as histamine, kinins, prostaglandins, and serotonin are also proposed mediators of the burn-induced hypovolemia (6). Testing the effects of antagonists of some of these agents led to the discovery that treatment of severe thermal injury in guinea pigs within 30 min with high-dose cimetidine decreased the necessary fluid replacement volume by 70%. It was also found that, in this case, cimetidine appears to be acting via mechanisms independent of its histamine type II (H_2) antagonism (7).

II. CIMETIDINE PROTECTION FROM BURN SHOCK

The last major advances in therapy for thermal injury occurred in the 1960s with the development of crystalloid and/or colloid solutions administered to maintain intravascular volume, thereby averting hypovolemia and burn shock. Additional problems arise with this treatment regimen. Although circulating blood volume may be normalized, the quantity of fluids necessary for volume maintenance can exacerbate burn wound and generalized edema (8). Burn edema develops in both burned and in remote normal tissue. It was in investigation of this phenomenon that cimetidine was first found to be beneficial.

A. Cimetidine Protection of Remote Edema Formation

Although cimetidine has been used in the latter stages of thermal injury for its protective gastrointestinal effects, Boykin et al. (9) reported the first studies of cimetidine given in high doses in the early phases following burn with an evaluation of cardiovascular effects. The purpose of these studies was to more clearly identify the mediators of remote edema formation in a mild scald injury in the hairless mouse. Of the interventions tested, cold water, high-dose cimetidine, and polymyxin B were effective in preventing remote edema formation. It was suggested that all three of these protective mechanisms involved blocking the histamine response. Agents which were ineffective in preventing remote edema included the cyclooxygenase inhibitor indomethacin, the histamine and serotonin inhibitor cyproheptadine, and histamine type I receptor antagonist mepyramine. These studies suggested that cimetidine was acting via a histamine type II receptor antagonism action.

B. Cimetidine Prevention of Burn Shock

Based on the remote edema studies, the effect of cimetidine on burn shock development was evaluated in a guinea pig model of severe scald injury (7). Cimetidine therapy (100 mg/kg) was delivered intraperitoneally at 30 min postscald and at 4 and 8 hr postinjury in conjunction with replacement fluids. The results of this study demonstrated that cimetidine at a high dose maintained cardiac output and mean arterial pressure at control levels, while significantly decreasing resuscitative fluid volume by 70%. It was also found that this effect was time dependent in that cimetidine administration beginning 1 hr following burn had no protective effect on hemodynamics. Upon further investigation, results from ranitidine studies, with ranitidine administered at equipotent doses at 30 min, 4 and 8 hours postinjury, implicated non-histamine type II receptor antagonist mechanisms involved with this effect, as ranitidine offered no protection of cardiovascular parameters.

III. MECHANISMS OF CIMETIDINE PROTECTION FROM BURN SHOCK

Some of the actions of cimetidine that are independent of its histamine type II receptor antagonism which could prove advantageous in preventing burn shock include: (1) inhibition of cytochrome P-450, (2) scavenging of oxygen free radicals when complexed with copper, (3) modification of arachidonic acid metabolite production, and (4) enhanced buffering capacity (1). Cimetidine's protection from burn shock could involve components of all or several of these mechanisms.

A. Inhibition of Cytochrome P-450

Thermal injury leads to an increase in cytochrome P-450 (CP-450) activity. Seccia et al. (10) report a 76% increase in the NADPH (nicotinamide adenine dinucleotide phosphate) reducible fraction of CP-450 within the first 6 hr following burn. This increase is transient and concentrations of this fraction of CP-450 return to control levels by 24 hr. The NADPH reducible fraction of CP-450 participates in two types of free radical generation process (11). First, the autoxidation of this cytochrome yields superoxide anion. In the presence of small amounts of iron, superoxide anion is rapidly converted via the iron-catalyzed Haber-Weiss reaction to the highly reactive and toxic hydroxyl radical. In addition, it metabolizes some endogenous compounds, such as steroids, forming toxic radical metabolites. With an increase in oxygen-derived or metabolite radicals, lipid peroxidation could be initiated resulting in increased microvascular permeability and endothelial cell damage (Fig. 2). Another effect of CP-450 which may be harmful to preservation of cardiovascular performance is the initiation of the arachidonic acid cascade. It has been shown that one mechanism of endothelium dependent relaxation of vascular smooth muscle entails initiation of the arachidonic acid cascade by CP-450 (12,13). In the face of circulatory shock, the peripheral vasodilator effect of arachidonic acid metabolites is deleterious.

Cimetidine competitively binds with high affinity to CP-450. In support of the strong interaction of cimetidine with CP-450 during thermal injury treatment, in the same time period that CP-450 increases, there is an increase of nonrenal metabolism of cimetidine as indicated by an increase of oxidative metabolites of cimetidine (14). Data from our laboratory support this finding, as we measured a 2.5-fold increase in the sulfoxide metabolite fraction of cimetidine within the first 2 hr following injury (unpublished observations).

Cytochrome P-450 inhibition by cimetidine or other antagonists should prevent the production of radical species from this source, although during this phase of thermal injury oxygen-derived radicals are also generated by activated neutrophils. Preliminary studies from our laboratory indicate that there is a peak

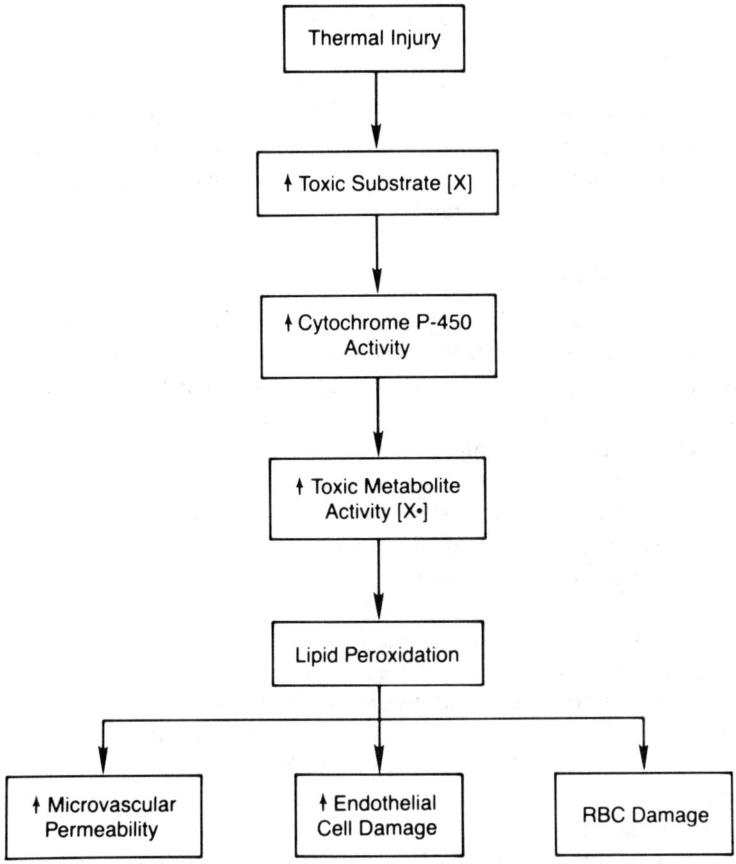

Figure 2 Suggested mechanisms of thermal injury. A major mechanism of thermal injury involves the activation of cytochrome P-450 to produce toxic metabolites, possibly radicals, which initiate lipid peroxidation. Increased lipid peroxidation may result in irreversible cellular membrane damage.

in conjugated diene activity, a measure of systemic lipid peroxidation, at 45 min following burn. Treatment with cimetidine has no effect on this peak, indicating that cimetidine protection probably does not involve this action of CP-450. Studies with SKF-525A and miconazole, also inhibitors of CP-450, have revealed an attenuation of edema formation and significant reduction of conjugated diene peak formation at 45 min after scald (unpublished observations).

As for the effect of CP-450 on the arachidonic acid cascade, cimetidine would be expected to block this action too. Cytochrome P-450 has been found and identified in endothelial cells of vascular smooth muscle (15). Inhibitors of CP-450 have been shown to inhibit the endothelium-dependent relaxation of muscle in response to arachidonic acid as well as to prevent the production of arachidonic acid metabolites (12,13). Specifically, SKF-525A inhibits acetylcholine and arachidonic acid-induced relaxation of the rabbit aorta. In the case of burn shock, cimetidine inhibition of this endothelium-dependent relaxation mechanism would be extremely beneficial.

B. Oxygen Free Radical Scavenger

The participation of free radicals in the pathophysiology of all types of circulatory shock has been a subject of debate. Proponents cite studies showing protection of pulmonary microvascular permeability following superoxide dismutase and catalase pretreatment as evidence of free radical participation. Opponents cite studies in which there is no change in mortality in sepsis models when superoxide dismutase and catalase are administered as evidence of lack of participation. It is generally agreed that oxygen free radicals play some role, if not a major one, in the pathophysiology of all types of circulatory shock. The effects of these radicals include lipid peroxidation, erythrocyte damage, microvascular damage, increased vascular permeability, increased platelet and neutrophil adherence to vessel walls, the promotion of production of arachidonic acid metabolites, and altered wound healing (5,16). The sources of oxygen free radicals following burn have been mentioned above and include activation of the NADPH reducible fraction of cytochrome P-450 and generation during the conversion of prostaglandin G_2 (PGG_2) to prostaglandin H_2 (PGH_2) in the arachidonic acid cascade (17).

Cimetidine action on oxygen free radical generation has been studied extensively by Kimura and coworkers (18). When copper is complexed with cimetidine the in vitro complex acts as an efficient superoxide anion scavenger. While cimetidine will scavenge superoxide anion when bound to divalent copper, large plasma proteins such as albumin have a much higher affinity for divalent copper in vivo than cimetidine. When albumin is added in these in vitro studies cimetidine loses its scavenging properties. Conversely, cimetidine binds very tightly to monovalent copper. Displacement of the monovalent copper-cimetidine complex is not significantly altered by plasma protein in vitro. The monovalent copper/cimetidine complex has been identified as having the highest measurable superoxide dismutase-like activity of any compound tested. For these reasons, the possible role of in vivo complexes of monovalent copper and cimetidine presented a unique and attractive scavenging mechanism which had not previously been observed following burn injury.

In our laboratory, serum copper levels following severe thermal injury in the guinea pig have been measured (unpublished observations). Serum copper levels increase significantly following severe untreated burn injury. Cimetidine treatment significantly lowers serum copper levels at 24 hr postinjury when compared to the burn group. It is possible that cimetidine complexing of the copper removes it from the measurable pool. If cimetidine does indeed act as a scavenger of oxygen free radicals, its ultimate action would be protection of membrane integrity and a prevention of microvascular injury which would contribute to preservation of intravascular fluid volumes. However, in light of the results of the conjugated diene studies following cimetidine treatment, it seems unlikely that a major part of cimetidine's protection arises from this mechanism.

C. Inhibition of Thromboxane Synthesis

Another protective mechanism of cimetidine in the treatment of thermal injury includes possible inhibition of thromboxane synthetase or an indirect inhibition of thromboxane generation. Thromboxane decreases coronary flow; therefore an inhibition of thromboxane synthesis would protect cardiovascular performance (19). The effect of cimetidine on thromboxane synthetase is questionable. In some laboratories, cimetidine appears to inhibit the enzyme (20). In others, there appears to be no effect on thromboxane synthesis (21). SKF-525A has been shown to inhibit thromboxane synthesis indirectly; that is, it does not appear to affect the synthetase enzyme (22).

While this effect of cimetidine has not been evaluated in our guinea pig model, Alexander et al. (23) have examined the effect of the thromboxane synthetase inhibitor ketoconazole in a thermal injury model. With ketoconazole pretreatment, the increase in microvascular permeability was prevented. Ketoconazole like cimetidine is a substituted imidazole with multiple effects in this model. It has recently been reported (24) that ketoconazole is also an inhibitor of CP-450, which like cimetidine blocks production of arachidonic acid metabolites, which are thought to be responsible for endothelium-mediated arachidonate-induced relaxation of vascular smooth muscle.

D. Buffer Action

A final suggested mechanism of protection of cimetidine in burn shock involves the buffering capability of cimetidine as a substituted imidazole. It has been reported that acidosis equivalent to that seen in the ischemic myocardium depresses myocardial sarcoplasmic reticulum calcium uptake (25). Compromise of the excitation-contraction coupling mechanisms would lead to impaired mechanical function. Cimetidine-mediated enhancement of acid-base homeostasis may contribute to the preservation of cardiovascular performance and microvascular integrity.

E. Summary of Protective Mechanisms

Of the above listed mechanisms, the most likely benefit of cimetidine treatment of burn shock promoting major protective effects is its inhibition of microsomal cytochrome P-450 enzyme systems. The consequences of increased activity of CP-450 are far reaching because of the multiple deleterious actions of the enzyme, including its free radical-related mechanisms and its capacity to increase the metabolism of arachidonic acid.

VI. CONCLUSIONS

The secondary effects of massive fluid resuscitation following thermal injury establish long-term complications which may impede patient recovery. Experimental results indicate that early administration of cimetidine leads to a 70% reduction in required resuscitative fluid volume. The mechanisms of this protection are currently under investigation. Of the mechanisms discussed here, the inhibition of cytochrome P-450 by cimetidine probably contributes the most to the protective effects. Preliminary data gathered using SKF-525A in the thermal injury model support this statement. The overall effects of CP-450 inhibition would be prevention of increased microvascular permeability with protection of intravascular fluid volume and prevention of arachidonic acid-induced endothelium-dependent vascular relaxation. These actions would help to maintain proper perfusion of vital organs thereby preventing shock and preserving cardiovascular performance. It is hoped that, in the future, cimetidine therapy could be established to promote a significant improvement in the overall recovery and rehabilitation of the severely burned patient.

REFERENCES

1. Boykin, J. V., Jr., and N. H. Manson, Mechanisms of cimetidine protection following thermal injury, Am. J. Med. 83(Suppl. 6A):76–81 (1987).
2. Bjornson, A. B., and H. S. Bjornson, Theoretical interrelationships among immunologic and hematologic sequelae of thermal injury, Rev. Infect. Dis. 6:704–714 (1984).
3. Jacob, H. S., P. R. Craddock, D. E. Hammerschmidt, and C. F. Moldoso, Complement-induced granulocyte aggregation: An unsuspected mechanism of disease, N. Engl. J. Med. 307:789–794 (1980).
4. Demopoulos, H. B., E. S. Flamm, D. D. Peitronigro, and M. L. Seligman, The free radical pathology and the microcirculation in the major central nervous system disorders, Acta Physiol. Scand. 492(Suppl.):91–119 (1980).
5. Till, G. O., J. R. Hatherill, and P. A. Ward, Lipid peroxidation products in experimental thermal injury. In Oxygen Free Radicals in Shock (Novelli, G. P., and Ursini, F., Eds.), Karger, New York, (1986), pp. 34–41.

6. Demling, R. H., Burns, N. Engl. J. Med. 313:1389–1398 (1985).
7. Boykin, J. V. Jr., S. L. Crute, and B. W. Haynes, Jr., Cimetidine therapy for burn shock: A quantitative assessment, J. Trauma 25:864–870 (1985).
8. Carlson, R. G., R. K. Finley, S. F. Miller, L. M. Jones, M. A. Morath, and S. Alkire, Fluid retention during the first 48 hours as an indicator of burn survival, J. Trauma 26:840–843 (1986).
9. Boykin, J. V. Jr., E. Eriksson, M. M. Sholley, and R. N. Pittman, Histamine-mediated delayed permeability response after scald burn inhibited by cimetidine or cold-water treatment, Science 209:815–817 (1980).
10. Seccia, A., C. Riberti, M. DeGennaro, and G. Flamini, Changes in cytochrome P450 levels in hepatic microsomes after burn injuries: Experimental study, Burns 6:174–180 (1979).
11. Ingelman-Sundberg, M., and A. L. Hagbjork, On the significance of the cytochrome P-450-dependent hydroxyl radical-mediated oxygenation mechanism, Xenobiotica 12:673–686 (1982).
12. Peach, M. J., H. A. Singer, and A. L. Loeb, Mechanisms of endothelium-dependent vascular smooth muscle relaxation, Biochem. Pharmacol. 34: 1867–1874 (1985).
13. Pinto, A., N. G. Abraham, and K. M. Mullane, Arachidonic acid-induced endothelial-dependent relaxations of canine coronary arteries: contribution of a cytochrome P-450-dependent pathway, J. Pharmacol. Exp. Ther. 240: 856–863 (1987).
14. Ziemniak, J. A., W. A. Watson, J. R. Saffle, I. L. Smith, J. Russo, Jr., G. D. Warden, and J. J. Shentag, Cimetidine kinetics during resuscitation from burn shock, Clin. Pharmacol. Ther. 36:228–233 (1984).
15. Abraham, N. G., A. Pinto, K. M. Mullane, R. D. Levere, and E. G. Spokas, Presence of cytochrome P-450-dependent monooxygenase in intimal cells of the hog aorta, Hypertension 7:899–904 (1985).
16. Hess, M. L., and N. H. Manson, Molecular oxygen: Friend and foe. The role of the oxygen free radical system in the calcium paradox, the oxygen paradox and ischemia/reperfusion injury, J. Mol. Cell. Cardiol. 16:969–985 (1984).
17. Kuehl, F. A., J. L. Humes, M. L. Torchiana, E. A. Ham, and R. W. Egan, Oxygen centered radicals in the inflammatory process. In Advances in Inflammation Research, vol. I. (Weissman, G., Ed.). Raven Press, New York (1979), pp. 419–430.
18. Kimura, I., T. Koike, Y. Shimizu, and M. Kodama, Complexes of the histamine H_2-antagonist cimetidine with divalent and monovalent copper ions, Inorg. Chem. 25:2242–2246 (1986).
19. Bach, M. K., The leukotrienes: Their structure, actions and role in diseases. In Current Concepts, Upjohn, Kalamazoo, pp. 1–15 (1983).
20. Mikhailidis, D. P., J. Christofides, M. A. Barradas, J. Y. Jeremy, J. Dilawari, and P. Dandona, The effect of cimetidine on platelet function: a study involving gastric fluid measurements, Agents Actions 19:34–41 (1986).

21. Compton, M. R., J. P. Seale, and J. Shaw, A possible mechanism in the anti-anaphylactic effect of beta-adrenoceptor agonists in guinea-pig lungs, Arch. Int. Pharmacodyn. Ther. 276:112–119 (1985).
22. Boeynaems, J. M., D. DeMolle, and A. VanCoevorden, Stimulation of vascular prostacyclin by SKF 525-A (Proadifen) and related compounds, Biochem. Pharmacol. 36:1637-1643 (1987).
23. Alexander, F., M. Mathieson, K. H. Teoh, W. V. Huval, S. Lelcuk, R. Valeri, D. Shepro, and H. B. Hechtman, Arachidonic acid metabolites mediate early burn edema, J. Trauma 24:709–712 (1984).
24. Capdevila, J., L. Gil, M. Orellana, L. J. Marnett, J. I. Mason, P. Yadagiri, and J. R. Falck, Inhibitors of cytochrome P-450-dependent arachidonic acid metabolism, Arch. Biochem. Biophys. 261:257-263 (1988).
25. Hess, M. L., N. H. Manson, and E. I. Okabe, Involvement of free radicals in the pathophysiology of ischemic heart disease, Can. J. Physiol. 60:1382–1389 (1982).

14

H_2 Antagonists and AIDS

NORBERT H. BROCKMEYER *University Clinic, Essen, Federal Republic of Germany*

I. DEFINITION OF AIDS

The generally accepted definition of AIDS (acquired immunodeficiency syndrome) was presented by the U.S. Centers for Disease Control in 1981 (1), and implies that there is

1. The presence of reliably diagnosed disease at least moderately indicative of cellular immune deficiency (e.g., Kaposi's syndrome [KS] in a patient less than 60 years of age or pneumocystis pneumonia infection)
2. An absence of known underlying immune deficiency and of any other reduced resistance reported to be associated with the disease (e.g., immunosuppressive therapy or lymphoreticular malignancy)

In 1985, this definition was revised to exclude patients in whom HIV-1 infection could not be proved either by serological methods or virus culture or in whom no normal helper cell counts could be found.

Acquired immunodeficiency syndrome was first described in 1981 by both Gottlieb et al. (2) and by Siegal et al. (3), who showed it to be a disease of the human immune system, which leads to the death of many affected patients by way of opportunistic infections or certain malignant tumors.

In 1982–1983, a cause of AIDS was discovered. Luc Montagnier, of the institute Pasteur Paris, isolated the lymphoadenopathy-associated virus (LAV) (4), and Robert Gallo isolated the human T-cell leukemia virus (HTLV-III) (5). These viruses were later proved to be identical. Thus we speak of the HTLV-III/LAV virus.

Later it was shown that the mechanism of action of the virus is to attack specific cells of the immune system (target cells are CD4 cells) (6,7), weakening the immune system and giving way to severe opportunistic infections and diseases.

II. THE VIRUS

HIV-1 (human immunodeficiency virus) is a lentivirus distantly related to HTLV-I and -II (which have been implicated in the pathogenesis of T-cell leukemias/ lymphomas). As a lentivirus, or slow virus, HIV-1 characteristically causes chronic, degenerating infections with a long incubation period.

The virus has the build-up of a typical retrovirus, which can only replicate after having transcribed its ribonucleic acid (RNA) genome into a double-strained deoxyribonucleic acid (DNA) copy, by a viral enzyme, called reverse transcriptase, a target of several drugs.

The specific structure of the virus shows it to be composed of an envelope consisting of glycoproteins, and a core, where the two strands of RNA, structural proteins, i.e., gp-24 and enzymes are located.

The envelope, which has several "spikes" on its surface, is composed of two glycoproteins (gp-120 and gp-41). This is the site of high-affinity binding to the CD4 molecule of the target cell, so that the virus can easily attack CD4-positive cells. It is also assumed that isolated gp-120 proteins can block the CD4 receptor of non-infected cells, thereby inhibiting their function.

III. VIRUS DETECTION

HIV-1 can be isolated and characterized or it can be indirectly detected by several tests, which measure the patient's antibodies in serum.

A. ELISA (Enzyme-Linked Immunosorbent Assay)

1. Antibody Detection

ELISA is used as an antibody screening test, consisting of a two-step process: First cleaned HIV-1 antigen, which is bound to a fixed phase is covered with the patients's serum. When specific antibodies are present they are bound to the antigens. If they are not present, they are washed out. In the second step, the complex of antigen and antibody (immunoglobulin) is covered by a solution containing antibody against human immunoglobulin coupled with an enzyme. In case of a positive first reaction, this additional antibody is bound to the patient's antibody. This complex can then be made visible by a color reaction owing to the coupled enzyme.

ELISA is a high sensitivity test, with false-positive results occurring in up to 20% of test subjects.

2. Western Blot

The Western Blot test has a higher specificity than ELISA, and is used to confirm the diagnosis of a HIV-1 infection. It is a reference test used when ELISA has displayed positive result. The method is to split HIV-specific proteins, e.g., p24 by polyacrylamid gel electrophoresis, according to their molecular weight (blot technique). After incubation with the patient's serum, the specific patient's antibodies are bound to the matching virus proteins and can be detected by a second antibody coupled with an enzyme.
Detection see ELISA.

B. HIV-1 Antigen Assay

The HIV Antigen Assay is a recently developed p24 HIV-1 viral antigen test which employs monoclonal antibodies, and thereby detects HIV-1 core proteins minimizing affections by nonspecific interferring substances.

IV. EPIDEMIOLOGY

Early cases of AIDS were reported in homosexuals, intravenous drug abusers, and recipients of blood products. A related disease is endemic in parts of Africa (9–11). Since the identification of the virus, HIV-1 infection rate has risen rapidly (12), showing an exponential, pandemic character in the United States and European countries (13). Whereas in the United States and Europe, mostly high-risk groups have been affected (i.e., homosexual/bisexual men in United States by 67%, and drug abusers by 16% in 1986), the African countries show a different picture with predominantly heterosexual transmission (14), involving large parts of the general population (15). As a third group, the Eastern countries are principally affected by way of infected blood or contact with infected travelers.

V. CLASSIFICATION AND CLINICAL PICTURE

There are two main coexisting classifications of AIDS: the Walter Reed (WR) classification proposed by the Walter Reed Institute, Washington, D.C., in January 1986 (16); and the Centers for Disease Control (CDC) classification, published in May 1986 (17).

In the Walter Reed classification, the lack or existence of lymph adenopathy, CD4 cell count less or more than 400 nl/, recall antigen reaction (= skin testing), candidiasis or opportunistic infections are common criteria for WR1-WR6.

The CDC classification uses the criteria:

I = Acute infection
II = Infection without symptoms
III = Persistent lymphadenopathy
IV = Other infections/diseases

It is important to note, that the CDC classification is fixed, whereas in the Walter Reed classification, a patient can be staged backward or forward according to the clinical picture.

Before AIDS becomes fullblown, the disease usually has different stages, referred to as:

Symptomless ARID (AIDS-related immune dysfunction)
LAS (lymphadenopathy)
ARC (AIDS-related complex), referring to symptoms such as weakness, night sweats, fever, diarrhea, and weight loss, with corresponding blood parameters
Progression to classic AIDS includes opportunistic infections of either viral, bacterial, or fungal origin or by protozoa; neoplasms such as KS, highly malignant lymphomas, or primary lymphoma of the central nervous system

VI. IMMUNOLOGY

When an antigen enters the body it is taken up by antigen-presenting cells especially macrophages, and split into smaller particles (antigens). The antigens are presented on the surface of the macrophage, thereby bound to human leucocyte antigens (HLA) of class I or II. The T cell, which has a corresponding receptor for this antigen-HLA-protein-complex, is then bound to the surface, and thereby activation occurs. T cells, which are to become cytotoxic cells ($CD8^+$), are cific B-cell receptor). T cells, which are to become cytotoxic cells ($CD8^+$), are associated with HLA proteins of class I, and helper cells ($CD4^+$) with HLA proteins of class II. When the macrophage and this special T cell ($CD4^+$ cell =

helper cell) come into contact, the macrophage releases cytokines, hormone-like substances which induces differentiation and division of the T cells.

The resulting, activated T-cells can now exhibit cytotoxicity or they can act as helper cells; i.e., allowing a faster immune response by contact with the same antigen, thereby inducing the division of activated B cells (plasma cells).

The plasma cells themselves release antigen-specific antibodies. T-helper cells are also involved in the stimulation of monocytes/macrophages, natural killer cells, killer cells, cytotoxic T cells, and T-suppressor cells (18).

Thus, as a decrease of the absolute T-helper cell population is the crucial finding in AIDS patients, several partial reactions are impaired, having devastating effects on the immune system:

1. T-helper cells: diminished reaction toward antigens, a disturbed regulation
2. T-suppressor cells: disturbed regulation
3. Cytotoxic T cells: less cellular toxicity
4. B cells: lack specific differentiation and therefore formation of plasma cells, unnecessary overreaction, increased immunoglobulin (Ig) production
5. Killer-cells: decreased activity
6. Monocytes/macrophages: diminished chemotaxis, spontaneous secretion of effector substances, less response to stimuli

It is easy to see that if the helper cells are functionally impaired, the immune system is out of control. Therefore, the examination of CD4 cells is an important laboratory evaluation aside from the enumeration of other parameters, which can be evaluated in laboratory diagnostics as neopterin, immunoglobulins, complement factors, and β_2 microglobulin (19-21).

VII. THERAPY

The acquired immunodeficiency syndrome first observed endemically in young men in San Francisco in the beginning of the 1980s was an up to this time unknown disease. In 1983, the virus isolation by both Luc Montagnier (4) and Robert Gallo (5) supported the assumption of a viral etiology. During the following months, the Henle-Koch postulates for an infectious disease were fulfilled (the virus has to be present in every patient, the isolation has to be successful, and the study of experimental infection in animals also has to be possible) (22,23). The presently valid statistics calculated an exponential logarithmic distribution of the HIV-1 infection with millions of people being infected worldwide (13). All antiviral agents on trial during this time, like suramin or HPA23, had the disadvantages of either impairing virus specificity, or of causing severe side effects; e.g., agranulocytopenia and the danger of carcinogenesis (24-29). For this reason, many teams chose the second of the two possible forms of therapy; i.e., the immunomodulation in HIV-1 infected patients. Many well-known new drugs or agents were tried (e.g., thymopentin, isoprenosine, interferons, and interleukins) (30,31).

Principally there are two forms of therapy:

1. Antiviral agents
2. Immunomodulating therapy

A. Antiviral Therapy

In order to appreciate the application of retroviral therapy, a knowledge of the replicative cycle of HIV-1 virus is important.

1. The first step in the cycle includes binding to specific cellular receptors, an epitope of the CD4 (T4) antigen that is expressed especially by T cells of the helper phenotype, but is also expressed by macrophages lungerhaus cells e.g.
2. After penetration of the cell, the virus is uncoated and reverse transcription of viral RNA into double-stranded DNA is initiated by the viral enzyme reverse transcriptase.
3. Posttranscriptional processing is the next step in the replication cycle, followed by translation of the new DNS strand.
4. The final stages are encapsulation of the newly secreted viral proteins, budding, and release.

Possible interactions of this cycle include interference with the interaction of the virus and target cells by monoclonal antibodies or peptides that bind to the CD4 receptor. This has been accomplished in vitro by antibodies directed against an epitope of the CD4 antigen (32). Another possibility includes the use of antibodies directed against the envelope protein (gp120) associated with receptor binding (33). The next possibility of interference is by means of antiviral agents inhibiting the enzyme reverse transcriptase, such as azidothymidine (AZT), a thymidine analog (23), 2′3′ dideoxy-nucleotides (34), suramin (35), phosphonoformate (36), antimoniotunstate (HPA23) (37), or ansamycin (38). Ribavirin interferes with the capping of the viral messenger RNA (39).

The side effects of these drugs differ:

1. AZT: anemia, granulocytopenia and neurotoxicity (40,41)
2. 2'3' Dideoxynucleotides: a severe dose-related neurotoxicity (42)
3. Suramin: fever, rash, increases SGOT levels and hepatotoxicity, proteinuria, neutropenia, paresthesias, and adrenal insufficiency (43)
4. Antimoniotungstate: potential nephrotoxicity in phosphonoformate; thrombocytopenia and hepatitis (44)
5. Ansamycin: hepatotoxicity and reversible neutropenia (45)
6. Ribavirin: depression of hemoglobin synthesis, headaches, and cognitive dysfunction (46)

1. Interferon-α and Interferon-β

Interferons are considered to possess an antiviral as well as an immunomodulating effect, and can therefore not be classified in one or the other category. Interferon-α is a protein that belongs to one of the three major classes of interferons (α, β, and γ). It has antiviral, immunomodulating, and antiproliferative effects. After binding to interferon receptors, interferon acts on the HIV-1-infected cell by inducing the production of several enzymes that most probably interfere with transcription/translation of the messenger RNA (mRNA), protein synthesis, assembly, and release of the virions. Side effects include flulike symptoms, central nervous system disturbances, leukopenia, thrombocytopenia, liver function abnormalities, and alopecia (47).

Interferon-β is produced by viral induction of fibroblasts, and has anti-HIV-1 as well as antitumor activity; the specific mechanism of action remains as yet, however, unclear. Adverse reactions are similar to those observed with interferon-α (48).

Therapy with interferon-α and -β have been reported to cause a regression of Kaposi's sarcoma and an improvement of the performance (40–52).

B. Immunomodulation

Interferon-γ lacks the anti-HIV-1 activity of interferon-α and -β. Since AIDS patients have been found to be deficient in interferon-γ, it is being administered in clinical studies (53). Drug-related flulike symptoms occur frequently. Other immunomodulating substances include isoprinosine, diphenylhydantoid, and cimetidine, which are thought to interfere positively with the immune system. Isoprinosine acts only on activated T cells and stimulates the differentiation of helper T cells, cytotoxic T cells, and monocytes, thereby initiating a cascade of cellular interactions leading to partial restoration of cell-mediated immune responses (54). The mechanism of action for diphenylhydantoid is not yet known.

Table 1 Effect of Cimetidine 800 mg day^{-1} on Absolute (Cells nl^{-1}) and Relatives (%) Number of CD4 and CD8 Lymphocytes and Total Skin Test Reactivity (mm) in Healthy Volunteers (mean ± SD)

Time (days)	CD4 absolute	CD4 relative	CD8 absolute	CD8 relative	CD4/CD8	Skin test
0	942 ± 142	42.91 ± 2.87	365 ± 63	16.09 ± 2.00	3.15 ± 0.50	13.8 ± 4.3
1	850 ± 121	42.90 ± 3.19	298 ± 46	15.09 ± 2.08	3.53 ± 0.67	ND[d]
2	879 ± 115	40.45 ± 2.99	307 ± 38	14.36 ± 2.49	3.73 ± 0.67	ND
4	874 ± 138	41.09 ± 3.30	302 ± 42	15.45 ± 2.02	3.43 ± 0.76	ND
7[a]	990 ± 123	44.82 ± 3.30	264[b] ± 64	12.70 ± 2.58	5.00[c] ± 1.14	24.8[c] ± 5.9
11	972 ± 149	44.09 ± 2.64	288 ± 53	13.73 ± 2.01	4.09 ± 0.80	ND

[a]Last day of cimetidine intake.
[b]$p < 0.05$, tested against value of day 0.
[c]$p < 0.01$, tested against value of day 0.
[d]ND not done.

Table 2 Effect of Cimetidine 800 mg day^{-1} on Blastogenesis in Healthy Volunteers (cpm 10^3; mean ± SD)

Time (days)	ConA	PHA		PWM	
day	1 ($\mu g\ ml^{-1}$)	0.2 ($\mu g\ ml^{-1}$)	0.4 ($\mu g\ ml^{-1}$)	0.1 ($\mu g\ ml^{-1}$)	0.4 ($\mu g\ ml^{-1}$)
0	26.6 ± 7.2	82.7 ± 14.0	66.5 ± 12.4	7.3 ± 2.7	8.8 ± 2.4
1	54.9 ± 11.3	175.6 ± 75.3	142.7 ± 48.5	18.2 ± 3.3	12.5 ± 3.0
2	39.9 ± 11.8	76.2 ± 11.4	75.8 ± 17.2	18.8 ± 3.4	13.3 ± 3.1
4	64.9 ± 13.3	134.9 ± 31.4	100.2 ± 18.1	18.1 ± 3.4	13.9 ± 3.1
7[a]	129.9[c] ± 14.9	177.7[c] ± 12.0	166.0[b] ± 15.7	27.6[b] ± 5.2	34.0[b] ± 8.3
11	55.6 ± 15.0	130.8 ± 11.9	105.5 ± 12.0	18.0 ± 5.2	18.2 ± 5.5

[a]Last day of cimetidine intake.
[b]$p < 0.05$, tested against value of day 0.
[c]$p < 0.01$, tested against value of day 0.

Table 3 Effect of Cimetidine 1600 mg day^{-1} on Blastogenesis in Healthy Volunteers (cpm 10^3; mean ±SD)

Time (days)	ConA (1 μg ml^{-1})	ConA (2 μg ml^{-1})	PHA (0.2 μg ml^{-1})	PHA (0.4 μg ml^{-1})	PWM (90.1μg ml^{-1})	PWM (0.4 μg ml^{-1})
0	10.5 ± 6.0	27.1 ± 14.6	50.9 ± 22.9	48.7 ± 19.0	6.1 ± 4.0	6.3 ± 3.6
7	38.7[b] ± 26.0	48.0 ± 26.7	85.6[b] ± 40.8	81.1[b] ± 38.5	15.0 ± 7.8	16.2[b] ± 11.7
21[a]	35.8[b] ± 23.8	83.2[b] ± 31.0	130.5[b] ± 70.9	133.5[b] ± 62.0	17.7 ± 3.7	18.9[b] ± 7.1
28	25.5[b] ± 11.8	59.2 ± 28.2	77.7 ± 30.5	71.0 ± 25.0	13.7* ± 10.2	15.2 ± 8.6
42	6.2 ± 5.7	25.3 ± 189.5	37.3 ± 26.9	37.6 ± 28.7	6.1 ± 4.2	7.0 ± 5.1

[a]Last day of cimetidine intake.
[b]$p < 0.05$, tested against value of day 0.

Table 4 Effect of Cimetidine 1600 mg day^{-1} on Absolute (cells nl^{-1}) and Relative (%) Numbers of CD4 and CD8 Lymphocytes and Total Skin Test Reactivity (mm) in Healthy Volunteers (mean ± SD)

Time (days)	CD4		CD8		Ratio CD4/CD8 +	Skin test
	absolute	relative	absolute	relative		
0	860.0 ± 327.3	41.5 ± 8.7	356.7 ± 187.8	17.9 ± 6.2	2.8 ± 2.1	18.4 ± 4.8
7	999.0 ± 457.1	45.1[b] ± 8.9	355.2 ± 205.1	17.1 ± 7.6	3.6 ± 2.8	21.9 ± 7.6
21[a]	1210.3[b] ± 303.0	56.3[b] ± 9.8	393.5 ± 155.5	19.1 ± 5.6	2.9 ± 1.8	17.2 ± 7.3
28	1373.5[b] ± 343.1	46.5[b] ± 9.3	592.6 ± 228.6	20.5 ± 5.8	2.6 ± 1.6	12.7 ± 5.5
42	1053.7 ± 278.1	46.3 ± 8.9	497.3 ± 241.6	20.8 ± 7.9	2.6 ± 4.7	ND[c]

[a]Last day of cimetidine intake.
[b]$p < 0.05$, tested against value of day 0.
[c]ND not done.

1. Therapy with Histamine Type II Antagonists

Therapy with immunomodulating substances generally is associated with the danger of an enhanced viral replication. In the beginning of an infection the HIV-1 virus is predominantly localized in immunocompetent cells carrying the CD4 receptor or similar molecular structures to this receptor (helper T lymphocytes, macrophages, Langerhans cells, or glia cells) (44). The immunomodulation leads to a change in cell activity and blastogenesis so that by an enhanced formation of immune cells there could also be an increased virus replication, as can, for example, be seen in the immunostimulatory effect observed after infections, or the immunomodulation by interleukin-2 (55–58).

We prefer the application of a histamine type II antagonist because we saw comparable results in healthy volunteers, as was previously described by White and Bellow for patients with hypogammaglobulinemia (59). Our evaluations were based on the histamine type II antagonist cimetidine, as all preliminary studies and indeed our own had shown that the major effect of cimetidine was that of a histamine type II antagonism, whereby the CD8-cytotoxic/suppressor cells had a key position (60–62).

Many immunological functions are inhibited by histamine via type II receptors. Owing to the action of histamine, CD8 cells are increased in number and secrete a humoral factor, histamin-induced suppressor factor (HSF) that reduces lymphocyte proliferation and lymphoblast transformation and diminishes the production of lymphokines such as migration inhibitory factor (MIF) and immunoglobulins.

In addition, B cells and leukocytes bear histamine type II receptors of their own and can directly respond to the inhibitory effect of histamine. Cimetidine addition to human lymphocytes in vitro results in decreased numbers and activities of CD8 (cytotoxic/suppressor) cells and augments in vitro mitogen stimulation with phytohaemagglutinin (PHA), pokeweed mitogen (PWM), and concanavalin A (Con A) (63,64).

a. Evaluation in Healthy Volunteers

The administration of 800 mg cimetidine over a period of 7 days leads to a significant decrease in CD8 cells in 12 healthy volunteers, and to a significant increase in the CD4/CD8 ratio from 3.15 to 5.0 and to a simultaneous smaller increase in CD4 cells (Table 1). These changes were reflected in an increase in blastogenesis measured by [^{3}H] thymidine incorporation of lymphocytes by the lymphocyte-transformation test via mitogenic lectins such as PHA, Con A, and PWM by 300% (Table 2).

Furthermore, a twofold increase over baseline of the delayed-type hypersensitivity skin test reaction (Merieux test) could be observed, as measured as a total diameter of skin induration due to the administration of *Trichophyton, Candida*, tetanus, diphtheria, *Streptococcus, proteus*, and tuberculin antigens

Table 5 Effect of Cimetidine 1600 mg day^{-1} on Immunoparameters Before and After Treatment in Healthy Volunteers (mean ± SD)

Parameters	Day 0	Day 21
WBCs (nl^{-1})	6.7 ± 3.1	7.7 ± 3.4
Lymphocytes (%)	31.6 ± 8.3	33.3 ± 11.7
Abs. Lymphocytes (nl^{-1})	2.0 ± 0.8	2.6 ± 0.8
Abs. B Lymphocytes (nl^{-1})	0.26 ± 0.1	0.34* ± 0.1
CD2 (%)	69.5 ± 6.0	77.8[a] ± 6.2
Abs. CD2 (nl^{-1})	1.4 ± 0.6	2.0[a] ± 0.6
CD3 (%)	64.0 ± 5.2	67.0 ± 6.2
Abs. CD3 (nl^{-1})	1.3 ± 0.03	0.28[a] ± 0.08
NK (%)	6.1 ± 3.8	6.9 ± 3.7
Abs. NK (nl^{-1})	0.12 ± 0.06	0.14 ± 0.06
Immunoglobulins (ml^{-1})		
IgG	1.1 ± 0.21	1.3[a] ± 0.25
IgA	0.17 ± 0.04	0.20[a] ± 0.05
IgM	0.13 ± 0.04	0.15 ± 0.05
Complement		
Total (titer)	1:141.5 ± 1:30.5	1:146.8 ± 1:24.3
C3 (mg 100 ml^{-1})	98.6 ± 25.2	118.7[a] ± 16.7
C4 (mg 100 ml^{-1})	19.6 ± 5.5	19.2 ± 5.7

[a]$p < 0.05$, tested against value of day 0.

(see Table 1). These results seemed to support the earlier observations that the effect of cimetidine is mainly achieved by a suppression of CD8 cells (65).

The effect of cimetidine in a reducing number of CD8 cells may be modulating the expression of the T8 antigen or lysis of these cells. We do not know what the mechanism is; however, it seems more reasonable to assume a modulating effect of this drug, since shortly after the end of drug administration CD8 cell numbers reached the starting value. The consequence of a diminished number of CD8 cells may lead to decreased suppressor-cell function. However, this seems unlikely, since a number of recent results question the role of CD8 cells as suppressor cells. Therefore, it can be suggested that the effect of cimetidine on T cells is a relative dominance of T-helper lymphocytes. The relative dominance of CD4 cells may reflect the systemic activation of the immune system.

Indeed, our results support this sytemic immune system activation. At first, Ficoll-Paque purified lymphocytes containing also macrophages and B-

Table 6 Effect of Cimetidine 800 mg day^{-1} on Zn and Mg amounts ($\mu g\ 10^{-6}$ cells) in T Lymphocytes in Healthy Volunteers (mean ± SD)

Time (days)	Zn	Mg
0	7.93 ± 2.41	37.9 ± 8.52
4	8.07 ± 2.46	39.2 ± 9.15
7[a]	11.81[b] ± 2.13	53.4[b] ± 10.40
11	8.46 ± 2.13	41.9 ± 9.91

[a]Last day of cimetidine intake.
[b]$p < 0.05$, tested against value of day 0.

lymphocytes showed an increased proliferation following activation by mitogens. After this short time interval of cimetidine administration, activation of the immune system seems to be limited to T cells, since the Ig production reflecting B-cell activation is unaltered. This result is in contrast to previous observations (66,67).

Subsequently we performed a dose-response study with the healthy volunteers of the previous study. We then administered 1,600 mg of cimetidine for a period of 3 weeks. In this study, there was also an increase in lymphocyte blastogenesis performed with PHA, Con A, and PWM by approximately 300% (Table 3). After 1 week and in a subsequent period, there was even an increase

Table 7 Effect of Cimetidine 1,600 mg day^{-1} on Zn and Mg Amounts ($\mu g\ 10^{6}$ cells) in T Lymphocytes in Healthy Volunteers (mean ± SD)

Time (days)	Zn	Mg
0	8.40 ± 2.86	39.0 ± 10.8
4	6.78 ± 2.43	34.4 ± 6.21
7	9.45 ± 3.90	42.7 ± 11.4
14	10.7 ± 4.47	49.3 ± 7.29
21[a]	13.9[b] ± 5.92	58.5[b] ± 10.1
28	13.0 ± 4.97	43.8 ± 13.2
42	10.1 ± 3.54	41.3 ± 9.95

[a]Last day of cimetidine intake.
[b]$p < 0.05$, tested against value of day 0.

Table 8 Cell Counts and Functions in Two Patients with the Acquired Immunodeficiency Syndrome, Before and After Cimetidine

	B (%)	CD2 (%)	CD3 (%)	CD4 (%)	CD8 (%)	CD4+/CD8+	PHA	Con A	PWM
Patient 1									
before cimetidine	9	14	66	48	21	2.3	Normal	Hyporeactive	Normal
after 1 week	8	18	56	35	10	3.5	Normal	Normal	Normal
Patient 2									
before cimetidine	28	38	30	7	26	0.3	Hyporeactive	Hyporeactive	Hyporeactive
after 1 week	19	50	28	15	17	0.9	Hyporeactive	Hyporeactive	Hyporeactive
after 2 weeks	22	76	32	13	17	0.8	Hyporeactive	Hyporeactive	Hyporeactive

Table 9 Effect of Cimetidine 1,200 mg day^{-1} on Humoral Factors of Immunity in ARC Patients (mean ± SD)

Time (weeks)	B lymphocytes (nl^{-1})	B lymphocytes (%)	IgG ($g\ ml^{-1}$)	IgA ($g\ ml^{-1}$)	C4 ($g\ ml^{-1}$)	β microglobulins (Ml^{-1})
0	239 ± 128	13.9 ± 7.1	1749 ± 490	161 ± 57	15.8 ± 6.2	2.5 ± 0.6
1	295 ± 191	15.2 ± 8.2	1742 ± 474	156 ± 59	17.1 ± 6.4	2.8 ± 1.5
3	285 ± 176	12.5 ± 6.3	1751 ± 595	164 ± 55	17.3 ± 4.5	2.2 ± 0.5
4	262 ± 162	14.1 ± 7.3	1662 ± 375	173 ± 49	16.8 ± 7.5	2.2 ± 0.7
8	275 ± 200	14.5 ± 9.5	1746 ± 426	175 ± 57	15.4 ± 4.1	2.3 ± 0.8
12	367[b] ± 323	16.5 ± 13.8	1849 ± 545	181[b] ± 58	18.1 ± 6.4	2.5 ± 0.7
15[a]	301 ± 189	17.4 ± 8.9	1851 ± 779	166 ± 62	16.2 ± 5.9	2.3 ± 0.5
21	441 ± 262	20.9[b] ± 9.2	2218[b] ± 749	198[b] ± 61	18.8[b] ± 6.1	2.4 ± 0.4

[a]3 weeks after discontinuation of drug intake.
[b]$p < 0.05$.

Table 10 Effect of Cimetidine 1,200 mg day^{-1} on Absolute (cells nl^{-1}) and Relative (%) Numbers of CD4 and CD8 Lymphocytes and Total Skin Test Reactivity (mm) in ARC Patients (mean ± SD)

Time (weeks)	CD4 absolute	CD4 relative	CD8 absolute	CD8 relative	CD4/CD8	Skin test
0	385 ± 143	21.1 ± 8.3	408 ± 416	26.8 ± 10.7	1.04 ± 0.38	9.8 ± 4.8
1	512 ± 242	30.6 ± 7.6	467 ± 265	24.0 ± 8.7	1.48 ± 0.76	ND[d]
2	598[b] ± 236	30.8[c] ± 9.2	512 ± 294	25.9 ± 10.6	1.40[c] ± 0.70	ND
4	603[c] ± 242	32.1[c] ± 7.5	458 ± 208	24.5 ± 7.8	1.47[c] ± 0.69	12.5[c] ± 4.8
8	627[c] ± 283	31.6[c] ± 8.2	498 ± 257	24.9 ± 8.3	1.42[c] ± 0.64	14.5[c] ± 6.4
12	779[c] ± 376	33.0[c] ± 8.7	498 ± 291	24.1 ± 7.6	1.53[c] ± 0.64	14.5[c] ± 6.4
15[a]	511 ± 250	27.0 ± 7.4	495 ± 303	25.4 ± 7.1	1.13 ± 0.37	10.4 ± 3.4
21[b]	693[c] ± 243	33.7[c] ± 6.8	447[c] ± 227	22.3[c] ± 6.7	1.65[c] ± 0.63	15.0[c] ± 4.5

[a]Three weeks after discontinuation of drug intake.
[b]Six weeks after reinstitution of cimetidine treatment.
[c]$p < 0.05$.
[d]ND not done.

in the CD8 cells, most apparent after 1 week of finishing cimetidine administration. On the other hand, a very distinct increase in the CD4 cells could be seen, rising from 860 to 1,210 cells/nl after 3 weeks (Table 4). This effect lasted even for the period when cimetidine had been stopped for over 7 days; there were 1,370 CD4 cells/ml. The CD4/CD8 ratio had not risen significantly from 2.8 to 3.6 after 1 week; thereafter, it remained at baseline levels.

B Lymphocytes also showed a significant increase by 31%, and the concentration of immunoglobulins G and A increased significantly. The complement subgroup C3 likewise changed from 98.6 to 118.7 mg 100 μl^{-1} (Table 5). All these changes, which account for a broad immunomodulation of cimetidine were at baseline levels again after 3 weeks. The measurement of the delayed-type hypersensitivity skin test reaction did not show a significant change during or after cimetidine intake. Therefore it seems, that a different drug concentration accounts for this lack of change in skin test results (68).

According to these results, the effect of cimetidine on the immune system is dose related and probably time related, and may include different types of cells according to their cimetidine responsiveness, and causes a systemic activation of the immune system, especially of the T lymphocytes. Activation of T cells via the T-cell receptor/CD3 complex (TCR) occurs after hydrolysis of membrane-associated phosphatidyinositol-4,5-biphosphate to form the two second messengers 1,4,5-triphosphate (IP_3) and 1,2-diacylglycerol (DG) (69). These two second messengers have different molecular targets within the cell, but they often act synergistically during the evocation of cell responses (70). 1,4,5-Triphosphate increases intracellular concentrations of the divalent cation Ca, liberating this ion from intracellular storage structures. 1,2-Diacylglycerol activates an intracellularly localized enzyme, protein kinase C, which phosphorylates the target proteins and increases the intracellular Ca^{2+} too. There is substantial evidence that a third molecule, inositol-1,3,4,5-tetrahisphosphate, promotes extracellular Ca^{2+} entry and has a synergistic effect with IP_3.

Besides TCR activation through antigen or Con A, transmembrane signaling occurs via the binding of ligands (lymphocyte function antigen [LFA-3], PHA) to the CD2 molecule. Transmembrane signaling via this "alternative" mechanism is mediated through the above-described intracellular pathway. This ubiquitous mechanism of transduction of signals from cell membrane receptors to lymphocyte nuclei triggers numerous physiologic responses, leading to lymphocyte proliferation. To establish the role of two other divalent cations, namely, Mg^{2+} and Zn^{2+}, we estimated the amounts of these ions in lymphocytes during the cimetidine therapy in healthy volunteers.

The effect of cimetidine on intracellular zinc and magnesium levels correlated well with the alterations in the lymphocyte blastogenic response in the two studies on healthy persons. After the first dose regimen (800 mg), the zinc levels

Table 11 Effect of Cimetidine on Blastogenesis in ARC Patients (cpm 10^3, mean ± SD)

Time (weeks)	ConA 2 (μg ml^{-1})	PHA 0.4 (μg ml^{-1})	PWM 0.4 (μg ml^{-1})
0	1.43 ± 0.61	1.53 ± 0.56	1.43 ± 0.61
1	1.54 ± 0.59	1.63 ± 0.65	1.63 ± 0.58
2	1.64 ± 0.56	1.76 ± 0.59	1.88[c] ± 0.52
4	1.67 ± 0.54	1.83 ± 0.37	1.74 ± 0.51
8	1.88[c] ± 0.43	1.84 ± 0.47	1.80[c] ± 0.50
12	1.78[c] ± 0.41	1.94[c] ± 0.40	1.78[c] ± 0.41
15[a]	1.17 ± 0.39	1.64 ± 0.49	1.47 ± 0.51
21[b]	1.56 ± 0.51	1.75 ± 0.44	1.68 ± 0.47

[a]Three weeks after discontinuation of drug intake.
[b]Six weeks after reinstitution of cimetidine treatment.
[c]$p < 0.05$, tested against value of week 0.

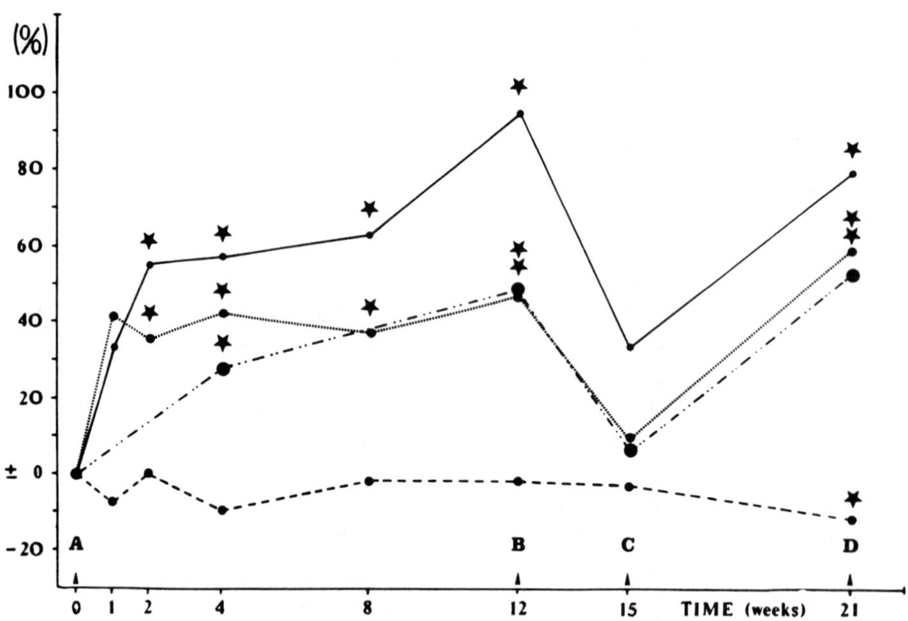

Figure 1 Relative change of cell mediated immunity during cimetidine intake. A = start of cimetidine therapy; B = therapy interruption; C = 3 weeks after therapy discontinuation; D = 6 weeks after reinstitution of cimetidine treatment; ——● = CD4 cells; – – – ● = CD8 cells; ---------● = CD4/CD8 ratio; – ·· – ·· – ● = delayed hypersensitivity skin test; significant *$p < 0.05$ correlation between CD4 and skin test ($r = 0.86$).

Table 12 Effect of Cimetidine on Clinical Data on AIDS and ARC Patients

		AIDS			ARC		
	Category	before		after	before		after
Performance status	I						5.8
	II	9.1		72.4	85.8		94.2
	III	36.3		27.6	14.2		
	IV	54.6					
	p<		0.05			0.05	
Body weight	I			18.2			
	II	12.5		81.8	59.0		100.0
	III	62.5			41.0		
	IV	25.0					
	p<		0.005			0.01	
Body temp.	I			23.2	47.1		94.1
	II	27.2		46.4	40.0		5.9
	III	9.1		30.4	12.9		
	IV	63.6					
	p<		0.02			0.005	
Infection	I						
	II			81.3	61.5		84.6
	III	50.0		18.7	38.5		15.4
	IV	50.0					
	p<		0.01			NS	
Lymphadenopathy	I	18.1		18.1			
	II			36.4			47.1
	III	72.7		36.4	91.2		41.1
	IV	9.1		9.1	8.8		5.8
	p<		NS			0.05	
Night	NO	18.2		72.4	26.5		100.0
	YES	81.8		27.6	73.5		
	p<		0.02			0.02	
Diarrhea	NO	36.3		63.7	20.5		100.0
	YES	63.7		36.3	79.5		
	p<		NS			0.01	

rose by 52% and the magnesium levels by 41% (Table 6). Following the second regimen (1,600 mg), there was an increase of 65% (Table 7) in zinc levels and 16% in magnesium levels after 3 weeks. In the first case, both parameters returned to baseline levels after 3 days, and in the second case after 3 weeks (71).

The central effect of zinc and magnesium on the function of the immune system has been shown in many studies. Most of them observed an impaired immune reaction in zinc and magnesium deprived patients or animals (72-77). For calcium, another dipolar cation, a higher lymphocyte concentration was observed when the lymphocytes were stimulated by mitogens or antigens. The three bivalent cations had a synergistic effect on protein and DNA synthesis in stimulated lymphocytes, blastogenic response, B cells, and immunoglobulin levels.

The variable results obtained by delayed hypersensitivity skin testing that was found in the different dose regimen studies could be explained by the effect of zinc and magnesium on mast cell membranes, which prevent induced histamine release from mast cells. Therefore it is likely that, besides the effect of Ca^{2+} on T-lymphocyte proliferation, the divalent cations Mg^{2+} and Zn^{2+} may also promote the activation and proliferation of these lymphocytes.

b. *Effect of Cimetidine on HIV-1-Infected Patients*

The immunomodulatory potency of cimetidine was investigated in 33 ARC and 11 AIDS patients in whom detailed immunological and clinical evaluations were carried out. All 44 patients entered into this trial were strongly reactive for HIV-1 antibodies. The patient population consisted of 36 males ranging in age from 18 to 54, and eight females from 18 to 24 years, all of them in the ARC group. The evaluation included a complete history, physical examination, detailed lifestyle questionnaire, and standard medical as well as extensive immunological tests. In this study, we administered cimetidine orally in daily doses of 1,200 mg, for a period of 5 months with an interruption of therapy after the first three months for an interval of 3 weeks. Cimetidine was well tolerated by all patients.

c. *Effect on Clinical and Immunological Parameters in AIDS Patients*

In a preliminary observation in an ARC and AIDS patients, we found a marked regression of CD8 cells after 1 and 2 weeks, respectively (Table 8). We administered cimetidine 1200 mg per day (78). In the expanded study, cimetidine administration resulted in a marked enhancement of immune function: B cells increased by 54%; comparable alterations were seen in serum IgA and IgG concentrations and complement C4 activity (Table 9). At the beginning of the study, the number of peripheral CD8 cells showed a small reduction. Six weeks

Table 13 Effect of Cimetidine 1,200 $\mu g\ day^{-1}$ in AIDS Patients (mean ± SD)

Time (weeks)	0	12	15[a]	21[b]
Abs. B Lymphocytes (μl^{-1})	208 ± 196	325 ± 196	167 ± 89	468[c] ± 282
B Lymphocytes (%)	15.7 ± 7.7	16.4 ± 11.9	14.3 ± 10.7	22.3 ± 10.4
Abs. NK (μl^{-1})	302 ± 214	263 ± 182	186[c] ± 108	417 ± 251
NK (%)	20.5 ± 9.7	15.6 ± 4.4	11.4[c] ± 4.7	23.3 ± 7.1
IgG ($g \times ml^{-1}$)	1513 ± 704	2115[c] ± 980	1689 ± 848	2357[c] ± 978
β_2 ($g \times ml^{-1}$)	3.0 ± 1.3	3.9 ± 1.6	4.0 ± 0.5	4.7 ± 0.4
Abs. CD4 (μl^{-1})	289 ± 155	433 ± 358	222[c] ± 167	327 ± 267
CD4 (%)	14.8 ± 9.7	20.4 ± 13.4	11.6[c] ± 7.8	14.8 ± 7.1
Abs. CD8 (μl^{-1})	581 ± 404	520 ± 439	550 ± 426	478 ± 315
CD8 (%)	36.1 ± 9.7	30.7 ± 14.0	34.0 ± 15.9	29.8 ± 10.3
CD4/CD8	0.4 ± 0.3	0.7 ± 0.5	0.4 ± 0.3	0.5 ± 0.3
Skin test (mm)	0.0 ± 0.0	4.3 ± 2.9	0.6 ± 1.3	3.5 ± 0.7

[a]Three weeks after discontinuation of drug intake.
[b]Six weeks after reinstitution of cimetidine treatment.
[c]$p < 0.05$, tested against value of week 0.

Table 14 Effect of Cimetidine 1,200 mg day^{-1} on Absolute (cells nl^{-1}) and Relative (%) Numbers of CD4 and CD8 Lymphocytes and Total Skin Test Reactivity (mm) in ARC Patients

Time (months)	CD4		CD8		
	absolute	relative	absolute	relative	CD4/CD8
0	264 ± 97	19.1 ± 6.3	463 ± 128	25.1 ± 8.2	0.74 ± 0.31
3	738[a] ± 186	32.7[a] ± 11.4	431 ± 197	24.8 ± 6.5	1.29[a] ± 0.43
12	468 ± 119	28.7[a] ± 8.5	367* ± 105	21.1 ± 7.2	1.31[a] ± 0.38
24	411 ± 89	26.4[a] ± 7.2	309[a] ± 99	20.5 ± 7.8	1.26[a] ± 0.35
36	402 ± 106	26.2[a] ± 7.9	341[a] ± 116	21.8 ± 7.6	1.23[a] ± 0.42

[a]$p < 0.05$, tested against value of month 0.

Table 15 Effect of Cimetidine 1,200 mg day^{-1} on Blastogenesis in ARC Patients (cpm 10^3; mean ± SD)

Time (weeks)	ConA 2 (μg ml^{-1})	PHA 0.4 (μg ml^{-1})	PWM 0.4 (μg ml^{-1})
0	68.4 ± 21.3	76.3 ± 25.6	31.6 ± 8.8
3	131.2[a] ± 42.7	138.2[a] ± 39.4	78.1[a] ± 18.9
12	126.9[a] ± 38.5	121.6[a] ± 37.8	65.3[a] ± 14.7
24	101.3[a] ± 48.6	124.1[a] ± 43.2	58.2[a] ± 13.9
36	114.3[a] ± 42.0	114.3[a] ± 31.5	50.9 ± 12.1

[a]$p < 0.05$, tested against value of week 0.

after reinstitution of cimetidine, the cells were significantly diminished. The number of CD4 cells reached an elevated level after 2 weeks of oral cimetidine intake, whereas lower values were recorded when the patient did not receive the histamine type II antagonist. The alterations in CD4/CD8 ratio paralleled those of the CD4 cells (Table 10). Also, the lymphocyte blastogenic response measured as [^{3}H] thymidine incorporation after PHA, Con A, PWM exposure and the delayed-type hypersensitivity skin reaction were significantly enhanced (Table 11). Furthermore, a positive correlation was found between CD4 cell numbers and the results of delayed hypersensitivity skin testing ($r = 0.86$; $p < 0.01$) (Fig. 1) and between CD4 cell count and the in vitro blastogenic response to mitogen stimulation (Con A, $r = 0.80$; PHA, $r = 0.84$; PWM, $r = 0.82$).

Clinical parameters of the ARC patients are presented in Table 12, the number of patients being classified in each category given as percentage values. All patients showed an improvement regarding their clinical data. Performance status ($p < 0.05$), body weight ($p < 0.01$), and fever ($p < 0.05$) were incluenced favorably. The frequency of diarrhea and the lymph node size were also diminished significantly. In this study, ARC patients showed a significant improvement of their clinical status after cimetidine administration. The amelioration of clinical parameters correlated well with the enhancement of delayed hypersensitivity skin reaction to seven recall antigens and the mitogen-stimulation response to PHA, PWM, and Con A. Peripheral B-lymphocyte counts, immunoglobulin concentrations, and complement concentrations were also increased compared to pretreatment values. Similar results were obtained concerning the ratio of CD4/CD8 cells. It appears that the improvement of clinical status in ARC patients by cimetidine depends on an effect on the immune system. Unexpectedly, a reduction in absolute and relative numbers of CD8 cells were only found after 6 weeks of reinstitution of cimetidine after an intervention of therapy of 3 weeks.

Table 16 Effect of Ranitidine 600 mg day^{-1} in ARC Patients

Time (weeks)	CD4		CD8		CD4/CD8
	absolute	relative	absolute	relative	
0	321 ± 109	17.1 ± 7.1	543 ± 198	29.5 ± 13.2	0.58 ± 0.32
4	236 ± 117	17.9 ± 7.4	496 ± 171	26.2 ± 9.8	0.64 ± 0.41
8	302 ± 95	16.5 ± 6.8	464 ± 189	28.3 ± 11.1	0.58 ± 0.37
12	286 ± 91	16.6 ± 6.2	508 ± 117	28.9 ± 12.4	0.56 ± 0.29

Table 17 Effect of Ranitidine 600 mg day^{-1} on Blastogenesis on ARC Patients (cpm 10^3; mean ± SD)

Time (weeks)	ConA 2 (μg ml^{-1})	PHA 0.4 (μg ml^{-1})	PWM 0.4 (μg ml^{-1})
0	83.3 ± 29.7	87.4 ± 26.3	26.2 ± 7.9
4	72.5 ± 21.8	79.6 ± 25.9	24.0 ± 6.1
8	91.7 ± 31.1	75.6 ± 23.0	32.4 ± 9.4
12	98.2 ± 29.6	81.2 ± 29.9	29.5 ± 8.6

In AIDS patients, small effects on the immune system due to cimetidine were observed. The CD8 cell counts showed a small but significant decrease and the CD4 cell counts showed an insignificant enhancement, but 3 weeks after therapy discontinuation there was a significant decrease in the numbers. The delayed-type hypersensitivity skin test reaction showed an enhanced response after 12 weeks (Table 13). The clinical data such as performance status, body weight, and fever were favorably influenced in these patients. In this study, the clinical data of AIDS patients showed a greater response than the immunological parameters (see Table 12) (80). In AIDS patients, all cells and functions of the immune system were disturbed, so it is possible that measurable effects on this impaired system are more difficult to evaluate than on a less deficient immune system. On the other hand, these studies are not double-blinded and considering the difficult emotional situation of AIDS and also ARC patients, a specific pharmacodynamic effect of therapy cannot be well separated from psychological influences.

d. Follow-up Observation

Eight ARC patients from the first study took cimetidine 1,200 mg/day^{-1} without interruption for a period of 36 months. Some of the 25 patients who did not take cimetidine over this period were heroin addicts, who interrupted therapy for this reason; others did not want therapy at all; and the main group were patients who had an additional Zidovudine (Retrovir®) therapy the previous year.

The eight patients who received cimetidine for 3 years did not want additional therapy, which included Zidovudine. The results of this group surely have to be interpreted cautiously, as it is a self-selected group.

There was no differences between the Zidovudine and cimetidine groups in terms of clinical staging; they were all in class WR III-V. In this group, a slightly positive, although not statistically significant enhancement, in levels of CD4 cells could be seen. During a period of 24 months over this time the CD8 cells showed a significant decrease and the CD4/CD8 ratio was increased over the whole observation period of 36 months (Table 14). The effect on the CD4/

Table 18 Immunologic Reaction Pattern of Two Different Histamine Type II Antagonists

	Cimetidine				Ranitidine
	Healthy volunteers		ARC	AIDS	
Immunologic parameter	800 mg 7 days	1,600 3 weeks	1,200 mg 21 weeks with 3 weeks of discontinuation of therapy		ARC 600 mg 12 weeks
Cell number					
CD8	<	=	<	=	=
CD4	=	>	>	=	=
CD4/CD8	>	=	>	=	=
B	-	>	>	>	=
B-cell function					
IgG	=	>	>	>	=
IgA	=	>	>	=	=
IgM	=	=	=	=	=
T-cell function					
PHA	>	>	>	=	=
Con A	>	>	>	=	=
PWM	>	>	>	=	=
Skin test	>	=	>	>	=

$>$ significantly ($p < 0.05$) increased
$<$ significantly decreased
= no significant alteration
\- unmeasured

CD8 ratio is on the one hand due to an increase in CD4 cells and on the other hand to the decrease in levels of CD8 cells. The effect on the blastogenic response was also clearly visible by increased lymphocyte proliferation with PHA, Con A, and PWM (Table 15). At the present time, it is known that 10% of the patients currently in state WR3-WR4 will progress to the fullblown AIDS in 3 years, these results obtained by the eight patients can be interpreted in a positive way. Here as in other studies, administration of low-dose cimetidine resulted in a reduction in levels of CD8 cells.

e. *Effect of Ranitidine on Immune Function in ARC Patients*

To evaluate the effect of ranitidine, another histamine type II antagonist, on the immune system of patients, 600 mg of ranitidine was given to six patients in stages WR3 and WR4 over a period of 3 months. The clinical and immunological status of the patients was measured according to the previous studies. For the immunological parameters, no significant changes in CD4 or CD8 cells pointing to an effect of the drug were seen (Table 16). Likewise, the CD4/CD8 ratio did not change. In addition, the blastogenic response measured as $[^3H]$ thymidine incorporation after stimulation with mitogens PHA, Con A, and PWM did not show any alteration (Table 17). No effect on the humoral factors of immunity were observed either. No effect was seen on the clinical status of the 6 patients.

In order to assess the effect of a drug on HIV-1 infection, a longer treatment period than 3 months and a larger number of patients than six would be needed. However, we decided (keeping in mind the efficacy of cimetidine) to interrupt this study.

Some studies have reported a positive in vitro effect of ranitidine on immunocompetent cells. Based on the inhibition of histamine-related human culture lymphoblast (HCL) production in the stomach, ranitidine has two- to threefold more potency on a molar basis than cimetidine. For this reason we chose a dose of 600 mg day^{-1}. There is however the possibility that the lack of response observed can be explained by an incorrect choice of dosage.

f. *Combined Therapy of Zidovudine and Cimetidine*

The preliminary results of a 1 year treatment in 50 HIV-1-infected patients in stages WR3 to WR5 in which 25 received Zidovudine only and 25 zidovudine combined with cimetidine, 1,200 mg, showed a clear-cut increase in levels of CD4 cells after 8-12 weeks of zidovudine therapy alone. The CD4 levels decreased their baseline value on zidovudine therapy alone but could be stabilized with combined therapy. Also, the positive effect on clinical status with combined therapy seems to be greater than on zidovudine treatment alone. An increase in side effects was not seen in patients receiving combined therapy. According to the now completed data, the histamine type II antagonist cimetidine seems to be an appropriate drug for the combined therapy with the antiviral agent zidovudine.

VIII. CONCLUSIONS

In summary, we would confirm that cimetidine is an immunomodulating agent with different effects depending on the dosage and duration of treatment chosen, but with the same efficacy in healthy and HIV-1-infected individuals

(Table 18). Whereas the lower dose decreases the number of CD8 cells, higher doses also influence the number of CD4 cells and B-function. In all regimens, changes in cell numbers are correlated with increased mitogen-induced activation and proliferation of T lymphocytes. Therefore, a theoretical concern is if activation causes increased proliferation of HIV-1 viruses in infected individuals as well. At the present time, we cannot answer this question directly, but in our experience, especially based on the results of 3-year follow-up of eight infected patients, increased virus replication seems unlikely, since no patient experienced a progression of the AIDS status. Since the overall immunomodulating capacity of cimetidine seems favorable for the clinical situation of HIV-1-infected individuals, further trials should resolve this unanswered question.

Presently, if combined therapy of cimetidine with a virostatic agent is administered, the danger of an increased virus replication by cimetidine can be neglected. In view of our concern about increased viral replication, we give 900 mg Zidovudine day^{-1} over a period of 8 weeks and then start the combined therapy. Cimetidine is a useful therapy in combination with Zidovudine. In our experience cimetidine is well tolerated and should be administered in combination with an HIV-1 antiviral agent so that a causal therapy combined with an immunodulating therapy would result.

I thank Ernst Krenzfelder for helpful comments and review.

REFERENCES

1. MMWR, 30:250–2 (1981).
2. Gottlieb, M. S., R. Schroff, H. M. Schanker, J. D. Weisman, P. T. Fan, R. A. Wolf, and A. Saxon, N. Engl. J. Med. 305:1425–1431 (1981).
3. Siegal, F. P., C. Lopez, G. S. Hammer, A. E. Brown, S. J. Kornfeld, J. Gold, J. Hassett, S. Z. Hirschman, S. Cunningham-Rundles, and D. Armstrong, N. Engl. J. Med. 305:1439–1444 (1981).
4. Barre-Sinoussi, F., J. C. Chermann, F. Rey, M. T. Nugeyre, S. Chamaret, J. Gruest, C. Dauguet, C. Axler-Blin, F. Vezinet-Brun, C. Rouzioux, W. Rozenbaum, and L. Montagnier, Science 20:220(4599):868–871 (1983).
5. Popovic, M., N. Flomenberg, D. J. Volkman, D. Mann, A. S. Fauci, B. Dupont, and R. C. Gallo, Science 226:459–462 (1984).
6. Klatzman, K., E. Champagne, S. Chamaret et al., Nature 312:763–767 (1984).
7. Gartner, S., P. Markovitz, D. M. Markovitz, M. H. Kaplan, R. C. Gallo, and M. Popovic, Science 233:215–219 (1986).
8. Müller, F., M. Gromm, and K.-H. Müller, Immun. Infekt. 16:(4/88).
9. Clumeck, N., J. Sonnet, H. Taelman, et al. N. Engl. J. Med. 310:492–497 (1984).
10. Clumeck, N., M. Robert-Guroff, van de Perre, et al., J.A.M.A. 254:2599–2602 (1985).

11. Piot, P., H. Taelman, and K. B. Minlangu, Lancet 2:65–69 (1984).
12. Masur, H., M. A. Michelis, J. B. Green et al., N. Engl. J. Med. 305:1431–1438 (1981).
13. Weekly Epidemiological Record 60:85–92 (1985).
14. Leads from the MMWR J.A.M.A. 256:20–25 (1986).
15. Mann, M., and J. Chin, AIDS: A Global Perspective, N. Engl. J. Med. 4(5): 319 (1988).
16. MMWR 35:334–339 (1986).
17. Redfield, R. R., D. C. Wright, and E. C. Tramont, N. Engl. J. Med. 9:131–132 (1986).
18. Stites, D. P., J. D. Stobo, H. H. Fudenberg and J. V. Wells, Basic and clinical immunology, Lange, Los Altos, California (1987), p. 6.
19. Gallo, R. C., M. Robert-Guroff, and F. Wong-Staal, et al., Int. Arch. Allergy Appl. Immunol. 82:471–475 (1987).
20. Yarchoan, R., R. Redfield, and S. Broder, J. Clin. Invest. 78:439–447 (1986).
21. Gartner, S., P. Markovits, D. M. Markovits et al., Science 233:215–219 (1986).
22. Rocklin, R. E., J. Clin. Invest. 57:1051–1058 (1976).
23. Shearer, G. M., K. L. Melmon, Y. Weinstein, and M. Sela, J. Exp. Med. 136: 1302–1307 (1972).
24. Cheson, B. D., A. M. Levine, and D. Mildval, J.A.M.A. 258:(10)1347–1351 (1987).
25. Rouvroy, D., J. Bogaerts, J.-B. Habyarimana, et al., Lancet 1:878–879 (1985).
26. Sandström, E. G., and J. C. Kaplan, Drugs 34:372–290 (1987).
27. HPA-23 Cooperative Study Group. Proceedings of The Third International Conference on AIDS, Washington, D.C., June 1–5 (1987), p. 99.
28. Vittecocq, D., J. Modai, R. Woerle, et al., Proceedings of the Interscience Conference on Antimicrobial Agents and Chemotherapy, October 4–7 (1987), p. 162.
29. Centers for Disease Control AIDS Weekly, November 9 (1987), p. 9.
30. Clumeck, N., and P. Hermans, Am. J. Med. 85(Suppl. 2A)165–172 (1988).
31. Palmisano, L., T. Chisesi, M. Galli, et al., Clin. Immunol. Immunopathol. 47:253–261 (1988).
32. McDougal, J. S., M. S. Kennedy, and J. M. Sligh, Science 231:382–385 (1986).
33. Mitsuya, H., K. Weinhold, P. Furmen et al., Proc. Natl. Acad. Sci. U.S.A. 82:7096–7100 (1985).
34. Mitsuya, H., M. Matsukura, S. Matsurshita, et al., J. Cell. Biochem. 10A (Suppl.):D21 (1986).
35. Mitsuya, H., M. Popovic, R. Yarchoan, et al., Science 226:172–174 (1984).
36. Sunquist, B., and B. Oberg, J. Gen. Virol. 45:273–281 (1979).
37. Chermann, J. C., F. Sinoussi, and C. Jasmin, Biochem. Biophys. Res. Commun. 65:1229–1236 (1975).

38. Anand, R., J. Moore, P. Feorino, et al., Lancet 1:97 (1986).
39. Goswami, D. B., E. Borek, and O. Sharma, Biochem. Biophys. Res. Commun. 89:830–831 (1979).
40. Hagler, D., and P, Frame, Lancet 2:1392 (1986).
41. Richman, D., M. Fischi, and M. Grieco, N. Engl. J. Med. 317:192–197 (1987).
42. Mitsuya, H., F. Jarrett, M. Matsukura, et al., Proc. Natl. Acad. Sci. U.S.A. 84:2033–2037 (1987).
43. Levine, A., P. Gill, L. Cohen, et al., Ann. Intern. Med. 105:32 (1986).
44. Sunquist, B., and E. Larner, J. Virol. 30:847–851 (1979).
45. Burger, H., B. Weiser, and F. Ness, Proceedings on the Third International Conference on AIDS, Washington, D.C., June 1–5 (1987), p. 202.
46. McCormick, J., S. Mitchell, and J. Gretchell, Lancet 1:1367–1369 (1984).
47. Friedland, G. H., S. H. Landesman, C. S. Crumpacker, et al., Proceedings of the Third International Conference on AIDS, Washington, D.C., June 1–5 (1987), p. 48.
48. Miles, S. A., E. Cortes, S. G. Marcus, et al., Proceedings of the Third International Conference on AIDS, Washington, D.C., June 1–5 (1987), p. 227.
49. Brockmeyer, N. H., L. Mertins, C. Daecke, and M. Goos, J. Invest. Dermatol. 92:776 (1989).
50. Gelman, E. P., O. Preble, R. Steis, et al., Clin. Res. 32:415–417 (1984).
51. Krown, S. E., F. X. Real, and S. Vadhan-Raj, Cancer 8 57(Suppl.):1662–1664 (1986).
52. Hutchinson, V., and J. M. Cummins, Lancet 2:1530–1531 (1987).
53. Wong, G. H. W., J. Krowka, D. P. Stites, and D. V. Goeddel, Proceedings of the Third International Conference on AIDS, Washington, D.C., June 1–5 (1987), p. 54.
54. Tsang, P., S. Yoshitatsu, and G. Bekesi, Clin. Immunol. Immunopathol. 45: 166–176 (1987).
55. Centers for Disease Control AIDS Weekly May 11 (1987), p. 16.
56. Centers for Disease Control AIDS Weekly November 9 (1987), p. 14.
57. Reuben, R., C. Gschwind, and E. M. Hersh, Proceedings of the Third International Conference on AIDS, Washington, D.C., June 1–5 (1987), p. 132.
58. Reuben, J., A. Rios, G. Brewton, et al., Proceedings of the Third International Conference on AIDS, Washington, D.C., June 1–5 (1987), p. 186.
59. White, W. B., and M. Ballow, N. Engl. J. Med. 312:198–202 (1985).
60. Rocklin, R. E., J. Immunol. 118:1734–1738 (1977).
61. Rocklin, R. E., and D. K. Greineder, Cell. Immunol. 44:404–415 (1979).
62. Rocklin, R. E., and Haberek-Davidson, J. Clin. Immunol. 1:73–79 (1981).
63. Jorizzo, J. L., M. W. Sams, B. V. Jegasothy, et al., Ann. Intern. Med. 92: 192–195 (1980).
64. Gifford, R. R. M., S. M. Hatfield, and J. R. Schmidtke, Transplantation 29: 143–148 (1980).

65. Brockmeyer, N. H., E. Kreuzfelder, C. H. Bluhm, et al., Br. J. Clin. Pharmacol. 21:567P (1986).
66. McGregor, C. G. A., A. J. Cochran, and L. J. Ogg, Lancet 122–123 (1977).
67. Raptopoulou, M. Gigi, P. Boura, N. Valcanos, and G. Goulis, Immunopharmacology 6:173–183 (1984).
68. Brockmeyer, N. H., E. Kreuzfelder, N. Chalabi, et al., The effect of cimetidine on immune parameters in healthy volunteers. In Proceedings of the Third World Conference on Clinical Pharmacology & Therapeutics, Stockholm, Sweden, July 26–August 1 (1986).
69. Isakov, N., and A. Altman, Immunol. Today 7:155–157 (1986).
70. Michell, B., Nature 324:613 (1986).
71. Brockmeyer, N. H., E. Kreuzfelder, N. Scheiermann, et al., Arbeitsgemeinschaft Dermatologische Forschung, Jahrestagung, Freiburg, Federal Republic of Germany (1986), p. 14.
72. Flynn, A., and B. R. Yen, J. Nutr. 111:907–913 (1981).
73. Prasad, A., Dermatology Immunology and Allergology, Julius Stone (1985), pp. 759–765.
74. Daeschner, C., Scand. J. Haematol. 35:186–190 (1985).
75. Allen, J. I., E. Neil, and E. Kay, Ann. Intern. Med. 95:154–157 (1981).
76. Elin, R., Proc. Soc. Exp. Biol. Med. 148:620–624 (1975).
77. McCoy, J. H., and M. A. Kenney, J. Nutr. 105:791–797 (1975).
78. Brockmeyer, N. H., E. E. Ohnhaus, E. Kreuzfelder, and E. Kuwert, Letter to the Editor, N. Engl. J. Med. 313:265–266 (1985).
79. Brockmeyer, N. H., E. Kreuzfelder, L. Mertins, et al., Clin. Immunol. Immunopathol. 48:50–60 (1988).
80. Brockmeyer, N. H., E. Kreuzfelder, W. Kirch, et al., Klin. Wochenschrift 64(Suppl. 5):106 (1986).

15

Immunomodulatory Effects of H_2-Receptor Antagonists in Transplantation and Malignancy

FRANCESCA T. AWEEKA, JOHN G. GAMBERTOGLIO, and MARVIN R. GAROVOY *University of California, San Francisco, California*

I. INTRODUCTION

Histamine type II (H_2) antagonists, such as cimetidine and ranitidine, are used in the treatment of peptic ulcer disease and for prophylaxis of a variety of gastrointestinal disorders. They account for a large percentage of the current prescription drug market. These agents compete with histamine for type II receptors, preventing stimulation of gastric acid secretion (1). Recently, studies have indicated that histamine type II antagonists have immunostimulatory properties. As early as 1978, anecdotal case reports suggested that renal transplant recipients treated with histamine type II antagonists have an increased incidence of acute allograft rejection (2,3). In addition, recent reports have suggested that these agents may provide some beneficial therapeutic effect in patients with immunosuppressive disorders such as patients with cancer (4-6).

The histamine type II antagonists are thought to oppose the immunosuppressive effects of histamine by competitive binding to type II receptors (7-12). As originally proposed by Beer and Rocklin, histamine interacts with histamine type II receptor-bearing lymphocytes leading to activation of suppressor T cells. Histamine type II antagonists block this activation, causing an immunostimu-

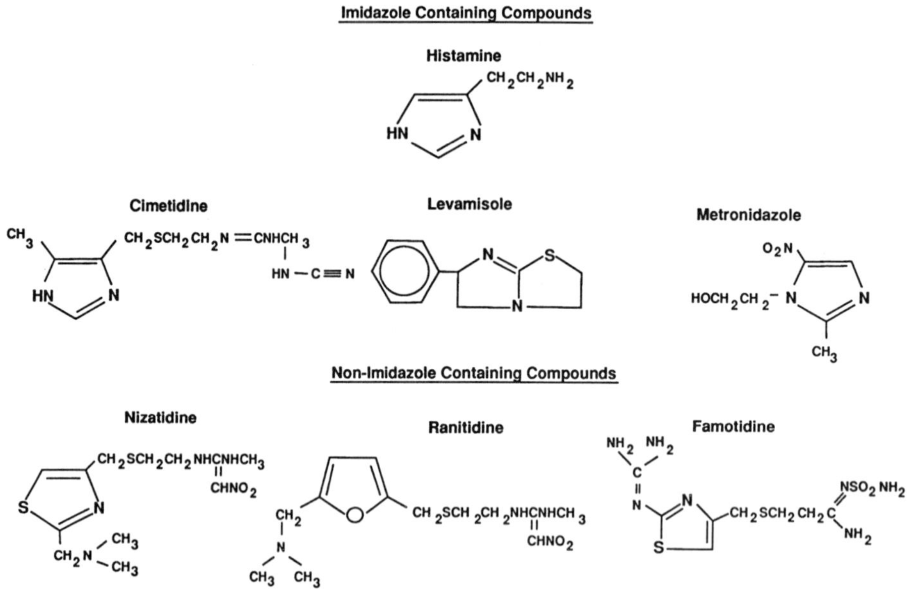

Figure 1 Chemical structures of histamine, histamine type II antagonists, and other similar immunomodulatory agents.

latory effect. Regarding structure-activity relationships, cimetidine is chemically similar to histamine in having an imidazole ring. However, ranitidine does not contain this ring. Levamisole, an antihelminthic agent with immunostimulatory effects, used in the treatment of pemphigus, contains an imidazole ring, though its effects on the immune system may be due to mechanisms other than histamine receptor antagonism (13–14). Thus, it remains unclear what role the imidazole ring plays in altering the immune response (Fig. 1).

II. ROLE OF HISTAMINE AND TYPE II ANTAGONISTS IN REGULATING SUPPRESSOR-CELL ACTIVITY AND THE IMMUNE RESPONSE

The immune system is highly complex and regulated by various cells, lymphokines, and cytokines. A number of cells such as T-helper cells can upregulate the immune system and play a central role in maintaining homeostasis. The macrophage stimulates the antigen-specific helper T cell by direct cell-to-cell contact, leading these cells to produce lymphokines such as interleukin-2 (IL-2) and interleukin-4 (IL-4) (15). Interleukin-2 is a major regulatory protein of the immune system and augments T and B cell activity, whereas IL-4 is an important component responsible for B-cell activation and immunoglobulin production.

Alternatively, there are a number of cells responsible for suppressing certain immunologic processes. Suppressor T lymphocytes play a regulatory role by inhibiting the growth and function of helper T lymphocytes through down regulation or negative feedback (16). The functions of suppressor T cells include suppressed proliferation of helper T cells, decreased stimulation of cytotoxic T cells, and suppressed antibody production from B cells. Suppressor T cells can be activated by various stimuli and involve other cells of the immune system such as monocytes, inducer T lymphocytes, and precursors of T-suppressor cells. Histamine is now believed to play an essential regulatory role in cellular immune reactions by acting as a positive signal for activation of the suppressor-cell network (7). Activation of these cells would therefore lead to immunosuppressive effects.

The mechanism underlying the interaction between histamine and the suppressor-cell network has been studied extensively by Rocklin and associates (7-12,17-20). Research from the 1970s revealed that a nondialyzable, soluble mediator, termed histamine-induced suppressor factor (HSF), was released into culture supernatant of guinea pig lymph node cells when these cells were incubated with histamine of concentrations of $10^{-5}-10^{-3}$ M(8). This factor when co-cultured with sensitized lymphocytes was shown to have an antiproliferative effect leading to suppression of various components of the immune system. When cells bearing histamine receptors were removed from culture, lymphocyte response to histamine was diminished (9). In addition, these studies showed that the antiproliferative effect seen in the presence of histamine was blocked by the type II receptor antagonist burimamide, but not by the type I antagonist chlorpheniramine. Furthermore, the release of HSF was stimulated in the presence of a histamine type II agonist (4-methyl histamine) and not a type I agonist (2-methyl histamine) when lymphocytes were incubated with both agents at low concentrations (10^{-5} M) (10).

Subsequent studies demonstrated that human suppressor T lymphocytes were responsible for HSF synthesis when incubated with varying concentrations of histamine (10^{-9}-10^{-4} M) (11,12). These cells expressed histamine type II receptors and were found within the CD8-positive population (17). In addition, studies have shown that the monocyte is necessary for proper activation and expression of suppressor cells by histamine. In vitro cultures of T lymphocytes containing less than 2% monocytes were unable to be activated by histamine to express suppressor activity (18,19). Furthermore, it has been shown that prostaglandins play a role in suppressor T cell activation, since the addition of indomethacin (a prostaglandin inhibitor) can block this histamine-induced suppression (18,20) (Fig. 2).

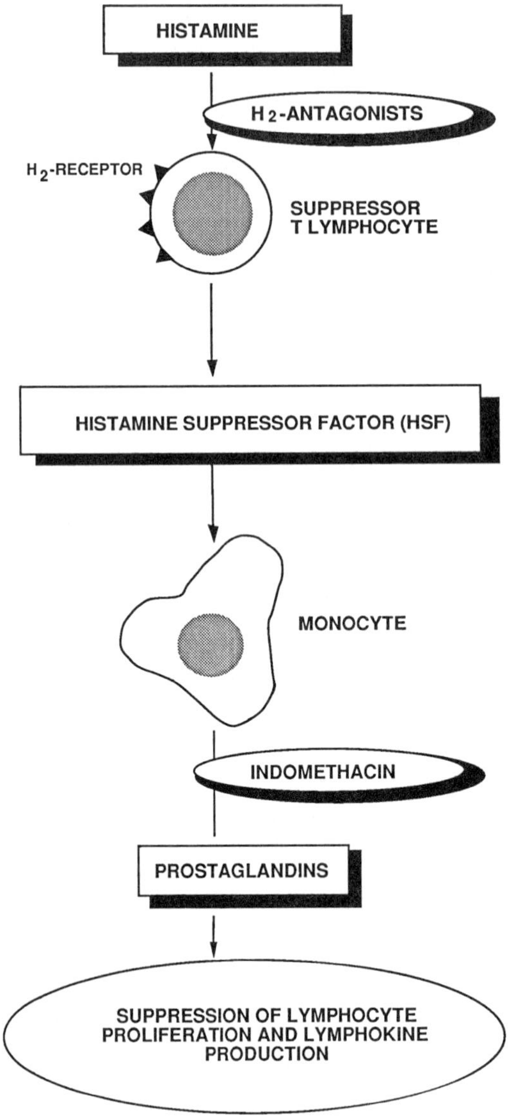

Figure 2 Proposed model of Rocklin et al (7) illustrating the interaction between T lymphocytes and monocytes. Histamine activates suppressor T lymphocytes to produce histamine-induced suppressor factor (HSF), which in turn stimulates monocytes to produce prostaglandins. Histamine type II antagonists are believed to block the effects of histamine by competitive binding to type II receptors.

Based on our understanding of how histamine interacts with type II receptor-bearing lymphocytes, further studies have been undertaken to better define how type II antagonists counteract the immunosuppressive effects of histamine.

III. IN VITRO STUDIES

A number of in vitro studies have been carried out to determine the effect of histamine type II antagonists on various immunologic parameters. Utilizing different in vitro models, histamine type II antagonists are capable of augmenting various elements of the immune response such as human lymphocyte blastogenesis, cell-mediated cytotoxicity, tumor formation and IL-2 production (Table 1). This may lead to an immune restorative effect in patients suffering from cancer, whereas on the other hand be detrimental for patients undergoing organ transplantation, since these patients require immunosuppressive therapy.

A. Human Lymphocyte Blastogenesis

Human lymphocyte blastogenesis, an in vitro technique commonly used to assess cellular immunity, measures the functional capability of T and B lymphocytes to proliferate following mitogenic or antigenic challenge. This test can be used to measure the immunocompetence of various patient populations such as renal transplant recipients and patients with immunodeficiency disorders (21). In addition, this test has been used to study the immunostimulatory properties of the histamine type II antagonists (22-27).

The most extensive research in this area has been carried out by Gifford et al., whose preliminary work determined the effect of cimetidine on the proliferative response of human lymphocytes to both mitogens and antigens (22). Using a similar model, this group proceeded to determine the effects of cimetidine on the proliferation of peripheral blood lymphocytes (PBLs) when incubated with other agents such as levamisole (23).

Initially PBLs were cultured with and without cimetidine at concentrations of 10^{-3}-10^{-8} M (22). Phytohemagglutinin (PHA) or pokeweed mitogen was added to the PBLs either simultaneously with the cimetidine or following 96 hr of preincubation with the drug. Following 3-5 days incubation, PBL activity was measured and cimetidine was shown to augment the PHA and pokeweed-stimulated response by 22 and 27%, respectively, following simultaneous addition. After 96 hr preincubation with cimetidine, the response increased by 59 and 52%, respectively. Similar amplification of PBL stimulation was observed when bacterial antigen (streptokinase-streptodornase) or alloantigen was used for activation.

Table 1 Immunostimulatory Effects of Histamine Type II Antagonists

	In vitro		
5-year period	Human lymphocyte blastogenesis	Cell-mediated cytotoxicity	Interleukin-2 production
1975–1980	Cimetidine and levamisole augment lymphocyte proliferation in response to mitogens (13,22,23). Cimetidine blocks activation of suppressor T cells in presence of PBLs and Con A (24).	Cimetidine augments murine cell-mediated cytotoxicity (29,30).	
1981–1985	Cimetidine did not reverse steroid suppression of PBL response (26).		
1986–1989		Cell-mediated lympholysis increased by cimetidine in normal and down-regulated murine splenocytes (31).	Cimetidine and ranitidine enhance IL-2 production of mitogen-activated murine splenocytes (32). Cimetidine reversed suppression of IL-2 production by CSA (33). Potentiation of IL-2 activity of T lymphocytes when exposed to other imidazole-containing compounds (levamisole and metronidazole) (14).

Using the same model, the immunostimulatory effects of cimetidine have been compared to levamisole, which causes significant augmentation of PHA-induced proliferation of human PBLs (23). Cimetidine approaches levamisole in terms of stimulatory effects. Cimetidine augments PHA and pokeweed mitogen–stimulated responses by 22 and 26%, respectively, whereas levamisole causes a 28 and 44% increase.

Additional work has been carried out by others to evaluate the effects of histamine type II antagonists on PBL stimulation. Osband et al. showed that concanavalin A (Con A) in the presence of PBLs activates suppressor T cells by provoking histamine release (24). This activation was blocked by cimetidine but not by the histamine type I antagonist diphenhydramine. When PBLs were

In vivo		
Tumor formation in animals	Human studies	Clinical studies
		Primack reported allograft rejection following treatment with cimetidine (2). Increased rejection in dogs treated with cimetidine (37). Others reported no effect (36).
Cimetidine reduced tumor formation and offered protection following tumor challenge in mice (34,35).	Augmentation of PBL stimulation by in vivo treatment with cimetidine and ranitidine in duodenal ulcer patients (25).	Immune restoration in cancer patients treated with cimetidine as measured by GVH reactions (41,42). Cimetidine/IFN combination therapy led to significant tumor regression in melanoma patients unresponsive to IFN therapy alone (4).
Prolongation of tumor immunity in tumor-bearing mice (31).	IL-2 and Ig increase following administration of cimetidine and ranitidine to healthy volunteers (39).	Cimetidine therapy alone led to 16% tumor response rate in melanoma patients (5). Partial reversal of suppression of IL-2 production by chemotherapy in patients with ovarian cancer (6).

incubated with Con A alone and in the presence of 10^{-3} M cimetidine mixed lymphocyte culture suppression decreased from 59 to 6%.

B. Cell-Mediated Lympholysis

Cell-mediated lympholysis (CML), or cell mediated cytotoxicity, an additional in vitro test designed to measure T-cell function, can be used to estimate histocompatibility and presensitization in clinical transplantation (28). In addition, since the T-cell response is crucial for suppressing antigenic tumor growth, this test can be used as a measure of immunocompetence for patients with cancer.

The cell-mediated lympholysis response, determined by mixing responding PBLs from a mixed lymphocyte culture (MLC) with PHA-stimulated ^{51}Cr-labeled target lymphocytes, is measured as the amount of ^{51}Cr released into the culture media. The effect of cimetidine on the CML response using mice splenocytes has been evaluated (29,30). The cell-mediated lympholysis response was measured in the presence and absence of cimetidine (10^{-4}-10^{-7} M) in vitro (29), and also after the mice were administered cimetidine orally for 6 weeks (30). In all cases, cimetidine consistently augmented cytotoxicity.

In addition, CML is also increased by cimetidine in normal and down regulated murine splenocytes (31). Cimetidine was shown to partially reverse CML suppression by suppressor cells generated in vitro. Furthermore, mixed tumor lymphocyte cytotoxicity of splenocytes from syngeneic tumor-bearing mice was increased by in vivo cimetidine treatment, resulting in prolongation of concomitant tumor immunity.

C. Interleukin-2

There is increasing evidence that IL-2 is an important regulatory signal of the immune system, and this parameter has been used to monitor the immunologic status of various patient populations. Therefore, the effects of the histamine type II antagonists on IL-2 production has been investigated using mitogen-activated normal murine splenocytes. Gifford et al. compared the effect of cimetidine and ranitidine on IL-2 production by incubating murine cells with 10^{-4}-10^{-6} M of each drug for 48 and 72 hr (32). In the presence of cimetidine (10^{-4} M), IL-2 activity increased to 8.8 U from a baseline of 1 U, whereas ranitidine increased IL-2 activity to 5.6 U. This work was the first demonstration that histamine type II antagonists are capable of increasing IL-2 production.

Using the same model, the effect of cimetidine on the inhibitory effects of cyclosporine (CSA) was evaluated (33). Murine spleen cells were incubated with cimetidine (10^{-4}-10^{-5} M) and/or cyclosporine (0.1-10.0 ng/ml). Cimetidine completely reversed the cyclosporine (0.1 ng/ml and 1.0 ng/ml)–induced 25 and 41% inhibition of IL-2 production, respectively. Using a higher concentration of cyclosporine (10 ng/ml), IL-2 production was reduced by 64%, with cimetidine only partially reversing this inhibition to 48%.

Based on these findings, an increasing interest in histamine type II antagonists as potential immunostimulators has developed. Subsequent research has been carried out to evaluate the use of these agents in a variety of patient populations by monitoring immunologic parameters as well as clinical outcome in renal transplant recipients and patients suffering from metastatic cancers.

D. Immunostimulatory Role of Other Imidazole-Containing Compounds

Other imidazole-containing compounds, such as levamisole, metronidazole (an antibiotic), and imidazole itself, have been shown to possess immunostimulatory effects. In one study, both levamisole and imidazole augmented PHA-induced proliferation of human PBLs, mouse thymocytes, and T cell–enriched splenocytes (13). These changes were believed to result from the effect of imidazole on lymphocyte cyclic nucleotide levels, particularly guanosine monophosphate (GMP). In addition, levamisole, metronidazole, and imidazole were shown to have a direct potentiating effect on IL-2–dependent proliferation of several T-lymphocyte clones (14).

III. IMMUNOLOGIC EFFECTS OF HISTAMINE TYPE II ANTAGONISTS IN VIVO

A. Animal Studies

Once it was established that cimetidine could increase cell-mediated lympholysis, studies to determine if the histamine type II antagonists may have a protective effect against tumors were carried out. Using a murine tumor model, in which suppressor-cell function has been shown to increase with advancing tumor burden, cimetidine was administered to mice following tumor transplantation. In two studies, cimetidine led to a significant reduction in tumor formation and increase in survival in mice challenged with two types of syngeneic tumor (34,35) (see Table 1).

B. Clinical Studies

A number of studies have been carried out in humans to evaluate the effects of histamine type II antagonists on various patient populations. In addition to an immunology study in patients with clinically active duodenal ulcers (25), additional work has suggested that these agents may counteract the immunosuppressive therapy required by transplant patients (36-39), or provide some clinical benefit when administered to immunosuppressed patients such as those with metastatic cancer (4-6) (see Table 1).

One of the first studies carried out in humans compared the effects of ranitidine and cimetidine on mitogen stimulation of PBLs in patients with clinically active duodenal ulcers (25). Subjects were treated with either cimetidine (800 mg daily) or ranitidine (320 mg daily) for 28 days. Stimulation of PBLs incubated with PHA, Con A, and pokeweed mitogen was measured on days 14 and 28. On day 14, increases in lymphocyte response in the cimetidine-treated group was 12, 14, and 16% for the three mitogens, respectively, whereas on day 28, the increases were 12, 8, and 4%. In all but the last case, these changes were significantly different from control values. Differences between measurements on days 14 and 28 may be attributed to the fact that blood sampling occurred soon after drug administration on day 14, as opposed to 14–16 hr following the

Table 2 Effect of Cimetidine on Allograft Rejection in Humans and Dogs

Human study		
PUD prophylaxis	Rejection episodes	Functioning grafts at 3 months
Antacids/anticholinergics (n = 46)	46 (1/patient)	38 (83%)
Cimetidine/antacids (n = 12)	9 (0.75/patient)	10 (83%)
Animal study		
	Onset of rejection (days ± SD)	Survival (days ± SD)
Immunosuppression alone	37 ± 23	42 ± 17
Immunosuppression plus cimetidine (300 mg b.i.d.)	15 ± 8 ($p < 0.01$)	20 ± 12 ($p < 0.02$)

last dose on day 28. In contrast, changes in PBL stimulation for the ranitidine-treated group were negligible.

C. Transplantation

Transplant recipients often receive histamine type II antagonists and steroids concomitantly, since these patients have an increased incidence of gastrointestinal ulceration owing to their immunosuppressive therapy. However early reports have suggested that the use of histamine type II antagonists in renal transplant recipients may lead to an increased incidence of allograft rejection (2,3,36-39). Primack et al. first reported two pediatric renal transplant recipients who were started on cimetidine on days 1 and 17 posttransplantation. Both patients experienced acute allograft rejection 4-5 days after initiating the drug. Owing to the severity of the rejection episodes and the similarity in timing, it was suggested that cimetidine may have contributed to the rejection by counteracting the concomitant immunosuppressive therapy required by these patients. Subsequent to this, however, a retrospective study reported no difference in rejection frequencies or graft function between two groups of patients (36). The first group received cimetidine for peptic ulcer disease (PUD) prophylaxis for 1 month posttransplant, whereas the second group received antacids and an anticholinergic agent for prophylaxis (Table 2).

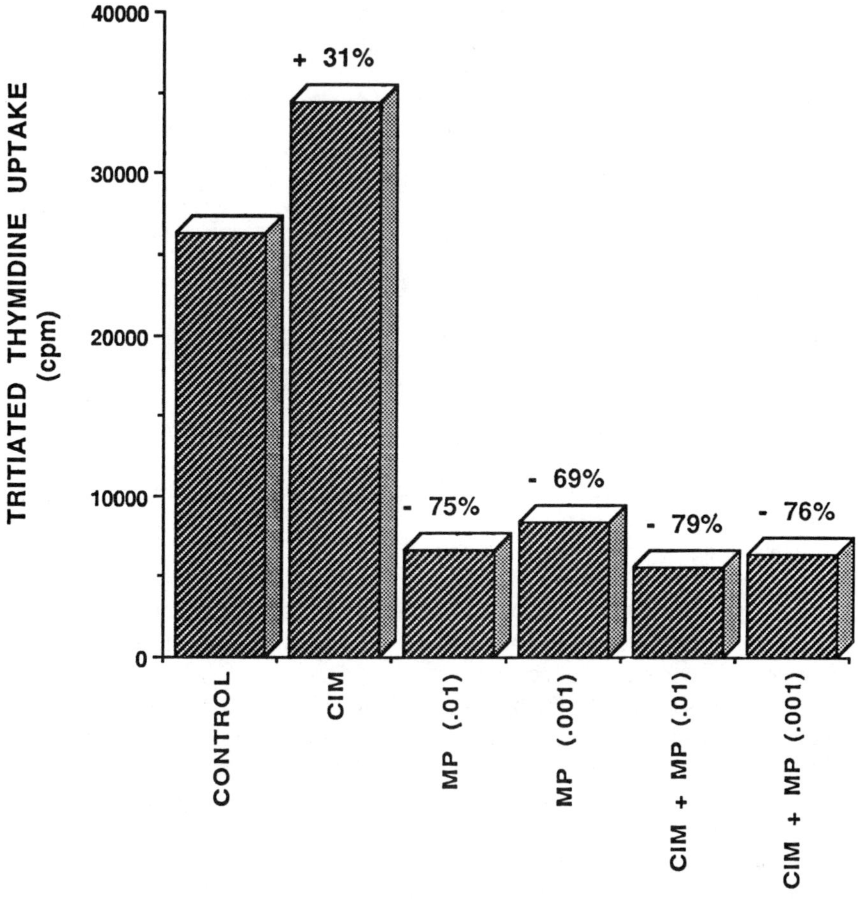

Figure 3 In vitro effects of cimetidine and methylprednisolone as compared to controls on proliferation of peripheral blood lymphocytes from healthy volunteers (measured by tritiated thymidine uptake). CIM = cimetidine (10^{-4}–10^{-7} M), MP = methylprednisolone (0.01–0.001 μg/ml).

An additional study was carried out looking at the timing of transplant rejection in dogs undergoing renal transplantation (37). Dogs receiving high-dose cimetidine (300 mg twice daily) showed a significant trend toward increased rejection when compared to those not treated with cimetidine (see Table 2).

Though the reports of changes in the frequency of allograft rejection are conflicting, an increasing interest arises regarding the possible counteracting

Table 3 Mean Percent Change (CPM) in PBL Stimulation[a] in Renal Allograft Recipients Following Incubation with Cimetidine

Patient group (No. patients)	Pooled plasma	p value	Autologous plasma	p value
All living related (14)	17.9		24.3	
vs.		$<.025$		$<.025$
all cadaver (10)	40		61.7	
Living related, rejection (4)	23.5		36.8	
vs.		NS		NS
living related, no rejection (10)	15.6		19.5	
Cadaver, rejection (5)	34.6		50.8	
vs.		NS		NS
cadaver, no rejection (5)	31.8		72.6	

[a]PBLs were incubated with 25% plasma (pooled or autologous) and irradiated stimulator cells.

immunologic effects of the histamine type II antagonists and immunosuppressive agents. Therefore, further studies have evaluated the possible interaction between these two classes of agents.

Gifford et al. studied the opposing in vitro effects of cimetidine and methylprednisolone on proliferation of peripheral blood lymphocytes from healthy volunteers (26). Following addition of 10^{-4}-10^{-7} M cimetidine alone, the allogeneic proliferative response increased by 31% over control values, whereas incubation with 0.01 and 0.001 μg/ml of methylprednisolone alone suppressed the MLC response by 69-75%. This suppressive effect was not reversed when PBLs were incubated with both agents together (-76% to -79%) (Fig. 3).

The effect of cimetidine on PBL proliferation was also determined in renal transplant recipients (27). The degree of cimetidine responsiveness was compared to the subjects' clinical immunologic status as determined by the incidence of allograft rejection. The data suggested that patients whose PBLs exhibited a high response when exposed to cimetidine in vitro (10^{-4}-10^{-7} M) had a greater incidence of rejection. For example, when incubating PBLs with autologous plasma, the low responsive group ($<+15\%$) had three rejections in nine patients (0.33 rejections/patient), and the high responsive group ($>+40\%$) had nine rejections in 11 patients (0.82 rejections/patient). However, when grouping patients in terms of donor source (living related vs. cadaver), PBLs from cadaver graft recipients responded significantly greater to cimetidine, which could par-

Table 4 Percentage Change of Immunologic Parameters from Baseline Following Cimetidine and Ranitidine Administration to Renal Transplant Recipients

	SI	MLC	CML	IgM	IgG
Cimetidine					
Mean	-6	-24	259	82	-4
SD	116	47	591	100	45
Ranitidine					
Mean	10	10	35	282	220
SD	81	48	103	386	222

SI = Stimulation index; MLC = Mixed lymphocyte culture; CML = cell-mediated lympholysis.

tially explain the findings. Furthermore, the responsiveness between rejectors and nonrejectors within the cadaver recipient group were not statistically significant (Table 3).

More recently, our group designed two studies to determine the effect of these drugs on specific immunologic parameters when administered to both renal transplant patients and healthy volunteers (38,39). Renal transplant recipients received cimetidine (300 mg four times daily) and ranitidine (150 mg twice daily) for 1 week, each separated by 1 week washout period. Immunologic studies, including mixed lymphocyte culture, cell-mediated lympholysis, and immunoglobulin production were determined.

Following stimulation of PBLs with x-irradiated cells, mixed lymphocyte culture (MLC) proliferation was measured on day 6. The stimulation index was defined as the ratio of proliferating cells exposed to the stimulating pool versus autologous cells. The cell-mediated lympholysis response was determined by mixing responding PBLs with PHA-stimulated ^{51}Cr-labeled target lymphocytes derived from HLA-DR–typed allogeneic-stimulating cells. The degree of cell-mediated lysis was measured as the amount of ^{51}Cr released into the culture media. In addition, a reverse hemolytic plaque assay was used to measure the number of immunoglobulin (Ig)–secreting lymphocytes generated in the MLC.

Table 4 summarizes the results of the effects of cimetidine and ranitidine on these various immunologic parameters. Mean values for MLC proliferation did not change significantly following treatment with cimetidine or ranitidine (-24% and +10% from baseline values, respectively). The stimulation index was also essentially unchanged with -6% and +10% from baseline values following treatment with both agents. However, cimetidine increased cell-mediated lympholysis more than ranitidine, with increases of +259 and +35% from baseline values,

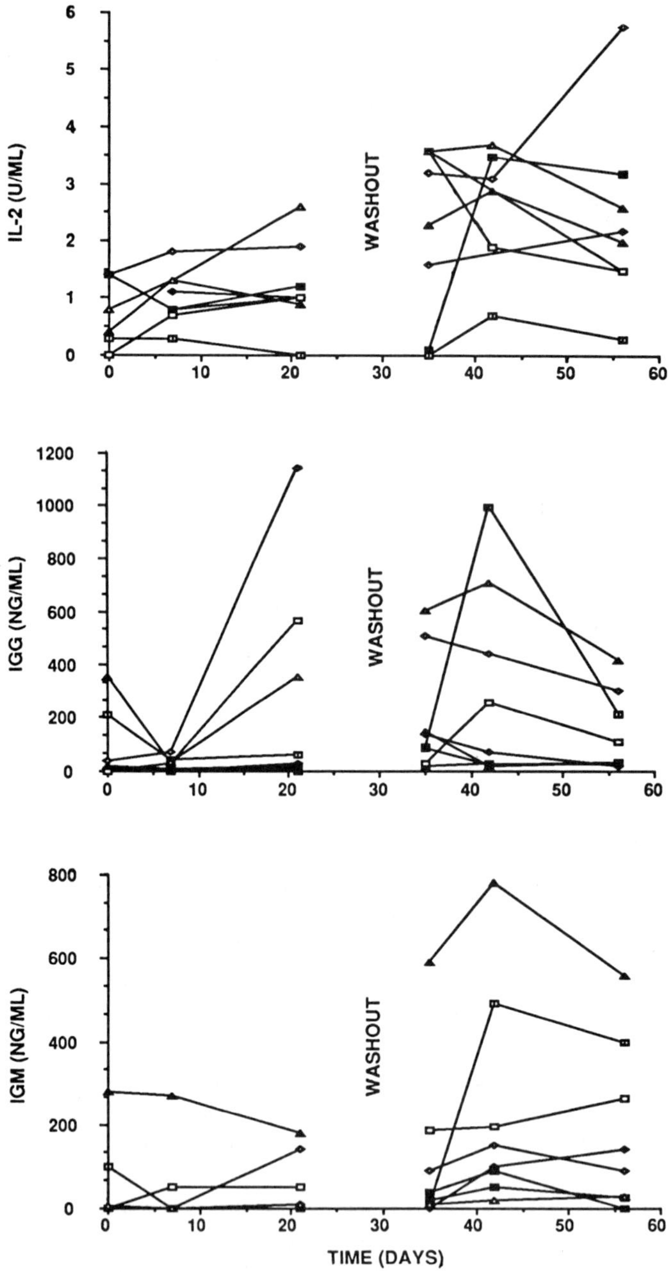

Figure 4 IL-2, IgG, and IgM levels following treatment with cimetidine and ranitidine (each for 3 weeks separated by a 2-week washout period). Data for all eight subjects is presented using a unique symbol for each volunteer.

respectively. Contrary to this, ranitidine had a greater effect on the plaque-forming cell response. Immunoglobulin M and IgG changes were +82 and -4% for cimetidine and +282 and +220% for ranitidine.

In general, few conclusions regarding the immunologic effects of these two histamine type II antagonists could be made based on this preliminary study. A large degree of interpatient variability was observed in our results, which may be attributed to the complex patient population studied and the amount of immunosuppressive therapy they received. In addition, treatment with each agent was limited to 1 week, and it appears that a longer period of drug exposure may be necessary.

A second study in healthy volunteers was carried out as a better model designed to determine the effects of histamine type II antagonists alone on specific immunologic parameters induced by MLC activation (39). Eight subjects were administered cimetidine and ranitidine for 3 weeks each, separated by a 2-week washout period with IL-2 and Ig levels measured throughout the study. Interleukin-2 levels were measured using an IL-2-dependent cytotoxic lymphoid line (CTLL) line, whereas IgG and IgM were quantitated by binding to anti-human Ig in an ELISA assay.

Individual values for IL-2, IgM, and IgG levels measured throughout the 8-week period are shown graphically in Figure 4. Mean values for all parameters increased steadily throughout the 8-week period despite the washout period, with significant increases on days 42 and 56 compared to baseline values. In addition, the effects of ranitidine and cimetidine were not significantly different as determined by separating the patients into two groups; those receiving ranitidine first and those receiving cimetidine first. The change in the mean IL-2 levels from baseline for the ranitidine-first group was 200% on day 42 (peak value) and 182% on day 56 for the subjects receiving cimetidine first. Changes in mean IgG and IgM (day 42) for the ranitidine-first group were 481 and 660%, respectively, whereas changes in these parameters for the cimetidine-first group were 173 and 286%.

This is one of the first studies to report that the histamine type II antagonists cimetidine and ranitidine increase IL-2 and Ig production in humans. This work continues to support the in vitro and animal work that indicates that these agents have potent immunostimulatory properties. More definitive studies should be carried out, however, in all organ transplant recipients as well as renal allograft patients to better determine the effects of these drugs in these patient populations.

D. Cancer

As described previously, cimetidine has increased survival time among tumor-bearing animals as well as increased their resistance to tumor challenge (34,35).

Table 5 Effect of Cimetidine on Local GVH Reactions in vitro

	Before cimetidine		After cimetidine	
	No. negative[a]	No. positive[b]	No. restored[c] (– to +)	No. augmented (> 50% in GVH RXN)[d]
Patients				
10^{-5} M Cimetidine (20)	11	9	6	3
10^{-4} M Cimetidine (23)	15	8	14	5
Normal donors				
10^{-5} M Cimetidine (19)	1	18	–	4
10^{-4} M Cimetidine (26)	1	25	–	5

Effect of Cimetidine Therapy (7 days) on Local GVH Reaction in vivo

	Before cimetidine		After cimetidine	
Patient group	No. negative	No. positive	No. restored (– to +)	
Cimetidine (20)	16	4	7	$p < 0.01$
Controls (9)	8	1	0	

[a]GVH nodules $<50\ mm^3$.
[b]GVH nodules $>50\ mm^3$.
[c]Conversion from negative to positive.
[d]Increase of 50% or more in the GVH reaction.

Increasing evidence that histamine type II antagonists have important immunomodulatory properties led to investigations of the efficacy of these agents in the treatment of cancer.

Initial work documented the immune restorative effect of cimetidine in cancer patients as measured by the local xenogenic graft-versus-host (XGVH) reaction. The XGVH reaction has been shown to be a useful bioassay for assessing T-lymphocyte function and immunocompetence among cancer patients (40). Positive XGVH reactions found in 99.5% of normal donors is only found in 70% of cancer patients with early-stage disease and 30% of cancer patients with metastatic disease.

Mavligit et al. used the XGVH reaction to study the effects of cimetidine in 43 cancer patients and 43 healthy controls (41). Using isolated mononuclear cells (MNCs), aliquots of these cells were incubated with either 10^{-5} or 10^{-4} M cimetidine or left untreated. They were then injected intradermally into partially immunosuppressed rats to stimulate local GVH reaction. Graft-versus-host nodules < 50 mm^3 were considered negative GVH reactions and were indicative of T-cell dysfunction, whereas GVH nodules ≥ 50 mm^3 were classified as positive and represented T-cell competence. Immune restoration was defined as conversion from negative to positive, whereas immune suppression was defined as the reverse. In addition, immunoaugmentation was defined as an increase of 50% or more in the GVH reaction.

Results for this study are summarized in Table 5. Immune restoration was achieved in 55% (6 of 11) and 93 percent (14 of 15) of GVH-negative cancer patients following MNC incubation with 10^{-5} M and 10^{-4} M cimetidine, respectively. In addition, the median GVH volume produced by the untreated cells and treated cells following incubation with 10^{-5} M cimetidine was 15 and 25 mm^3, respectively, whereas the GVH volume produced for the two groups was 17 and 85 mm^3 when the concentration used was 10^{-4} M. The differences between the two groups were statistically significant. Furthermore, augmentation was observed in 33 and 62% of GVH-positive cancer patients following MNC incubation with the two concentrations of cimetidine. All but one normal donor was GVH positive at the onset of the study, and augmentation in this group was not significant.

Using the same model, GVH response was evaluated in 29 cancer patients; 20 were treated with 1200 mg cimetidine daily, whereas nine remained untreated (42). A significant change in GVH reaction was observed in the cimetidine-treated group, with total response before treatment measured as 33 ± 21 versus 50 ± 46 mm^3 after treatment. As expected, no significant change was observed in the control group (30 ± 14 vs 28 ± 17 mm^3). In addition, 44% of the cimetidine-treated patients initially characterized as negative converted to positive compared with 0 of the untreated controls (see Table 5).

Subsequent to these reports that used GVH reactions to evaluate the effect of histamine type II antagonists on the immunocompetence of cancer patients, a number of studies determined whether these agents provide clinical benefit to patients with metastatic cancers. Patients with metastatic malignant melanoma and ovarian cancer were studied following addition of cimetidine to standard chemotherapeutic regimens (4-6).

Flodgren et al. administered cimetidine to 20 patients with metastatic malignant melanoma who had experienced no objective tumor regression following therapy with interferon alone (4). Twelve of the patients had failed therapy for prior relapse, whereas eight patients were studied at the time of first relapse. Following treatment with 1000 mg of cimetidine daily in addition to the interferon therapy, five of eight patients with skin metastasis had complete tumor regression. Though four of the five patients continued in complete remission at 100, 54, 24, and 19 weeks at the time of publication, one patient relapsed after 82 weeks.

The effects of cimetidine alone in treating patients with malignant melanoma was also monitored in a subsequent study (5). Nineteen patients were treated with cimetidine 1200 mg daily. A response was defined as a decrease of $> 50\%$ in the size (product of longest perpendicular diameters) of the largest cancerous lesion. Sixteen percent of patients responded.

Patients with advanced ovarian carcinoma were also treated with cimetidine (6). Thirty-eight patients received six courses of combination chemotherapy consisting of cisplatin, adriamycin, and cyclophosphamide. In addition, each patient received cimetidine 1000 mg daily either concomitantly with the chemotherapy or following treatment completion. Peripheral blood lymphocytes were collected and assayed for T-cell subsets, IL-2 production, and IL-2 receptor expression. Though chemotherapy alone markedly depressed IL-2 production, the addition of cimetidine significantly counteracted this effect and led to a significant increase in CD4-positive cells. When cimetidine was administered following completion of chemotherapy, IL-2 production was restored to the level exhibited by control patients.

IV. CONCLUSIONS

The majority of these provocative studies all point to an immunostimulatory effect of histamine type II antagonists. Whether this effect can significantly alter allograft survival in transplant recipients remains to be determined. An increasing amount of evidence, however, suggests that these agents are useful for the treatment of malignancies. Clinically, the challenge remains to identify the circumstance under which the immunostimulatory effect of the histamine type II antagonists can be optimized and regulated for the treatment of these patients and others with immunosuppressive disorders. Clearly, only by further, well-controlled studies can their full potential benefit be realized.

REFERENCES

1. Goodman, L. S., and A. G. Gilman, The Pharmacological Basis of Therapeutics, 7th ed., Macmillan, New York (1985), pp. 624–625.
2. Primack, W. A., Cimetidine and renal-allograft rejection, Lancet 1:824 (1978).
3. Ahonen, J., Cimetidine and ranitidine in renal transplantation, Scand. J. Gastroenterol. 17(S78):196 A779 (1982).
4. Flodgren, P., S. Borgstrom, P. E. Jonsson, C. Lindström, and H. O. Sjögren, Metastatic malignant melanoma: Regression induced by combined treatment with interferon [HiIFN-a(Le)] and cimetidine, Int. J. Cancer 32:657–665 (1983).
5. Morton, R. F., E. T. Creagan, S. A. Cullinan, J. A. Mailliard, L. Ebbert, M. H. Veeder, and M. Chang, Phase II studies of single-agent cimetidine and the combination N-phosphoacetyl-L-aspartate (NSC-224131) plus L-alanosine (NSC-153353) in advanced malignant melanoma, J. Clin. Oncol. 5:1078–1082 (1987).
6. Kikuchi, Y., I. Kizawa, K. Oomori, I. Iwano, T. Kita, M. Miyauchi, and K. Kato, Effects of cimetidine on interleukin-2 production by peripheral blood lymphocytes in advanced ovarian carcinoma, Eur. J. Cancer Clin. Oncol. 24: 1185–1190 (1988).
7. Beer, D. J., and R. E. Rocklin, Histamine induced suppressor-cell activity, J. Allergy Clin. Immunol. 73:439–452 (1984).
8. Rocklin, R. E. Histamine-induced suppressor factors (HSF): Effect of migration inhibitory factor (MIF) production and proliferation, J. Immunol. 118:1734–1738 (1977).
9. Rocklin, R. E., D. Greineder, B. H. Littman, and K. L. Melmon, Modulation of cellular immune function in vitro by histamine receptor-bearing lymphocytes. Mechanism of action, Cell. Immunol. 37:162–173 (1978).
10. Rocklin, R. E., D. K. Greineder, and K. L. Melmon, Histamine-induced suppressor factor (HSF): Further studies on the nature of the stimulus and the cell which produces it, Cell. Immunol. 44:404–415 (1979).
11. Garovoy, M. R., M. A. Reddish, and R. E. Rocklin, Histamine-induced suppressor factor (HSF): Inhibition of helper T cell generation and function, J. Immunol. 130:357–361 (1983).
12. Rocklin, R. E., J. Breard, S. Gupta, R. A. Good, and K. L. Melmon, Characterization of the human blood lymphocytes that produce a histamine-induced suppressor factor, Cell. Immunol. 51:226–237 (1980).
13. Hadden, J. W., R. G. Coffey, E. M. Hadden, E. Lopez-Corrales, and G. H. Sunshine, Effects of levamisole and imidazole on lymphocyte proliferation and cyclic nucleotide levels, Cell. Immunol. 20:98–103 (1975).

14. Redondo, J. M., J. A. Lopez-Guerrero, and M. Fresno, Potentiation of interleukin-2 activity by levamisole and imidazole, Immunol. Lett. 14:111–116 (1986).
15. Rocklin, R. E., K. Bendtzen, and D. Greineder, Mediators of immunity: Lymphokines and monokines, Adv. Immunol. 31:1 (1980).
16. Dorf, M. E., and B. Benacerraf, Suppressor cells and immunoregulation, Ann. Rev. Immunol. 2:127–158 (1984).
17. Damle, N., and S. Gupta, Autologous mixed lymphocyte reaction in man. II. Histamine-induced suppression of the autologous mixed lymphocyte reaction by T-cell subsets defined with monoclonal antibodies, J. Clin. Immunol. 1:241–249 (1981).
18. Beer, D. J., L. J. Rossenwasser, C. A. Dinarello, and R. E. Rocklin, Cellular interactions in the generation and expression of histamine-induced suppressor activity, Cell. Immunol. 69:101–112 (1982).
19. Beer, D. J., C. A. Dinarello, L. J. Sossenwaser, and R. E. Rocklin, Human monocyte derived soluble product(s) has an accessor function in the generation of histamine and concanavalin A-induced suppressor T cells, J. Clin. Invest. 70:393–400 (1982).
20. Rocklin, R. E., I. Kiselis, D. J. Beer, P. Rossi, F. Maggi, and J. A. Bellanti, Augmentation of prostaglandin and thromboxane production in vitro by monocytes exposed to histamine-induced suppressor factor (HSF), Cell. Immunol. 77:92–98 (1983).
21. Stites, D. P., J. D. Stobo, and J. V. Wells, Chapter 18 Clinical Laboratory Methods for Detection of Cellular Immune Function in Basic and Clinical Immunology, 6th ed., Appleton and Lange, Norwalk, Connecticut (1987), pp. 293–295.
22. Gifford, R. R., S. M. Hatfield, and J. R. Schmidtke, Cimetidine-induced augmentation of human lymphocyte blastogenesis by mitogen bacterial antigen and alloantigen, Transplantation 29:143–148 (1980).
23. Gifford, R. R., and J. R. Schmidtke, Cimetidine-induced augmentation of human lymphocyte blastogenesis: Comparison with levamisole in mitogen stimulation, Surg. Forum 30:113–115 (1979).
24. Osband M, D. Gallison, B. Miller, R. P. Agarwal, and R. McCaffrey, Concanavalin A activation of suppressor cells is mediated by the release of histamine and is blocked by cimetidine. Clin. Res. 28:356A (1980).
25. Peden, N. R., A. J. Robertson, E. J. S. Boyd, R. A. Brown, J. H. Gibbs, R. C. Potts, K. G. Wormsley, and J. Swanson Beck, Mitogen stimulation of peripheral blood lymphocytes of duodenal ulcer patients during treatment with cimetidine or ranitidine, Gut 23:398–403 (1982).
26. Gifford, R. R., S. M. Hatfield, J. R. Schmidtke, R. M. Fergunson, Effect of cimetidine on steroid suppression of normal human lymphocytes, Curr. Surg. 38:65–67 (1981).
27. Gifford, R. R., J. R. Schmidtke, and R. M. Ferguson, Cimetidine modulation of lymphocytes from renal allograft recipients, Transplantation Proc. 13:663–666 (1981).

28. Stites, D. P., J. D. Stobo, and J. V. Wells, Chapter 18 Clinical Laboratory Methods for Detection of Cellular Immune Function in Basic and Clinical Immunology, 6th ed., Appleton and Lange, Norwalk, Connecticut (1987), pp. 297–298.
29. Gifford, R. R., C. E. Gamble, J. R. Schmidtke, et al., Cimetidine augmentation of in vitro generated cell-mediated cytotoxicity, Surg. Forum. 31:379–382 (1980).
30. Gifford, R. R., and D. A. Vallera, Cimetidine induced augmentation of murine cell mediated cytotoxicity after in vitro and in vivo treatment. Fed. Proc. 39:924 (1980).
31. Gifford, R. R., B. V. Voss, J. R. Schmidtke, and R. M. Ferguson, Histamine type 2 receptor antagonist immune modulation. I. Increased cell-mediated cytotoxicity in normal and in down-regulated systems, Surgery 103:184–192 (1988).
32. Gifford, R. R., and A. F. Tilberg, Histamine type-w receptor antagonist immune modulation II. Cimetidine and ranitidine increase interleukin-2 production, Surgery 102:242–247 (1987).
33. Gifford, R. R., and A. F. Tilberg, Cimetidine reduces cyclosporin inhibition of interleukin-2 production, J. Surg. Res. 45:276–280 (1988).
34. Gifford, R. R., R. M. Ferguson, and B. V. Voss, Cimetidine reduction of tumor formation in mice, Lancet 1:638–639 (1981).
35. Gifford, R. R., B. V. Voss, and R. M. Ferguson, Cimetidine production against lethal tumor challenge in mice, Surgery 90:344–351 (1981).
36. Charpentier, B., and D. Fries, Cimetidine and renal-allograft rejection, Lancet 2:1265 (1978).
37. Zammit, M., and L. H. Toledo-Pereyra, Increased reduction after cimetidine treatment in kidney transplants, Transplantation 27:358–359 (1979).
38. Aweeka, F. T., J. Birnbaum, W. Amend, P. Lizak, M. Garovoy, J. Gambertoglio, Immunomodulatory effects of H2-antagonists in renal transplant recipients (unpublished data).
39. Aweeka, F. T., P. Lizak, M. Garovoy, W. Amend, J. Birnbaum, M. A. Gumbert, J. Gambertoglio, Interleukin-2 and immunoglobulin increases with H2-antagonists in humans, Transplant. Proc. 21:1718–1721 (1989).
40. Mavligit, G., Y. Ishii, Y. Patt, and W. Wong, Local xenogeneic graft-vs-host reaction: A practical assessment of T cell function among cancer patients, J. Immunol. 123:2185–2188 (1979).
41. Mavligit, G. M., D. B. Calvo, Y. Z. Patt, and E. M. Hersh, Immune restoration and/or augmentation of local xenogeneic graft versus host reaction by cimetidine in vitro, J. Immunol. 126:2272–2274 (1981).
42. Talpaz, M., J. E. Medina, Y. Z. Patt, H. Goepfert, O. M. Guiliamondegui, W. Wong, and G. M. Mavligit, The immune restorative effect of cimetidine administration in vivo in the local graft-versus-host reaction of cancer patients, Clin. Immunol. Immunopathol. 24:155–160 (1982).

Part IV
Future Trends: Congeners of Autacoids as Immune Modulators

16

Autacoids as Tissue- and Receptor-Specific Immune Modulating Drugs

KENNETH L. MELMON *Stanford University School of Medicine, Stanford, California*

I. INTRODUCTION

As was discussed in Chapter 3, autacoids appear to have the potential to play modulating roles in the immune response. The net of the in vitro data on histamine (as one example) appears to be suppression of immunity by a variety of mechanisms. If the same suppression occurred in vivo, such results would help to explain why in spite of the fact that inflammation must generate foreign antigens and release histamine, the process usually is not followed by detrimental immune responses. Thus, the locally released amine and other autacoids instead of simply being modulators of inflammation actually might prevent responses to the antigens generated during inflammation; i.e., modulate immunity.

The extent of in vivo modulation of the immune response by any given autacoid is not known. But by the examples given in Chapter 3, we know that receptors particularly for histamine, but also to other autacoids including lymphokines, are not equally distributed on different effector cells. We also know

---

This chapter is based substantially on references 25 and 26.

that expression of receptors to various autacoids is changed on distinct subtypes of lymphocytes by a variety of stimuli (e.g., mitogens, the mixtures of cell types in the site of the immune response, the various lymphokines in the environment, and the stage of the immune response).

Of the known autacoids, we have focused our studies on histamine. The focus may be justified because the amine is stored in tissues very frequently associated with the immune response; some lymphokines that are released by immune stimuli release histamine; a variety of other immune-related stimuli release histamine; of the autacoids, histamine seems to exert control on release of histamine-induced suppressor factor (HSF), soluble immune response suppressor (SIRS), some chemoattractants, and lymphocyte migratory inhibiting factors. In some cells, response to histamine may be linked to compartmentalized adenylate cyclase or cAMP; and histamine seems capable of regulating T-cell surface antigens (see Chap. 3). In short, cellular responses to histamine seem exquisitely controlled by localized mechanisms of amine release as well as local factors that impact on receptor distribution and expression. The latter is under unusual control mechanisms related to cell-cell interactions and the state of participation of the cells in the immune response. Thus, the biologic environment of the immune response seems particularly well orchestrated to modify and organize the responses to histamine in biologically and immunologically meaninfgul ways. So far, the same controls and functions have not been defined for response of immunocytes to catecholamines and prostaglandins, although in time it would not be surprising to find that some control on the nonrandom distribution of β-adrenergic and prostaglandin E receptor occurs.

Autacoids generally can be synthesized in diverse tissues, and theoretically they can produce effects in many cell types. The localization and specificity of effects of autacoids rest largely on their site and mechanism of release as well as the ability of most tissues to biologically inactivate them. If autacoids are released in excessive amounts, or if pharmacologically effective amounts are infused intravenously, they distribute more widely than is physiologic and have widespread and diverse pharmacologic effects in most of the tissues they reach. Widespread effects of infused histamine or other autacoids in humans produce clinical chaos. Histamine, for instance, can cause hypotension and shock, tachycardia, capillary fragility and leaking, and bronchospasm as can be seen in some patients with mastocytosis or in some with severe hypersensitivty to drugs. Thus, there have been few if any serious proposals to use an autacoid like histamine or epinephrine as a drug that could specifically or dominantly modify immunity.

We have synthesized derivatives of histamine (congeners and conjugates), catecholamines, and beta blockers in an attempt to alter their pharmacokinetics and tissue distribution, and thereby modify their pharmacodynamics and even their tissue selectivity. We reasoned that if the drugs could be made tissue and/or

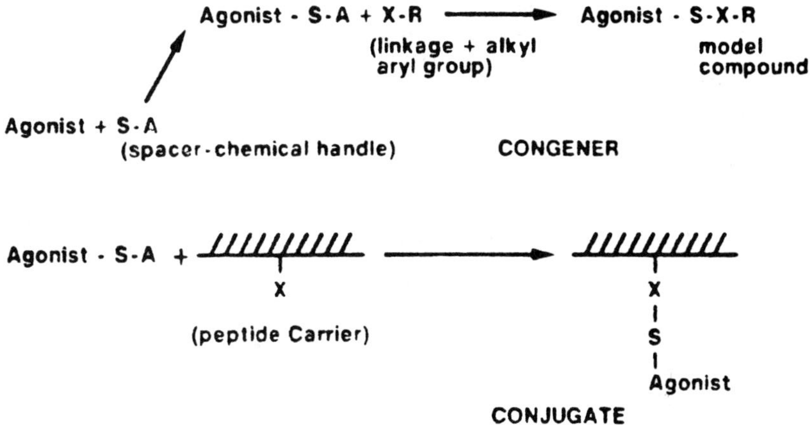

Figure 1 Congener approach to drug-conjugate design. (From Ref. 25, used with permission.)

effect specific, the derivatives could be used as probes to define the specific physiologic and pathologic roles of their progenitors. We also believed that effect- and tissue-specific catecholamines, histamine, or their antagonists ultimately could have interesting therapeutic potential (1-5). We have found more than we bargained for. The compounds can do what we had expected, and beyond that, even develop receptor specificity. The mechanisms of these changes remain largely unknown.

Chronologically, our approach first was to modify the β-adrenergic amines and their antagonists. We initiated our synthetic program using catecholamines for two reasons. The known structure-activity relationships of the catecholamines allowed modification of the amino moiety without total loss of pharmacologic activity and the screening strategy for the new congeners and conjugates was simple. β_1 and β_2 cardiovascular versus other tissue specificity would be relatively easy to discern. We derivatized the norepinephrine molecule by using its amino end and adapting the molecule (congener) so that it could be linked to monodisperse oligopeptides, and even to proteins such as albumin and monoclonal antibodies (conjugates) (Fig. 1) (1-5). We assumed that the chemical characteristics of the pharmacologically inert ligands attached to the pharmacophore would produce major net chemical alterations of the new molecule as opposed to the chemical characteristics of the progenitor compound. We had planned to systematically synthesize and test the effects of added ligands on the alterations

Table 1 Structure Predicts Pharmacologic Novelty

STRUCTURE	ISOPROTERENOL (Type I)	PROPRANOLOL (β_2) (Type II)	PRACTOLOL (β_1) (Type II)	HISTAMINE (Type III)
METHYLENE CHAIN				
C_2	⬇	⬇	—	↓
C_3	↓	⬇	↓	⬆ H_1-Lymph
C_4	⬆	⬆	⬆	⬆ H_1,H_2-Lymph
C_5	↓	↓	↓	↓
BRANCHED METHYLENE CHAIN	↑	↑	↑	↑
TOLUIDIDE MOIETIES				
P-methyl	↑ β_1 (Heart vs Lung-TS))	↑ β_1 (Fat vs Heart) RS & TS	↑ β_1 RS & TS	⬆ RS-H_1 & TS-lymph
P-trifluo-romethyl	⬆ OA; TS [Peripheral vs Coronary Metabolic, Skeletal Muscle (Glycogen)]	↓ β_1 (Fat vs Heart)	↑ β_2 RS & TS	⬆ RS-H_1 & TS-lymph
Ortho	↓	—	—	↓
Meta	↔	—	—	—
AMINO ACID	↑ β_1 (TS, RS)	↑ β_1 (TS, RS)	↑ β_1 TS, RS	—
DIPEPTIDE	↑ OA; (TS, RS)	↓ Fat vs Heart	—	TS - Heart vs lymph RS-H_2
LONGER PEPTIDE	↔ or ⬇	—	—	—

Histamine derivatives not active on heart (type II) can be vasoconstrictive (type I).
OA = Oral activity, TS = Tissue selectivity. NT = No Tachyphylaxis in heart.
RS = Receptor selectivity, — = not tested.

that they would cause in pharmacokinetics, tissue distribution, and thereby pharmacodynamics of the congeners and conjugates compared to the unaltered progenitor (6). We hoped for localized pharmacologic effects in one tissue or another and for different durations of effect than those of the native amines. If the experiments with catecholamines were successful, our ultimate aim was to design histamine compounds that were tissue and receptor specific. If such compounds could be made, we planned to use them to study immunomodulation.

We found that we could chemically modify both amines. We obtained remarkable changes in potency and some unexpected tissue, receptor, and effect specificity. For instance, we developed catecholamine congeners that could almost exclusively affect the heart. Even in that tissue, inotropic effects were greatly augmented, whereas chronotropic effects were almost nil (7-9,22). The congeners that affected the heart had almost no systemic (i.e., metabolic or hormonal) effects. Many congeners were magnitudes more potent and some were magnitudes less potent than the progenitor drug. Some of the congeners could be given orally to dogs and rabbits and were active even though two were peptide derivatives (9). To our surprise, the altered pharmacology of the catecholamine congeners, for example, could not be explained by their pharmacokinetics or metabolism (6). What was more interesting was that all of the effects produced by our derivatives appeared to employ the same classic mechanisms of agonism or antagonism as was used by their progenitors.

This chapter will first report the data on congeners and conjugates of catecholamines, then on a similar parallel series made with the β-adrenergic antagonists propranolol and practolol, and finally on a parallel series of congeners and conjugates made with histamine. We have found that often similar derivatives of each antagonist and of histamine showed remarkably predictable parallels in potency, tissue selectivity, and receptor specificity as was seen with the catecholamines (10,11) (Table 1). The primary purpose of this chapter is to summarize the methods of synthesis and the effects of some of our derivatives and to describe the congeners of histamine as potential immune modulators.

II. SYNTHESIS AND CHEMICAL EVALUATION OF CONGENERS AND CONJUGATES

The methods for synthesis of the catecholamine congeners and conjugates (up to octapeptides); propranolol and practolol congeners and conjugates, and histamine congeners and conjugates (up to dipeptides); their purification and characterization have been described and only will be briefly summarized for the histamine derivatives in this chapter (2,4,5,9-18).

The attachment of drug modifiers to histamine was explored by acylation and alkylation of the side chain primary amine (19). Figure 1 illustrates the

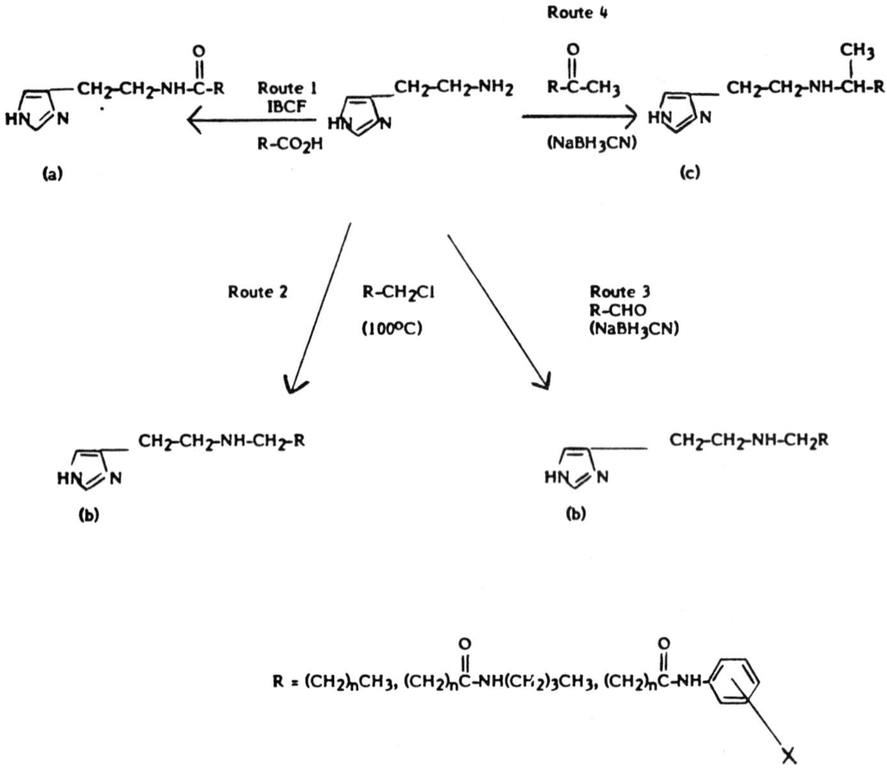

Figure 2 The derivatives of histamine. (From Ref. 19, used with permission.)

general methods used to make modifications of each of the pharmacophores. Figure 2 illustrates the more specific routes of histamine congener and conjugate syntheses. Initially, several alkyl analogs were prepared in order to study the effect of the mode of attachment on histaminergic activity. Subsequently, aromatic amide groups also were used to modify the histamine (Table 2).

The acyl derivatives of histamine (Table 2, compounds 3 and 4) were synthesized from histamine and the appropriate acid by the mixed anhydride method (Fig. 2, route 1). For the unbranched derivatives (Table 2, compounds 1 and 2), the alkylation of the primary amino group on histamine was achieved by reductive amination with the appropriate aldehyde (Fig. 2, route 3), or by S_N2 displacement of chlorine from the appropriate chloro compound (Fig. 2, route 2). The most efficient route for the synthesis for compound 1 was found to be the reductive amination of hexanal and histamine with sodium cyanoborohydride as the reducing agent. Other routes such as reductive amination via hydrogenation with platinum dioxide or displacement reaction with 1-chlorohexane resulted in low yields. In the case of the nonbranched toluide derivative (compound 2), the displacement reaction gave an acceptable yield.

The synthesis of all the branched histamine derivatives (Table 2, compounds 5–19) were accomplished by reductive amination (Fig. 2, route 3). These reactions never proceeded to completion even though the presence of the initial reactants could be verified by thin-layer chromatography and excess reducing agent was still present.

Crude purifications to remove side products and starting materials were carried out by a series of extractions at pH ~ 2 and 9 with $CHCl_3$. In most cases, the product was isolated as the HCl salt, where final purifications usually involved recrystallization from EtOH/ether or flash chromatography with CH_2Cl_2/MeOH/AcOH as eluent. For the isolation of the histamine dipeptide (Table 2, compound 15), semipreparative HPLC (52% methanol/0.01 M NH_4HCO_3, pH 8.5) was found to be the most effective method.

III. PHARMACOLOGIC TESTING OF CONGENERS OF CATECHOLAMINES AND HISTAMINE

The pharmacologic testing for each of the derivatives of the β-adrenergic agonist and antagonist included binding and displacement assays on whole-cell and membrane preparations of S-49 mouse lymphoma cells (β_2 receptors), turkey erythrocytes (β_1 receptors), rat adipocytes (β_1 receptors), rat heart (β_1 receptors), and rat lung (β_2 receptors). Biologic activity of the agonist progenitors and their derivatives were first measured by cyclic adenosine monophosphate (cAMP) accumulation assays. Inhibition of isoproterenol induced cAMP accumulation was the assay used for the antagonists. More complex effects were assessed in vitro using preparations of intact heart, papillary muscle from the heart, bronchial tissue, and the tissues mentioned above that were used for the membrane preparations. In vivo tests ranged from simple measurements of heart rate and blood pressure in anesthetized rats to complex measurements of cardiac contractility, chronotropic actions, coronary vasodilation, and systemic metabolic and hormonal effects ordinarily expected of catecholamines on rats, rabbits, and dogs.

The biologic functions of the derivatives of histamine were tested by accumulation of intracellular cAMP in murine lymphocytes (histamine type II [H_2] receptor effect) (11) and in mixed lymphocyte reaction (MLR) preparations (histamine type I [H_1] receptor effects) (11). Other assays were adenylate cyclase activation in the guinea pig myocardium (a histamine type II receptor effect) and vasoconstriction of the rabbit aorta (type I receptor effect) (19).

Table 2 Yields and Microchemical Analyses of Histamine Derivatives

Compound	X	yield (%)	mp (°C)
1	$(CH_2)_5$-CH_3	16	229–231
2	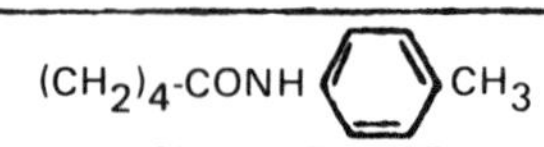	35	225–227
3	$\overset{O}{\overset{\Vert}{C}}$-$(CH_2)_4$-$CH_3$	47	128–129
4	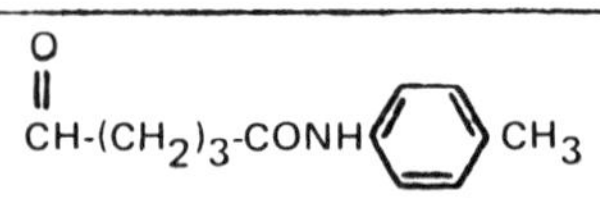	53	175–176.5
4 (n = 1) 6 (n = 2) 7 (n = 3) 8 (n = 4) 9 (n = 5)	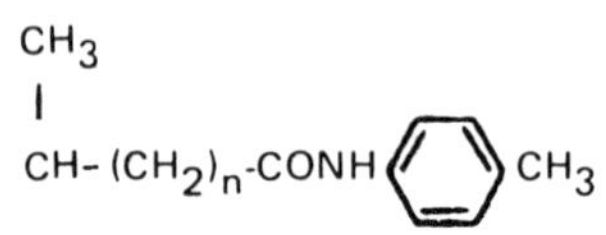	40 22 27 10 50	hygroscopic >80 (dec) hygroscopic 152–155 144 (dec)
10 (n = 1) 11 (n = 2) 12 (n = 3) 13 (n = 4)	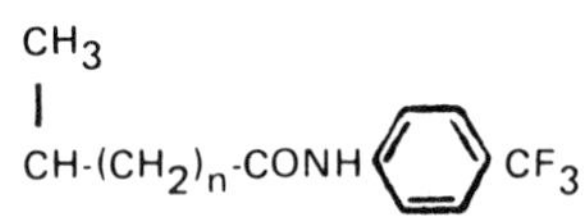	32 26 20 37	hydroscopic 105 (dec) hygroscopic hygroscopic
14	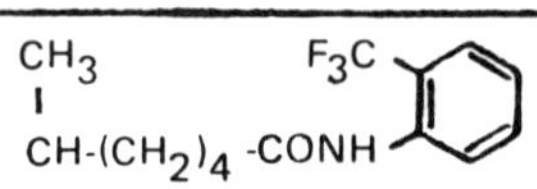	47	195–199
15 (n = 2) 16 (n - 3) 17 (n = 4)	CH_3	CH-$(CH_2)_n$-CONH	Boc-Phe-Gly-$NHCH_3$	9 9 30	>80 (dec) >85 (dec) hygroscopic
18	CH_3	CH-$(CH_2)_4$-CONH-$(CH_2)_3CH_3$	51	hygroscopic
19	CH_3	CH-$(CH_2)_4CH_3$	66	194–195.5

Purification methods	solvents	Elemental analysis ($C_1 H_2 N$)
Recrystallization	EtOH	$C_{11}H_{23}N_3Cl_2$
Recrystallization	$EtOH/Et_2O$	$C_{17}H_{26}N_4OCl_2$
Recrystallization	EtOH	$C_{11}H_{19}N_3O$
Precipitation	H_2O	$C_{17}H_{22}N_4O_2$ $1.5H_2O$
Flash chromatography	$CH_2/Cl_2/MeOH/AcOH$ 70:30:10	$C_{16}H_{24}N_4OCl_2$ H_2O
Flash chromatography	$CH_2Cl_2/MeOH/AcOH$ 6:3:1	$C_{17}H_{26}N_4OCl_2$
Recrystallization	$CHCl_3/Et_2O$	$C_{18}H_{25}N_4OCl_2$ H_2O
Recrystallization	$EtOAc/Et_2O$	$C_{19}H_{30}N_4OCl_2H_2O$
Recrystallization	$EtOH/et_2O$	$C_{20}H_{32}N_4OCl_2$
Flash chromatography	$CH_2Cl_2/MeOH/AcOH$ 70:10:3	$C_{16}H_{21}N_4OCl_2F_3$ H_2O
Flash chromatography	$CH_2Cl_2/MeOH/AcOH$ 6:3:1	$C_{17}H_{23}N_4OCl_2F_3$ 0.5 H_2O
Recrystallization	$CHCl_3/Et_2O$	$C_{18}H_{25}N_4OCl_2F_3$ $5H_2O$
Recrystallization	$EtOH/Et_2O$	$C_{19}H_{27}N_4OCl_2F_3$ H_2O
Recrystallization	$EtOH/Et_2O$	$C_{19}H_{27}N_4OCl_2F_3$ $0.5H_2O$
Flash chromatography	$CH_2Cl_2/MeOH/AcOH$ 6:3:1	$C_{27}H_{43}N_7O_5Cl_25$ H_2O
Flash chromatography	$CH_2Cl_2/MeOH/AcOH$ 6:3:1	$C_{25}H_{45}N_7O_5Cl_26$ H_2O
Semipreparative HPLC Whatman Partisil Magnum 10/25 ODS-3, 1cm x 25cm flow rate 1.0 ml/min retention time 15 min	52% MeOH/0.01 M NH_4HCO_3 pH 8.5	
Recrystallization	$EtOH/et_2O$	$C_{16}H_{32}N_4OCl_2$
Recrystallization	$EtOH/Et_2O$	$C_{12}H_{25}N_3Cl_2$

Table 3 In Vitro Biological Activity of Congeners and Model Derivatives of Isoproterenol

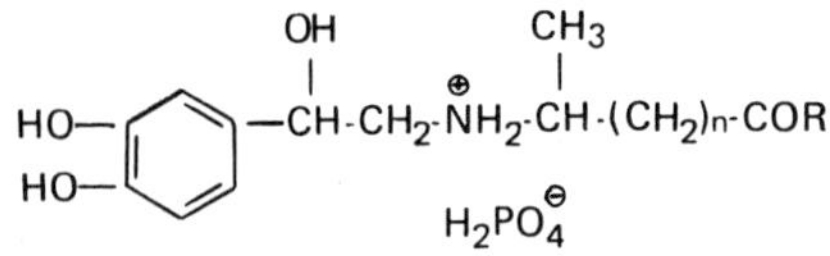

Compound	*R*	n[a]	Activity relative to isoproterenol
1. Carboxylic acid	—OH	4	1.6×10^{-4}
2. p-Toluide	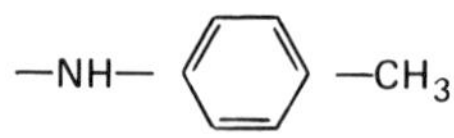	4	5.4×10^{1}
3. p-Trifluoromethylanilide	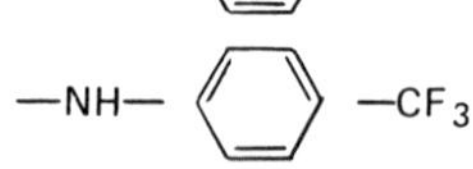	4	8.6×10^{2}
4. m-Trifluoromethylanilide	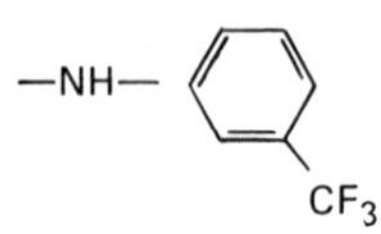	4	9.8×10^{-1}
5. o-Trifluoromethylanilide	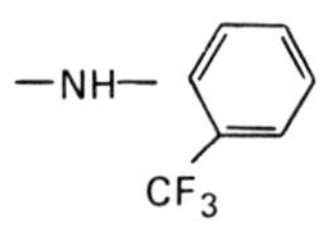	4	2.5×10^{-4}
6. p-Butylanilide	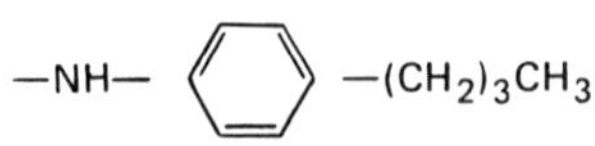	4	3.2×10^{3}
7. p-Methoxylanilide	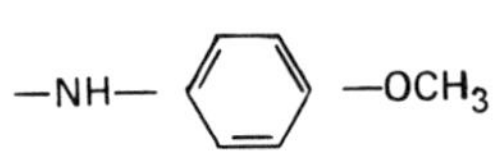	4	3.1
8. p-Toluide	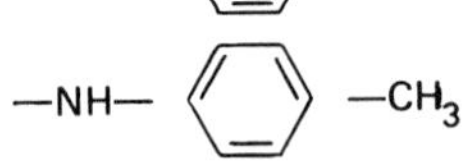	2	7.1×10^{-3}
9. p-Toluide	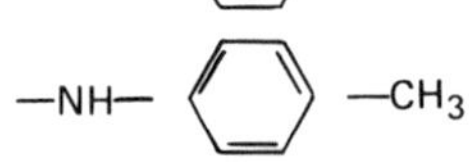	3	3.6×10^{-1}
10. p-Toluide	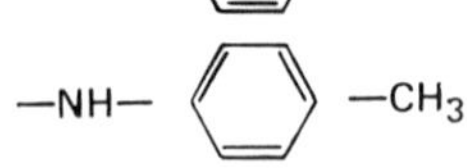	5	1.9×10^{-1}

Biological activity was measured by cyclic AMP acculululation in S-49 cells. Relative activity is expressed as the ratio of the K_a for isoproterenol to K_a for the test compound

[a]n = Number of methylene groups in the spacer group.

Source: From Ref. 8, used with permission.

A. Pharmacologic Results

1. Catecholamines

About 150 derivatives of the catecholamine norepinephrine, the β-adrenergic blockers propranolol and practolol, and histamine have been characterized. Because we focused on the branched chain substitutions made on the amino end of norepinephrine, comparisons of the pharmacologic effects of the congeners and conjugates were made with isoproterenol rather than norepinephrine. As can be seen in Table 3, the potency of the congeners tested on S-49 cells' intracellular accumulation of cAMP showed the most striking changes when the lenghts of the methylene chain varied from 2-5 carbons, and when different substituents were added to the aromatic moiety. The most profound increase in potency was obtained from the C_4 methylene chain with a p-trifluoromethyl substitution on the toluidide group. This component (Table 3, compound 3) and its p-methyl toluidide partner (Table 3, compound 2) became key derivatives for comparison with like derivatives using the beta-blocking and histamine pharmacophores. Tables 2 and 3 illustrate the important shifts in potency by simple position changes of the trifluoromethyl group on the toluidide moiety (Table 2, compounds 13 and 14; Table 3, compounds 3-5).

Peptide conjugates ranging from a dipeptide with phenylalanine-glycine that was four times more potent than isoproterenol to an octapeptide that still maintained classic β-adrenergic actions also were studied (20).

In general, the compounds were selective in the tissues that they affected. Even within a single tissue and a presumed similar receptor derived effect, the effects of the congener could be shifted to only one of the effects mediated through a common receptor. For instance, despite the fact that chronotropic and inotropic effects of beta mimetic amines seem to go hand in hand, compound 3 (Table 3) was close to five times more potent as an inotropic agent, but only two and four-tenths times more potent as a chronotropic agent when tested on the guinea pig atrial muscle (8,16). The dichotomous effects on inotropism vs chronotropism also was seen in vivo in rabbits and dogs (21).

The in vitro data indicated that compound 3 could not be easily washed from the heart tissue, an action that corresponded to, but may not have fully explained, the very long duration of the drug effect as compared to isoproterenol when given in vivo (8). Furthermore, the compound was a much more potent and efficacious coronary vasodilator than isoproterenol, but had no effect in reversing histamine-induced bronchoconstriction in guinea pig bronchi (8) or provoking systemic metabolic changes as isoproterenol did. Finally, a dipeptide conjugate of the norepinephrine that had most of the selective effects shown by compound 3 as well as compound 3 were pharmacologically active when given orally (9,21)–an action not seen with isoproterenol.

Table 4 Relative Potencies of β-Adrenerigic Antagonist Derivatives[a]

		S-49/Lung	Fat cells/Heart	S-49/Fat cells	Lung/Heart[b]
	Propranolol	0.54	1	0.1	0.77
1	$CH(CH_3)-(CH_2)_4-C(=O)-NH-(CH_2)_3-CH_3$	0.1	25	0.003	10
4	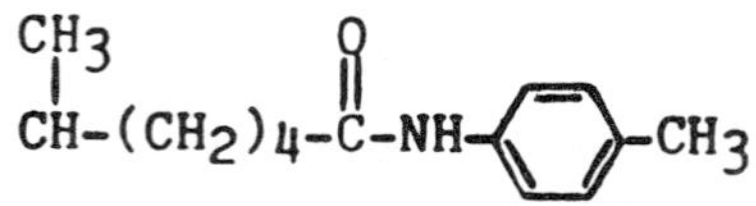	0.0054	15	0.0005	1.3
6	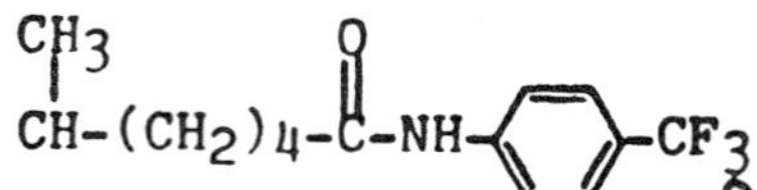	0.05	414	0.0003	2.5
9	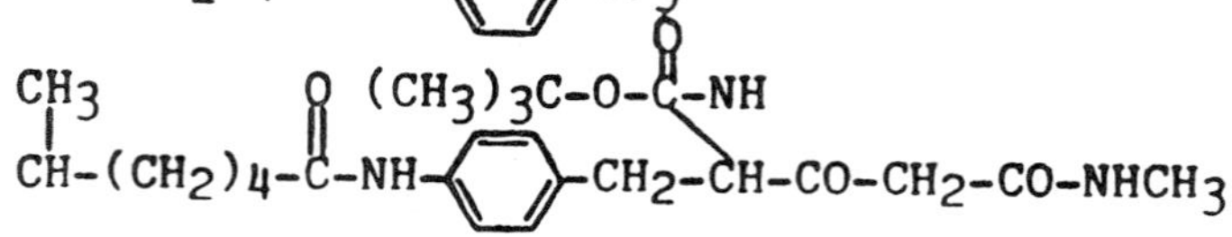	0.26	3.0	0.13	1.5
	Practolol	0.25	0.81	0.91	14.5
14	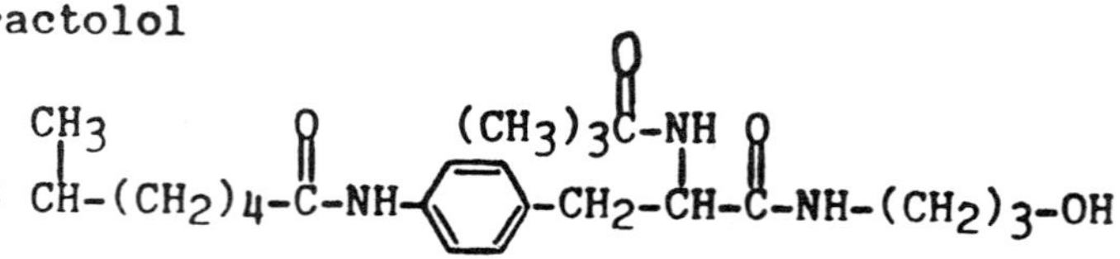	0.048	1.45	1.39	42

[a]Taken from inhibition constants (K_i).
[b]Rat lung and heart contain 15–20% β_1 and β_2 receptors, respectively.
Source: From Ref. 10, used with permission.

We were impressed that in spite of its prolonged effects in vivo, the pharmacokinetics of compound 2 was generally indistinguishable from isoproterenol (6). However, early studies have shown a much higher relative affinity of compound 3 for β_1 receptors of turkey erythrocytes than isoproterenol. Nevertheless, the tissue selectivity of the compound may not be explainable on this single feature of altered affinity for the receptor itself (22,23). In fact when compound 3 was incubated in vitro with guinea pig atrial muscle its effects were competitively blocked by propranolol. But when the bath was changed and the propranolol was washed free of the preparation compound 3 induced changes in contractility returned without adding additional drug (9,21). Thus, simple binding to receptors per se could not have accounted for the complex in vivo response described. We believe that binding to an unidentified portion of the microenvironment of the receptor may play a role in the receptor specificity of some of our compounds.

We next asked whether the potential value of making tissue- and effect-specific β agonists could also apply to β antagonists, and whether the ligands that had been used to create the most interesting skews from the progenitor pharmacophore in potency and effect specificity with the agonist would do the same with antagonists.

B. β-Adrenergic Antagonists

Table 4 samples propranolol derivatives analogous to those made with isoproterenol. While a number of comprisons between like derivatives of the agonist and antagonist series show analogy as well as differences in the changes of potency and tissue effect specificity in the two series, note compounds 4-4 and 4-6 correspond with compound 3-2 and 3-3 of the agonists (10). Table 4 reveals the remarkable tissue and effect specificity of the two antagonist derivatives. We now have congeners of propranolol that are several magnitudes more potent than propranolol. Some have selective anti-β_1 effects with 400-fold more affinity to the β_1 receptor of heart as opposed to that in adipose tissue. Other congeners appear to be selective for adipose tissue and may be among the first competitive blockers of the atypical beta receptor on adipocytes (12 and unpublished results). The specificity predicted by the in vitro tests was bourne out when the compounds were tested in vivo (12). A full description of these effects can be found in recent reports (10,12). In one of those reports we also identified a peptide conjugate of propranolol that became one of the most potent selective β_1 antagonists of the series and was far more potent in this selective effect than practolol or any of its congeners and conjugates (10).

The data confirmed the fact that the same pharmacologically inert ligands when linked to β antagonists had imparted altered potency, and allowed only selected effects of the progenitor to be expressed by the new congener or conju-

Table 5 Comparative Potencies of Similar Isoproterenol and Histamine Congener Derivatives on S–49 Cells (Beta II Receptors) Lymphoma and Natural Suppressor Cells (Histamine Type II Receptors)

Compound[a]		Activity relative to isoproterenol	Activity relative to histamine
7	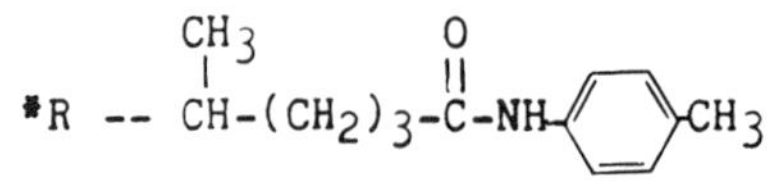	3.11×10^{-1}	3.0×10^{3}
8	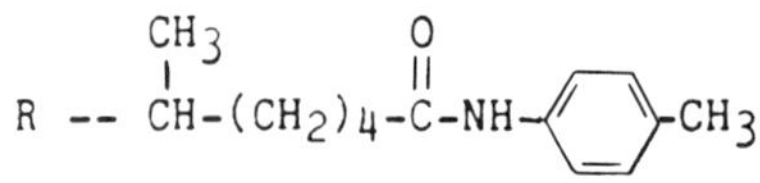	4.40×10^{1}	0.30×10^{1}
9	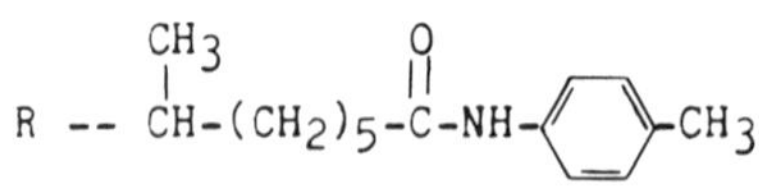	1.11×10^{-1}	0.20×10^{1}
10	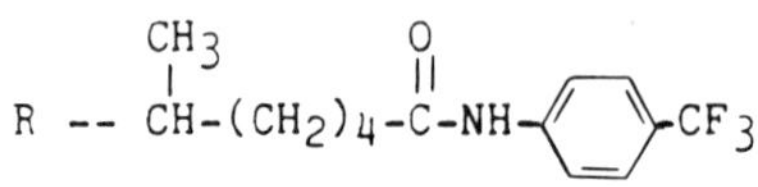	8.60×10^{2}	4.2×10^{4}
14	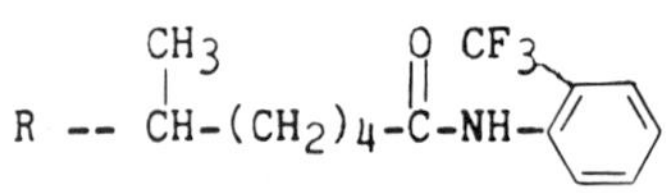	2.6×10^{-4}	Inactive
17	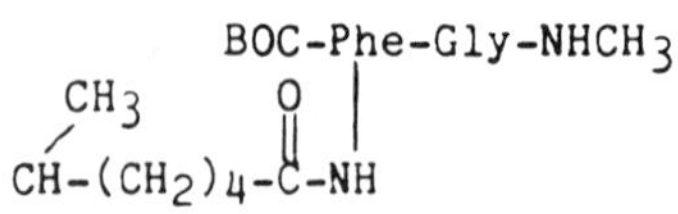	0.4×10^{1}	Inactive
18	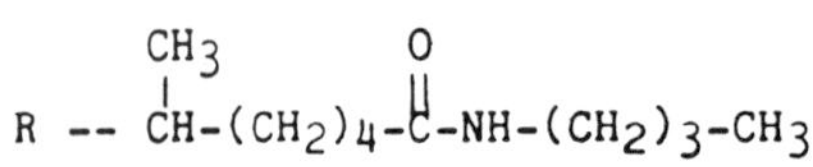	2.5×10^{-1}	Inactive

Biological activity was measured by cAMP accumulation in a mouse natural suppressor cell for the histamine-related compounds and in S-49 cells for the isoproterenol-related compounds. Relative activity is expressed as the ratio of K_a for histamine or isoproterenol to K_a for the test compound.

[a]Structures described in Table 2 for histamine congeners and conjugates.

*R= 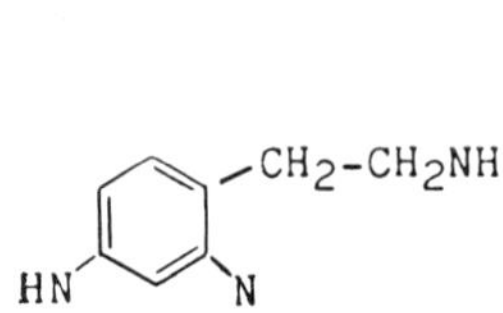 or 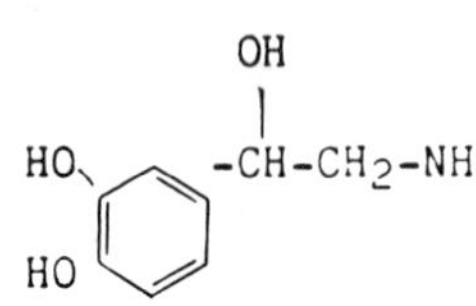

Source: From Ref. 25, used with permission.

gate. Yet as with the catecholamines, all the effects of these congeners or conjugates were mediated by classic drug-receptor interactions.

Although the progenitor agents in the two series were related pharmacologically, they were not chemically similar. The next question we asked was whether pharmacologically and chemically unrelated progenitors would develop unusual changes in potency and selection of effects when prepared in another parallel series. Histamine was the progenitor in this fourth series of congeners and conjugates. The only remaining obvious property shared by four progenitors used in this work was that each of their actions is mediated by well-defined interactions with receptors on the surface membrane of cells.

C. Histamine

1. In Vitro Effects

Once again the length of the aklyl chain of the congeners and conjugates was a key determinant of their potency as well as whether they would gain histamine type I or type I plus type II receptor specificity. The histamine type II effects of selected derivatives of histamine on lymphocytes can be seen in Table 5. The qualitative actions of the derivatives were similar to those of histamine, but the potency of the histamine congeners and conjugates varied from the progenitor as the derivatives in the previous three series varied from their progenitor. As an example of similar changes in potency in the congeners and conjugates, a comparison of the potency of similar derivatives of isoproterenol with histamine congeners is made in Table 5 to show how the pairs of congeners generally change potency in the same direction.

When chain length of the histamine congener ranged from C_1–C_3, the effects on lymphoid cells were predominantly type I. The C_3 trifluoromethyl derivative (see Table 2, compound 12) was the most potent and lacked any ability to affect the rabbit aorta, the guinea pig myocardium, or even the histamine type II receptors on lymphocytes (11,19). An unusually striking finding was the fact that the paratrifluoromethyl derivative of histamine with C_4 methylene chain possessed both type I and type II effects (see Table 5, compound 3). It is remarkable that the deletion of a single methyl group resulted in a total loss of histamine type II activity (Table 6, compounds 12 and 13). These two derivatives of histamine (see Table 2, compound 13 [type I and type II agonists] and Table 2, compound 12 [type I agonist]) were lymphocyte specific, and receptor-specific agonists that could be used as tools for determining the relative roles of type I and type II plus type II agonists on lymphocytes alone as modifiers of in vitro and possibly in vivo immunity. When the trifluoromethyl group was moved from the para position, the potency of the histamine congener fell dramatically, as it had with the "isoproterenol" congener (see Table 5, compound 14).

Table 6 The Effects of the Congener Derivatives and Conjugates of Histamine on Peripheral Vasculature, Natural Suppressor (type I) Cells, and Guinea Pig Myocardium

Compound[a]	[b]Percent change in contractility (H_2)	[c]Relative potency in NS (H_2)	[c]Relative potency in GMP (H_2)
Histamine	284 ± 38 $P < 0.05$	1	1
1	93 ± 23 $P < 0.05$	5	0
2	0	2	0.09
3	0	0	0
4	0	4.4	0
5	0	0	NT
6	0	0	NT
7	90 ± 29 $P < 0.05$	4000	0.01
8	0	3	0.07
9	0	2	0.02
10	0	0	NT
11	0	0	NT
12[d]	0	0	0
13	?	40,000	0
14	0	0	0
15	0	0	0
16	0	0	0
17	0	0	0.0007
18	0	0	0.01
19	0	0	0

[a]Compound numbers correspond to those structures in Table 2.
[b]Average ± SEM was calculated from at least three independent experiments.
[c]Biological activity was measured by cAMP assay in natural suppressor cells (NS) (i.e., histamine type II effects) and in guinea pig myocardium (GPM) by adenylate cyclase stimulation assay. Relative potency is expressed as the ratio of EC-50 for histamine to EC-50 for the derivatives. Inactive compunds were given a relative potency = 0. Inactive compounds did not cause any accumulation cAMP or the stimulation of adenylate cyclase. The relative potencies were calculated from EC-50 values which were average of at least three different determinations. The coefficient of variability was $<10\%$.
[d]Compound 12 was as potent as compound 13 in stimulation of histamine type I receptors on the natural suppressor cells.
Source: Modified from Ref. 19, used with permission.

Only when we made a dipeptide conjugate of histamine (analogous to the dipeptide conjugate of isoproterenol that had selective cardiac effects) did we see some retention of the cardiac stimulatory actions of histamine (see Table 5 and Table 6, compound 18). This cardiac effect was the only agonist effect that we were able to detect using the dipeptide; i.e., this drug had become quite tissue specific.

2. In Vivo Effects of Two Lymphocyte-Specific Histamine Type I and Type I plus Type II Agonists

Compounds 12 (a lymphocyte-specific highly potent histamine type I agonist by in vitro testing) and 13 (a lymphocyte-specific highly potent type I plus type II agonist by in vitro testing) recently have been synthesized in sufficient quantities to examine their effects in vivo. Three models of T cell–dependent immune responses in the mouse were selected for initial tests performed at Hoffmann-La Roche, Inc. in Nutley, New Jersey, by Drs. Bruce Devens, William Benjamin, and Denise Faherty. The in vivo models included antibody response to sheep red blood cells, cytolytic T-cell response to alloantigen and oxazolone-induced delayed-type hypersensitivity response. Doses of the drug ranged from 10 to 100 mg/kg/day given intraperitoneally daily for from 1 to 10 days starting 2 days before the administration of the antigen.

The two compounds produced no obvious systemic effects in the mice. Thus, the severe hypotension and/or bronchospasms expected of histamine were not obvious with the congeners. The data are consistent with the tissue specificity predicted for compounds 12 and 13 by the in vitro tests. In contrast, the toxicity of histamine at far less than the easily tolerated doses of compounds 12 and 13 was considerable. In fact, the pharmacologic data obtained in vitro from each series of congener and conjugate derivates have predicted the unusual receptor, effect, and tissue specificity that the drugs would develop in vivo.

More exciting was the fact that compound 12, the histamine type I agonist, had no effect on any of the three models, whereas compound 13 significantly and profoundly suppressed the cytolytic response and antibody production in a dose-dependent manner. At 100 mg/kg, compound 13 suppressed antibody production by 95%. These early results are consistent with the finding that histamine type II effects are likely to be suppressive and type I effects contrasuppressive (32), and that the suppression actions of histamine are blocked by type II antagonists (33). Histamine itself, given up to doses that produced unacceptable toxicity, did not show any qualitative ability to modify immunity as did compound 13.

IV. CONCLUSIONS

There are more questions than answers produced by the early in vivo experimental results using congeners of histamine. For instance, did compound 13 truly work by its histaminelike quality? If the compound truly worked as a histamine agonist, what are the optimal doses, dosage ranges and dose intervals? Did compound 13 work by both histamine type I and type II agonism? Why did not a pure histamine type I agonist have affects on any of the models? Could the pure histamine type I agonist be contrasuppressive? Were pharmacokinetics and metabolism factors in the absence of compound 12's effects? What would histamine type II antagonists do to the effects of compound 13 (would compound 13 then "work like" the ineffective compound 12)? What would histamine type I antagonists do to the effects of compound 13? Would histamine type II antagonists do anything to the response to compound 12? Do the actions of compound 13 begin to help to define the mechanisms by which other in vivo models appear to show immune enhancement caused by antihistamines (25-31)? Can lymphocyte-specific antihistamines be constructed? Would the suppression produced by compound 13 in one animal be transferable to a second animal naive to the exposure to and direct effects of compound 13? What cell types are involved in the suppression? Were they the same cell types in each model? Why was the model of delayed-type hypersensitivity unaffected by the drug? Would lymphocyte-specific β agonists show effects similar to compound 13?

Regardless of how many questions cannot be answered, we are beginning to answer two questions. Is the hypothesis that mediators of inflammation may modulate immunity a valid hypothesis? Our in vivo data using compounds 12 and 13 go a ways to support that hypothesis. And yes, it is possible to construct lymphocyte-specific agonists and possibly antagonists of some of the mediators of inflammation to be used as probes of the direction and mechanism of their effects on the immune response. Whether the same agents might be useful in prospectively nonspecifically modifying models of human immunity remains a third very important question to answer.

Although there are differences in the changes in pharmacologic properties (potency, tissue selectivity, and receptor specificity) when pairs of like derivatives from different series of agonists or antagonists are compared, there were striking and important similar changes in a narrow band of pairs taken from all four series (see Table 1). Some structural changes predicted pharmacologic novelty in each series (see Table 1). Furthermore, the work of Jacobsen et al. extends this generalization by testing a similar series of derivatives of adenosine antagonists (24). Therefore, using the ligands to create congeners and conjugates of other pharmacophores perhaps even peptides and proteins that work on the cell surface seems feasible and worthwhile. The approach might lead to useful investigative tools and therapeutic agents, some of which might even be orally active.

The mechanisms of altered potency, tissue, and receptor specificity of the derivatives are not clear, but must relate to the pharmacologically inert ligands. Although our leads toward explaining the altered pharmacologic effects of the derivatives are quite limited, early data point more toward some altered interaction with the microenvironment of the receptors than with simple drug-receptor interactions. Altered pharmacokinetics is unlikely to explain the useful changes in the pharmacologic profile of our derivatives. Defining the exact mechanisms of alteration of the pharmacologic properties of our derivatives is feasible and attractive. Such information might help us design tissue- and effect-specific derivatives of other pharmacophores with otherwise ubiquitous pharmacologic effects.

In the meanwhile, our approach might apply to the concerns of molecular biologists who are grappling with means to focus pharmacologic effects of the new larger molecular weight substances. Amont the strategies to limit the immunogenicity of the new large molecules, small peptides are being sought that possess most of the pharmacologic actions of the progenitor protein. But this approach is likely to lead to drugs that still possess most of the wide spectrum of biological effects that the unmodified proteins had. As long as the drugs are widely distributed and have an inherent spectrum of pharmacologic potential, then the modification will not change the breadth of the effects. Application of our approach may focus the pharmacologic profile of these drugs.

ACKNOWLEDGMENTS

This work was supported in part by NIH HL 26340 and AI 23463.

I am grateful to my collaborators, particularly Drs. Brian Hoffman, Manzoor Khan, Quan Ming Zhu, Julie Bauer, Andrea Wilson, and Karen Keaney at Stanford University; Drs. M. Goodman, M. Verlander, K. Jacobson, and D. Leisy at the University of California, San Diego; and Drs. B. Devens, W. Benjamin, and S. Faherty at Hoffmann-La Roche, Nutley, New Jersey.

We also thank Sara Fisher for her excellent editorial assistance in both of our chapters in this book.

REFERENCES

1. Melmon, K. L., Y. Weinstein, H. R. Bourne, T. Poon, G. Shearer, and N. Castagnoli, Jr., The pharmacological effects of conjugates of pharmacologically active amines to complex or simple carriers: A new class of drug, Mol. Pharmacol. 12:701-710 (1976).
2. Melmon, K. L., M. S. Verlander, L. Krasny, M. Goodman, N. Kaplan, N. Castagnoli Jr., and P. Insel, The chemistry and pharmacology of catecholamines and other low molecular weight ligands conjugated to carriers. In the

Fourth International Catecholamine Symposium: Catecholamines: Basic and Clinical Frontiers, vol. 1, Pergamon Press, (1979), pp. 474–476.

3. Rosenkranz, R. P., K. A. Jacobson, M. Goodman, M. Verlander, and K. L. Melmon, *In vitro* and *in vivo* betamimetic activity of congeners of isoproterenol, Proc. West. Pharmacol. Soc. 25:19–23 (1982).
4. Jacobson, K. A., R. P. Rosenkranz, M. S. Verlander, K. L. Melmon, and M. Goodman, Conjugates of catecholamines III. Synthesis and characterization of monodisperse oligopeptide conjugates related to isoproterenol. Int. J. Pept. Protein. Res. 22:284–304, 1983.
5. Verlander, M. S., K. A. Jacobson, R. P. Rosenkranz, K. L. Melmon, and M. Goodman, Some novel approaches to the design and synthesis of peptide-catecholamine conjugates, Biopolymers 22:531–545 (1983).
6. Ferraiolo, B. L., M. M. Halldin, Y. Asscher, Y. Akita, K. L. Melmon, L. Benet, and N. Castagnoli, Pharmacokinetics and excretion of unique beta adrenergics agonists, Pharmacology 34:157–166 (1987).
7. Rosenkranz, R. P., K. A. Jacobson, M. S., Verlander, M. Goodman, and K. L. Melmon, Betamimetic activity of peptide catecholamine conjugates, Proc. West. Pharmacol. Soc. 26:381–385 (1983).
8. Rosenkranz, R. P., B. B. Hoffman, K. A. Jacobson, M. S. Verlander, L. Klevans, M. O'Donnell, M. Goodman, and K. L. Melmon, Conjugates of catecholamines. II. Pharmacologic activity of N-alkyl functionalized carboxylic acid congeners and amides related to isoproterenol, Mol. Pharmacol. 24: 429–435 (1983).
9. Marki, H. P., Y. Crameri, R. Eigenmann, A. Krasso, H. Ramuz, K. Bernauer, M. Goodman, and K. L. Melmon, Optically pure isoproterenol analogues with sickle chains containing an amide bond: Synthesis and biological properties, Helvet, Chemica Acta 71:320, 1988.
10. Khan, M. M., D. Leisy, M. Verlander, B. Hoffman, M. Goodman, and K. L. Melmon, *In vitro* pharmacologic activity of congener derivatives and model conjugates of propranolol and practolol, Biochem. Pharmacol. Vol. 36, No. 13, pp. 2175–2182, 1987.
11. Khan, M. M., D. Leisy, M. Verlander, M. R. Bristow, S. Strober, M. Goodman, and K. L. Melmon, The effects of derivatives of histamine on natural suppressor cells, J. Immunol. 137:308–314 (1986).
12. Zhu, Q. M., C. H. Lee, C. Laughton, M. M. Khan, and K. L. Melmon, Tissue selectivity of propranolol derivatives in vivo, Biochem. Pharmacol. Vol. 38, No. 10, pp. 1563–1567, 1989.
13. Jacobson, K. A., M. S. Verlander, R. P. Rosenkranz, K. L. Melmon, and M. Goodman, Conjugates of catecholamines III. Synthesis and characterization of monodisperse oligopeptide conjugates related to isoproterenol, Int. J. Pept. Protein Res. 22:284–304 (1983).
14. Goodman, M., M. S. Verlander, K. L. Melmon, K. A. Jacobson, A. B. Reitz, J. P. Taulane, M. A. Avery, and N. O. Kaplan, Characterization of catecholamine-polypeptide conjugates, Eur. Polym. J. 19:997–1004 (1983).

15. Rosenkranz, R. P., K. A. Jacobson, M. S. Verlander, L. Klevans, M. O'Donnell, M. Goodman, and K. L. Melmon, Conjugates of catecholamines. IV. *In vitro* and *in vivo* pharmacological activity of monodisperse oligopeptide conjugates, J. Pharmacol. Exp. Ther. 227:267–273 (1983).
16. Verlander, M. S., K. A. Jacobson, A. B. Reitz, R. P. Rosenkranz, K. L. Melmon, and M. Goodman, Application of the congener approach to the design and synthesis of peptide-catecholamine conjugates, Proceedings of the International Symposium on Polymers in Meicine, Porto Cervo, Sardinia, Italy, Polym. Med. 57–75 (1984).
17. Reitz, A. B., E. Sonveaux, R. P. Rosenkranz, M. S. Verlander, K. L. Melmon, B. B. Hoffman, Y. Akita, N. Castagnoli, and M. Goodman. Conjugates of catecholamines. 5. Synthesis and beta-adrenergic activity of N-(aminoalkyl) norepinephrine derivatives. J. Med. Chem. 28:634–642 (1985).
18. Reitz, A. B., M. A. Avery, R. P. Rosenkranz, M. S. Verlander, K. L. Melmon, B. B. Hoffman, Y. Akita, N. Castagnoli, and M. Goodman, Conjugates of catecholamines. 6. Synthesis of beta-adrenergic activity of N-(hydroxyalkyl) catecholamine derivatives, J. Med. Chem. 28:642–647 (1985).
19. Khan, M. M., D. Leisy, M. Verlander, M. Egli, S. Lok, M. Goodman, and K. L. Melmon, Congener derivatives and conjugates of histamine: Synthesis and tissue and receptor selectivity of the derivatives, J. Med. Chem. 30: 2115–2120 (1987).
20. Fakuda, M., C. M. Beecham, M. Verlander, M. Goodman, M. M. Khan, and K. L. Melmon, Conjugates of catecholamines. VII. Synthesis of beta adrenergic activity of peptide catecholamine conjugates, Int. J. Pept. Protein Res. 29:300–317 (1987).
21. Eigenmann, R., W. B. Burkard, M. Holck, H. P. Marki, W. Osterrieder, M. Goodman, and K. L. Melmon, In vitro pharmacological properties of a series of isoprenaline derivatives, Arzneimittelforschung, 39(11), 842–847 (1989).
22. Eimerl, S., M. Schramm, S. Lok, M. Goodman, M. Khan, and K. L. Melmon, The four stereoisomers of a high potency congener of isoproterenol, Biochem. Pharmacol. 20:3523–3527 (1987).
23. Schramm, M., S. Eimerl, M. Goodman, M. S. Verlander, M. M. Khan, and K. L. Melmon, High potency congeners of isoproterenol: binding to beta-adrenergic receptors, activation of adenylate cyclase and stimulation of intracellular cyclic AMP synthesis, Biochem. Pharmacol. 35:2805–2809 (1986).
24. Jacobson, K. A., K. L. Kirk, W. L. Padgett, and J. W. Daly, A functionalized congener approach to adenosine receptor antagonists: amino acid conjugates of 1,3-dipropylxanthing, Mol. Pharmacol. 29:126–133 (1986).
25. Melmon, K. L., M. M. Khan, and M. Goodman, Like congeners and conjugates (including peptidylation) of catecholamines, beta antagonists and histamines produce unusual pharmacologic selectivity. In The Pharmacology and Toxicology of Proteins, Alan R. Liss, New York (1987), pp. 113–129.

26. Melmon, K. L., and M. M. Khan, Histamine and its lymphocyte-selective derivatives as immune modulators, TIPS 8:437–441 (1987).
27. Jorizzo, J. L., W. M. Sams, B. V. Jegasothy, and A. J. Olansky, Cimetidine as an immunomodulator: Chronic mucucutaneous candidas as a model, Ann. Int. Med. 92:192–195 (1980).
28. Nordlund, J. J., and P. W. Askenase, The effect of histamine, antihistamine, and a mast cell established in the growth of Cloudman melanoma cells in DBA/2 mice, J. Invest. Dermatol. 81:28–31 (1983).
29. Converse, P. J., R. M. Mshama, and G. J. Bjune, Cimetidine inhibits suppressor factor production in Ethiopian leprematous leprosy patients, Int. J. Leprosy, 55:548–551 (1986).
30. Gorczynski, R. M., M. Kennedy, and A. Ciampi, Cimetidine reverses tumor growth enhancement of plasmacytoma tumors in mice demonstrating conditional immunosuppression, J. Immunol. 134:4261–4266 (1985).
31. Eisenthal, A., J. Monselise, R. Zinger, and A. Adler, The effect of cimetidine on PBL from healthy donors and melanoma patients: Augmentation of T cell response to TCGF mitogens and alloantigens and of TCGF production, Cancer Immunol. Immunother. 11:141–147 (1986).
32. Siegel, J. N., A. Schwartz, P. W. Askenase, and R. E. Gershon, T cell suppression and contrasuppression induced by histamine H_2 and H_1 receptor agonists, respectively, Proc. Natl. Acad. Sci. U.S.A. 79:5052–5056 (1982).
33. Bealieu, L., J. Beaudoin, M. Jobin, and J. Hebert, Effects of H_1 and H_2 receptor agonists on nonspecific proliferative response of human peripheral blood lymphocytes, Int. Arch. Allergy Appl. Immunol. 79:249–252 (1986).

Index